Payne's
handbook of relaxation
techniques

DATE DUE

MAY 06 2013			

D1295677

Publisher: Sarena Wolfaard
Development Editor: Sally Davies
Project Manager: Srikumar Narayanan
Cover Design: Charles Gray
Page Design: Stewart Larking
Illustration Manager: Merlyn Harvey

FOURTH EDITION

Payne's handbook of relaxation techniques

a **practical guide** for the **health care professional**

Edited by

Rosemary A. Payne BSc(Hons) Psychology MCSP
Chartered physiotherapist and tutor in relaxation training, Cardiff, UK

Marie Donaghy BA(Hons) PhD FCSP FHEA
Professor of Physiotherapy; Dean, School of Health Sciences,
Queen Margaret University, Edinburgh, UK

Foreword by

Ilora Finlay FRCP FRCGP
Baroness Finlay of Llandaff, Professor of Palliative Medicine, Cardiff University,
President of the Chartered Society of Physiotherapy, London, UK

Photographs by

John Sheerin
Forth Photography, Edinburgh, UK

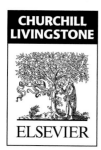

CHURCHILL
LIVINGSTONE

ELSEVIER

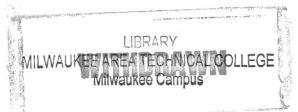

Edinburgh London New York Oxford Philadelphia St Louis Sydney Toronto 2010

CHURCHILL LIVINGSTONE
ELSEVIER

First Edition © Longman Group 1995
Reprinted © Harcourt Brace and Company Limited 1998
Second Edition © Harcourt Publishers Limited 2000
Third Edition © Elsevier Limited 2005
Fourth edition © 2010, Elsevier Limited. All rights reserved

ISBN 978-0-7020-3112-0

British Library Cataloguing in Publication Data
A catalogue record for this book is available from the British Library

Library of Congress Cataloging in Publication Data
A catalog record for this book is available from the Library of Congress

Notice
Neither the Publisher nor the Authors assume any responsibility for any loss or
injury and/or damage to persons or property arising out of or related to any use of the
material contained in this book. It is the responsibility of the treating practitioner,
relying on independent expertise and knowledge of the patient, to determine the
best treatment and method of application for the patient.

The Publisher

ELSEVIER your source for books,
journals and multimedia
in the health sciences
www.elsevierhealth.com

Working together to grow
libraries in developing countries

www.elsevier.com | www.bookaid.org | www.sabre.org

ELSEVIER   BOOK AID International   Sabre Foundation

The
Publisher's
policy is to use
**paper manufactured
from sustainable forests**

Printed in China

Contents

Relaxation is often seen as a panacea for stress. As such, it has given rise to many different approaches designed to cope with everyday stressors.

When people are ill, however, stress and tension mount; sleep is affected and other body systems negatively influenced. Some people with a chronic pattern of stress-related behaviour can find it very difficult to unlearn these behaviours and adopt a calmer lifestyle.

Many relaxation techniques are presented in this book. They have been selected with particular criteria in mind: that they should be easily learned and applied without requiring expensive equipment or specialized expertise. Their transferability is also important in that they can be adopted by small groups as well as individuals, and in a wide variety of settings across different age groups. Certain specialized techniques such as yoga are not covered in this book precisely because they require specific training or because, like biofeedback, they rely on special equipment.

An excellent introduction to the topic can be found in this book with its jargon-free style and its readability. Although addressed to health care professionals, it does not demand particular health care knowledge or specific previous training, and therefore has wide applicability. The book takes us through different aspects of relaxation, starting with a discussion on physiological and cognitive dimensions of stress and leading into a chapter containing coping techniques. In our society, where back pain is a major cause of absenteeism, the link between stress, muscle tension and perceptions of illness becomes particularly relevant.

The book then moves through a variety of somatic approaches including progressive muscle relaxation, breathing re-education, physical activity and passive relaxation. Cognitive approaches include imagery, visualizations, autogenics, meditation and some simple cognitive–behavioural techniques.

A common format running through the chapters makes this book easy to dip in and out of and allows the easy comparison of one technique with another. The final chapters relate to issues around measurement, a topic which is essential for any kind of audit. There is also a chapter indicating which conditions are likely to benefit from particular techniques. The book is essentially a practical manual with a step-by-step approach, allowing the reader to feel in touch with the practicality of each technique.

If you are feeling stressed, then this is the book to pick up. Its pages will make you feel both more relaxed and more in control.

Ilora Finlay FRCP FRCGP
Baroness Finlay of Llandaff, Professor of
Palliative Medicine, Cardiff University; President
of the Chartered Society of Physiotherapy,
London, UK

Preface to the fourth edition

For this fourth edition, the book has moved from single to dual authorship. This has allowed a more comprehensive review of the literature which has informed the evidence for practice outlined in the book. In accordance with earlier editions, the aim has been to produce a book containing a broad range of techniques which may be found useful by practitioners and students whose backgrounds lie in a wide variety of professional fields.

The book is addressed primarily to health care professionals such as nurses, occupational therapists, physiotherapists, speech and language therapists and social workers. General practitioners and psychologists also may find it useful. It can equally be used by lay people since it is written in a jargon-free style.

It focuses on methods which do not require specialized expertise or elaborate equipment but consist of simpler approaches which can be applied in the stressful situation. The division between somatic and cognitive is, to some extent, an arbitrary one, and one which has no place in the holistic context to which the authors subscribe. However, for the purpose of organizing material in the book, such a presentation has been adopted.

As in previous editions, the book is structured in four parts. Section One sets the scene, describing the states of relaxation and stress and providing guidance on preparing for relaxation. Sections Two and Three guide the reader through 21 somatic and cognitive approaches, each occupying a separate chapter. The book ends with an introduction to assessment followed by a chapter devoted to recent research on conditions and disorders, where best treatment, as determined by the evidence, is suggested.

Two chapters are completely new: one on mindfulness meditation, which has been included to reflect the growing interest and popularity of this approach, and the other on choice of technique for 35 specific conditions. Assessment, cognitive therapy and physical activity chapters have all been substantially rewritten. The book has also been restructured in the sense that chapters have been moved around to create a more convenient order and it is illustrated with a new set of photographs in keeping with changing fashion.

It was felt that a relatively slim volume would be of advantage. Consequently, certain chapters such as 'Other techniques' and 'Childbirth' have been removed. Evidence sections throughout have been updated and given a new emphasis, but the early work has not been entirely eliminated since it provides a useful historical context for understanding the different approaches. It is hoped readers will find this arrangement helpful.

It is not intended that health care professionals should, on the strength of reading this book, consider themselves teachers of autogenics or the Alexander technique. Such methods require lengthy training. These two methods are, however, included to indicate the importance of their contribution to the field; they are described for interest and for the applicability of their central ideas. For example, images of warmth and heaviness (autogenics) are relaxing in any context, and postural advice (Alexander technique) helps to promote a sense of well-being. Such concepts have universal value.

Like its forebears, this new edition is essentially a practical manual, easy to follow and conveniently sized to carry around.

Rosemary Payne
Marie Donaghy
2009

A few years ago, when giving a talk on relaxation techniques, I was asked by a social worker if the techniques I was describing could all be found in one publication. I said I knew of no book which contained them all. Since then, other healthcare professionals have, on different occasions, put similar questions to me. Is there a book which focuses on the practical side of relaxation training? Can the detail of the methods be found under one cover?

Many books mention relaxation techniques but tend not to present them in any depth, unless the entire work is devoted to a single method. It seemed that there was a gap which needed to be filled.

It is estimated that 80% of modern diseases have their beginnings in stress (Powell & Enright 1990) and that stress-related illness accounts for at least 75% of GP consultations (Looker & Gregson 1989). As concern about the safety, efficacy and cost of psychotropic drugs grows (Sibbald et al 1993), there is increasing interest in non-drug treatments, of which relaxation training is an example.

The book is addressed to healthcare professionals such as nurses, occupational therapists, physiotherapists, speech and language therapists and social workers; GPs and psychologists also may find it useful. It can equally be used by lay people since it is written in a jargon-free style.

Factors of practicality have governed the selection of methods. Thus, techniques which require expensive equipment or specialized expertise are not included, while the methods chosen are those which lend themselves to presentation in small group settings.

The book begins with a review of some of the theory surrounding stress and relaxation. This is followed by a chapter on general procedure which is applicable to all methods. Chapter 2 discusses stress, beginning with a further passage of theory and moving on to consider a variety of practical coping skills. The following 21 chapters deal with specific techniques: 12 chapters are, broadly speaking, concerned with physical or muscular techniques and nine deal with mental or psychological methods. There follows a chapter concerning 'on-the-spot' techniques for dealing with stressful situations, using skills drawn from earlier lessons. Assessment is addressed in Chapter 25* and the final chapter takes a look at a few topics not so far discussed: the relation between the approaches themselves, some ways in which they can be combined, and a brief reference to approaches which are not included. Physical and psychiatric disorders are not within the scope of this work.

Techniques whose main purpose is to promote relaxation are termed primary. The 'muscular' methods belong in this category, as does autogenic training. Where relaxation is not the main purpose, the technique can be seen as secondary: visualization, meditation and the Alexander technique fall into this category. Other approaches which enhance relaxation may be still further removed. These include cognitive techniques such as uncovering irrational assumptions and modifying automatic thoughts. Here, relaxation can be seen as a side-effect rather than a goal (Fanning 1988).

It is not intended that healthcare professionals should, on the strength of reading this book, consider themselves teachers of autogenics and the Alexander technique. These two methods are included to indicate their contribution to the field; they are described for interest and for the applicability of their central ideas. For example, images of warmth and heaviness (autogenics) are relaxing in any context, as also is postural advice (Alexander technique). Such concepts have universal value.

Indications of the effectiveness of the techniques are included but the book does not set out to review the evidence from the scientific literature. Other works do that, for example Lichstein (1988). Pitfalls associated with some methods are listed at the end of the relevant chapters.

The word 'relaxation' is used in two ways here, as it is in other works: first, in a general sense where it signifies a global state of rest; and second, as a technique such as progressive relaxation. It is difficult to

---

* To avoid confusion, the chapter numbers have been changed to match the chapter numbers in the fourth edition rather than the first. Please also note that some chapters have been deleted since the first edition.

avoid both meanings in a book of this sort; however, efforts are made throughout the work to distinguish the meanings wherever ambiguity arises.

The author is aware of the implications of gender-weighted language. She is also aware of the cumbersome phrasing that can result from a determination to avoid sexist forms of speech. In an attempt to avoid both traps and for the sake of clarity, it has been decided to refer throughout the book to the trainer as female. The trainee is referred to as male in Chapters 2–15 and as female in Chapters 16–27.

The words 'trainer' and 'instructor' are both used, the choice being largely determined by the nature of the method: for example, in autogenics, progressive relaxation and behavioural relaxation training the word 'trainer' is often used, while in imagery, meditation, Alexander technique and Mitchell's approach, the word 'instructor' seems more appropriate. The word 'therapist' is also used where it seems fitting.

A number of people have helped in the making of this book. One important contributor is Keith Bellamy, whose photographs have done so much to make the book what it is, not forgetting Sarah McDermott, who acted as the model. With regard to the text, Ian Hughes has given invaluable help in his careful reading and refining of the chapter on measurement. I would also like to mention those who have read other chapters and to whom I am indebted for their helpful suggestions. Alexandra Hough, Wendy Mair, Margaret Polden and Jim Robinson have all been kind enough to do this, and Christopher Rowland Payne undertook to read the whole manuscript. Thanks also go to Michael Adams, Joyce Gibbs, Olga Gregson, Andrzej Kokoszka, Brenda MacLachland, Pat Miller, Alison Ough, Stuart Skyte, Dinah Thom, June Tiley and Elizabeth Valentine. Finally, a word of appreciation for the members of all the groups with whom I have worked. Without them, this book would never have been written.

Rosemary Payne
Cardiff 1994

Acknowledgements

First of all, I want to thank Marie for agreeing to join me as an author of this fourth edition. She has improved the book in many ways and her work has been greatly appreciated. Thanks also go to Michele Hipwell who gave advice over the chapter on mindfulness and Ian Hughes whose guidance in earlier editions continues to stand out. I am also grateful to Dee Jenkins, my computer engineer, who has so often come to my rescue when my own computer skills proved inadequate. Helen Taylor, Anne Pitman and Danuta Ramos have also helped in different ways and I am indebted to them and others. Finally, a word of thanks to our publishers who have supported us throughout.

Rosemary Payne

I would like to acknowledge colleagues, students, friends and family who have made huge contributions to my thinking over the years and who have helped shape my view of health, relaxation, physical activity, and mind–body integration. I would like to thank in particular Nanette Mutrie for her friendship and wise counsel over the years. My thanks to the staff in the School of Health Sciences at Queen Margaret University who have encouraged and supported my research activities. To Michael, Claire, Kirsteen, Neil, James and Mirrin, my thanks for all the fun and joy you bring to our lives. Finally I would like to thank Rosemary for inviting me to co-author this fourth edition of her book. Her guidance has been invaluable.

Marie Donaghy

Section **One**

Setting the scene

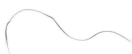

Introduction

It could be said that relaxation is doing nothing (Beck 1984). In spite of this. many people find it difficult to relax. Doing nothing, it seems, is not as easy as it sounds and the existence of a wealth of relaxation techniques appears to endorse this view.

For many people a hobby provides a source of relaxation. As an occupation devoid of deadlines, the hobby allows the mind to freeflow in an unconstrained manner, inducing a sense of inner calm. Activities which give pleasure tend to fall into this category. Some of these require moderate to high levels of physiological arousal such as active non-competitive sport, while others, such as listening to music or watching the waves breaking on a favourite beach, do not. Both, however, are characterized by an absence of stress.

It is when these activities fail to relieve stress that formal relaxation training can play a useful role. Such a training programme can help to lower a stress-induced high physiological arousal level, thereby protecting the organs from damage. It can also help to make the body's innate healing mechanisms more available. On a cognitive level, relaxation training can calm the mind and allow thinking to become clearer, and on a philosophical level, as practised in some Asian countries, it can bring an increased awareness of the self (Donaghy et al 2008).

The word 'relaxation' is often used with reference to muscles where it signifies release of tension and the lengthening of muscle fibres, as opposed to the shortening which accompanies muscle tension or contraction. Such a definition could be applied to the methods described in the early chapters of this book. However, since relaxation has a mental as well as a physical dimension, this definition is too restricted for our purposes.

A more comprehensive view comes from Ryman (1995) who defines relaxation as 'a state of consciousness characterized by feelings of peace and release from ... anxiety and fear' as well as tension. This includes psychological aspects of the relaxation experience such as the pleasant sensation it induces and the diminishing presence of stressful thoughts.

Thus, the word 'relaxed' is used to refer either to lax muscles or to peaceful thoughts. It is assumed that a link exists between them since an apparently general state of relaxation can be induced by using either physical or cognitive methods.

Purpose of the book

The book seeks to provide a compendium of different relaxation techniques and to describe them in relation to their underpinning rationales. Their selection has been governed by factors of practicality such as the following, that the method should:

- be easily learned and applied
- not require specialized expertise on the part of the trainer
- not require elaborate equipment
- be portable and capable of being used without attracting attention

- be convenient for use with individuals and small groups
- be suitable for all ages.

It is addressed principally to healthcare professionals and students who are not familiar with the topic of relaxation or to those who want to extend their knowledge about relaxation techniques. The book may also be helpful to people with chronic conditions such as rheumatoid arthritis, multiple sclerosis or enduring mental illness who wish to teach themselves relaxation as a personal coping mechanism.

Relaxation training has certain advantages which may make it particularly attractive to some people, such as being non-invasive and giving the client a sense of being in control. Benefits to employers and organizers include its low financial cost.

Structure and content

A variety of methods and techniques are presented, with one chapter devoted to each. The techniques are drawn from recognized sources and appear in slightly paraphrased versions of the originals. Each method is described and presented in a step-by-step manner. Rationale is contained in a short paragraph and there is a section on evidence of effectiveness. However, evidence to support the techniques is limited and cannot in all cases be used to inform the rationale. For this reason the rationale has been kept separate from the evidence.

Each chapter directs the reader to available research but it is beyond the scope of this book to provide a systematic review of the literature. Where appropriate, the reader is referred to other works such as the narrative review of Kerr (2000) whose paper covered progressive relaxation, the Mitchell method, massage, the Alexander technique, Benson's relaxation response and hatha yoga.

Chapter topics feature somatic and cognitive approaches. The present authors write from a firmly holistic position where any kind of division runs counter to their philosophy. However, for descriptive purposes it was found convenient to separate techniques with a cognitive focus from those with a somatic focus. Such a division is however, largely artificial.

Somatic approaches presented in this work are:

- breathing awareness
- Jacobson's progressive muscular relaxation
- Bernstein and Borkovec's modified version

- Everly and Rosenfeld's passive relaxation
- Madders' release-only
- Ost's applied relaxation
- Poppen's behavioural relaxation training
- the Mitchell method
- the Alexander technique
- differential relaxation
- stretchings
- exercise.

Cognitive approaches presented here are:

- cognitive–behavioural methods
- self-awareness
- imagery
- goal-directed visualization
- autogenic training
- meditation
- Benson's relaxation response
- mindfulness meditation.

A table summarizing the principles of each method and suggesting applications for its use may be found in Appendix 1.

The range of methods is not comprehensive since it does not include those methods which require long training periods, such as hypnosis, yoga and advanced autogenics, or elaborate apparatus, such as biofeedback. However, some of these methods are referred to for interest and background information. In the case of yoga, as taught in the West, the component parts of breathing, stretchings and meditation may be found in separate chapters.

Most methods described here are claimed to be relaxation techniques. However, there are a few which induce an indirect relaxation effect by increasing the sense of well-being. The Alexander technique is one of these.

There is a difference between methods which create 'deep' relaxation and those which create 'brief' relaxation. Deep relaxation refers to procedures which induce an effect of large magnitude and which are carried out in a calm environment with the trainee lying down, e.g. progressive relaxation and autogenic training. Brief relaxation refers to techniques (often contracted versions of the above) which produce immediate effects and which can be used when the individual is faced with stressful events, the object being the rapid release of excess tension. Thus, whereas deep relaxation refers to a full process of total-body relaxation, brief relaxation applies these procedures in everyday life.

1

Relaxation: what is it?

CHAPTER CONTENTS

Relaxation suggests a state of ease which is characterized by limited body tension and freedom
from unnecessary worries and fears. It is associated with feelings of warmth and tranquillity and
a sense of being at peace with oneself. Thus, the
state of relaxation involves a complex interplay
of psychological and physiological systems which
include the nerves, muscles and major organs such
as the heart, lungs, kidneys, liver and spleen.

Mechanisms thought to be responsible for
bringing about the state of relaxation have been
explored, giving rise to a number of theories.
Some of these emphasize physiological aspects such
as autonomic activity and muscle tension while
others focus on psychological elements such as self
perceptions and interpretation of life events.
The major theories are briefly described below.

Physiological theories

Body systems related to the states of stress and
relaxation include the autonomic and endocrine
systems on the one hand and the skeletal system
on the other. An integrated response of all these
systems occurs in the presence of stress.

The autonomic nervous system and the endocrine system

Physiological arousal is governed chiefly by the
autonomic nervous system. This has two branches:
the sympathetic, which increases arousal when the
organism is under threat, and the parasympathetic,
which restores the body to a resting state. Their
actions are involuntary and designed to enable the
organism to survive (Fig. 1.1).

Organs involved in activating these changes
include the adrenal glands, situated above the
kidneys (Fig. 1.2). These glands consist of an inner

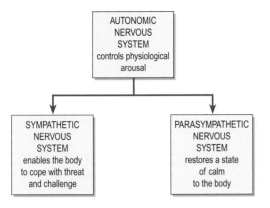

Figure 1.1 • The autonomic nervous system.

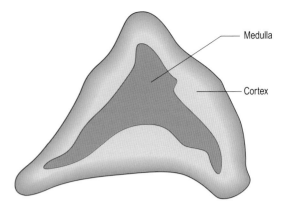

Figure 1.3 • Cross-section of an adrenal gland.

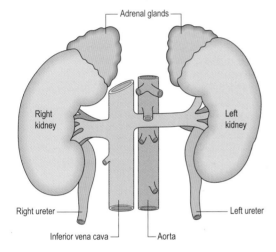

Figure 1.2 • The positions of the adrenal glands and some of their associated structures. (From Wilson 1990 with permission.)

part or medulla and an outer part or cortex (Fig. 1.3). Receiving directions from the hypothalamus via the spinal cord, they release hormones which modify the action of the internal organs in response to environmental stimuli.

When a situation is perceived as challenging, the brain immediately responds via the spinal ganglia, by stimulating the adrenal medulla to release catecholamines such as adrenaline and noradrenaline into the bloodstream. The function of these neurotransmitters is to prepare the organs for action in a manner which has been collectively

known as the 'fright/fight/flight' response. It is characterized by an increase in heart rate and a redistribution of the blood from the viscera to the voluntary muscles. Blood pressure and respiratory rate are also increased, alertness and sensory awareness are heightened, muscle tension is raised and there is a mechanism for losing body heat. These factors enable the individual to make a physical response. The autonomic systems and their actions are shown in greater detail in Figures 1.4 and 1.5.

Some of the changes which occur as a result of sympathetic stimulation produce noticeable symptoms, for example, faster breathing, stomach cramps and sweating. States such as fear and anger illustrate this and underline the link between emotion and the internal organs. When the changes are pronounced and occur frequently, the organs concerned can become fatigued and this has given rise to the concept of psychosomatic illness.

Closely associated with the autonomic system but acting in the longer term, the pituitary gland releases the adrenocorticotrophic hormone (ACTH). This stimulates the adrenal cortex to produce substances, the most important of which is cortisol which helps to maintain the fuel supply to the muscles. In this way it supports the action of the catecholamines (Waugh & Grant 2006). There is also evidence suggesting that the stimulation of normal levels of cortisol enhances the immune system (Jefferies 1991). High levels of cortisol such as those created by prolonged stress or by pharmacological doses are, however, associated with a suppressed immune system.

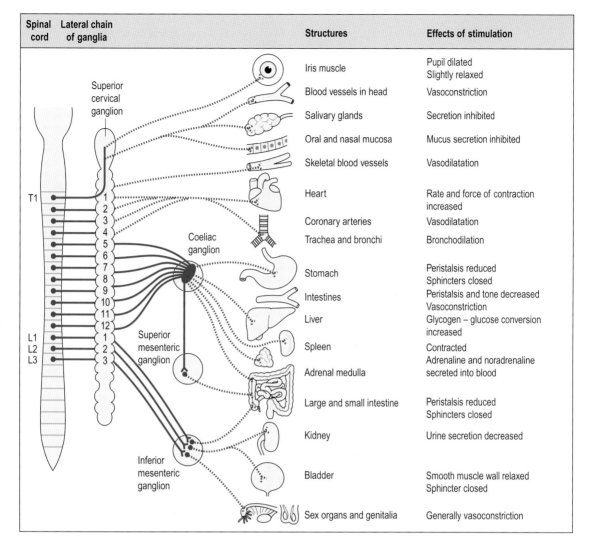

Spinal cord	Lateral chain of ganglia		Structures	Effects of stimulation
	Superior cervical ganglion		Iris muscle	Pupil dilated Slightly relaxed
			Blood vessels in head	Vasoconstriction
			Salivary glands	Secretion inhibited
			Oral and nasal mucosa	Mucus secretion inhibited
			Skeletal blood vessels	Vasodilatation
T1			Heart	Rate and force of contraction increased
			Coronary arteries	Vasodilatation
	Coeliac ganglion		Trachea and bronchi	Bronchodilation
			Stomach	Peristalsis reduced Sphincters closed
			Intestines	Peristalsis and tone decreased Vasoconstriction
			Liver	Glycogen – glucose conversion increased
L1 L2 L3	Superior mesenteric ganglion		Spleen	Contracted
			Adrenal medulla	Adrenaline and noradrenaline secreted into blood
			Large and small intestine	Peristalsis reduced Sphincters closed
			Kidney	Urine secretion decreased
	Inferior mesenteric ganglion		Bladder	Smooth muscle wall relaxed Sphincter closed
			Sex organs and genitalia	Generally vasoconstriction

Figure 1.4 • The sympathetic outflow, the main structures supplied, and the effects of stimulation. Solid lines, preganglionic fibres; broken lines, postganglionic fibres. (From Waugh & Grant 2006, Fig. 7.42, p171, with permission.)

Under challenge, all the above hormones are released (Fig. 1.6). When the situation of challenge passes and the stress response is no longer needed, neurotransmitters are released to restore balance to the autonomic system. The organs which were previously stimulated now weaken their hold and their actions subside as a state of equilibrium settles on the body metabolism. A shift occurs away from sympathetic dominance towards parasympathetic dominance. If the products of sympathetic activity are not burnt up in physical activity, they lie in the bloodstream, where they can irritate other organs and promote the development of

vascular deterioration (Gill 2008). It is important, therefore, to reduce their impact and this can be done either by controlling the stressor or by introducing a method of relaxation. The relaxation response method of Benson aims to counteract the effects of sympathetic activity by promoting the action of the parasympathetic, thereby exploiting the reciprocal nature of the two parts of the autonomic nervous system (see Ch. 22).

Activity of the parasympathetic, however, is not always benign (Poppen 1998). Asthma is exacerbated by bronchial constriction and gastric ulcers by acid secretion. Both bronchial constriction and

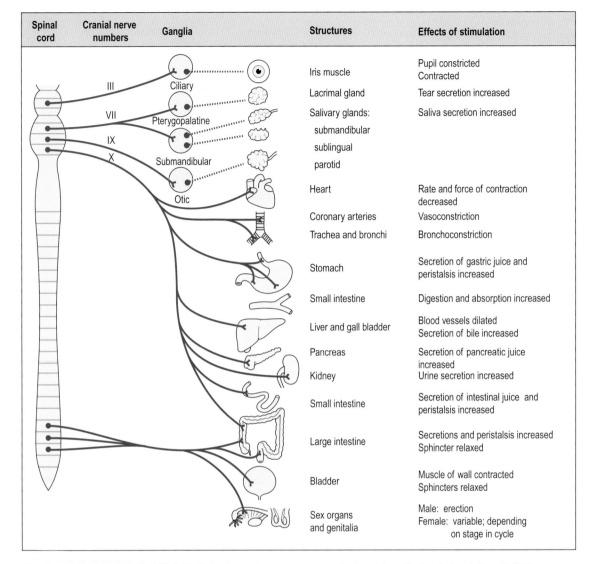

Spinal cord	Cranial nerve numbers	Ganglia	Structures	Effects of stimulation
	III	Ciliary	Iris muscle	Pupil constricted Contracted
			Lacrimal gland	Tear secretion increased
	VII	Pterygopalatine	Salivary glands: submandibular sublingual parotid	Saliva secretion increased
	IX			
	X	Submandibular		
		Otic	Heart	Rate and force of contraction decreased
			Coronary arteries	Vasoconstriction
			Trachea and bronchi	Bronchoconstriction
			Stomach	Secretion of gastric juice and peristalsis increased
			Small intestine	Digestion and absorption increased
			Liver and gall bladder	Blood vessels dilated Secretion of bile increased
			Pancreas	Secretion of pancreatic juice increased
			Kidney	Urine secretion increased
			Small intestine	Secretion of intestinal juice and peristalsis increased
			Large intestine	Secretions and peristalsis increased Sphincter relaxed
			Bladder	Muscle of wall contracted Sphincters relaxed
			Sex organs and genitalia	Male: erection Female: variable; depending on stage in cycle

Figure 1.5 • The parasympathetic outflow, the main structures supplied and the effects of stimulation. Solid lines, preganglionic fibres; broken lines, postganglionic fibres. (From Waugh & Grant 2006, Fig. 7.43, p172, with permission.)

acid secretion are associated with parasympathetic dominance, yet the conditions of asthma and gastric ulcer are often relieved by relaxation and aggravated by stress. The theory is not consistent (p155 and p164).

Psychological theories

Three types of psychological theory concerning relaxation are discussed in this section:

• cognitive

• behavioural
• cognitive–behavioural.

Cognitive theories

'Our thoughts define our universe,' writes Piero Ferrucci in *What we may be* (1982). The way we view what happens to us determines how we feel about it. This idea epitomizes the cognitive approach which sees feeling as a function of thought. Interpretations, perceptions, assumptions and

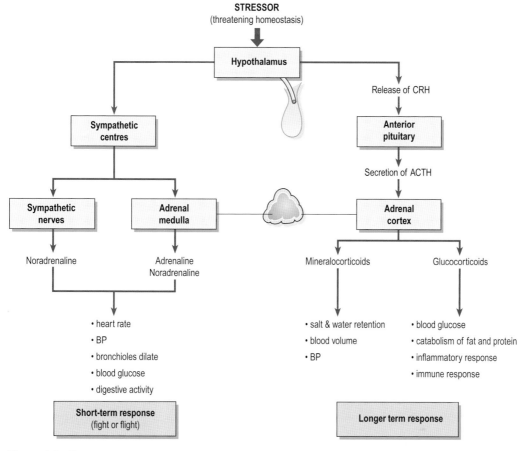

Figure 1.6 • Responses to stressors that threaten homeostasis. CRH, corticotrophin-releasing hormone; ACTH, adrenocorticotrophic hormone. (From Waugh & Grant 2006, Fig. 9.12, p224, with permission.)

conclusions will all give rise to particular feelings, which in their turn govern our behaviour. This means that our experience of stress and anxiety is related to the way we interpret events in our lives: we may, for example, appraise situations in ways which make them appear unnecessarily threatening (Lazarus & Folkman 1984).

Ellis (1962, 1976), a psychotherapist, attributes much anxiety to the irrational responses made by individuals, and cites the following example:

If person X puts me off, it must mean she doesn't like me, and if she doesn't like me it's probably because I'm unlikeable.

In this example the individual is basing his view of himself on one isolated event. Ellis also indicates that such a person tends to think in terms of absolutes, for example: 'I must be liked by everyone,

otherwise I'll feel worthless'. An individual locked into this pattern of thinking is doomed to disappointment and anxiety because of the impossible standards he has set for himself.

Treatment consists of identifying the irrational beliefs, challenging them and considering more rational alternatives. These ideas form the basis of Ellis's rational emotive therapy.

Beck (1984), a contemporary psychiatrist, also sees anxiety (and depression) as stemming from wrong thinking. To Beck, the distress is created by faulty thinking patterns which allow the individual to have a distorted view of events. For example:

- an individual blames himself whenever something goes wrong although he is not responsible
- he feels he is unemployable after one job rejection

- he blows up a minor mistake into a catastrophe: accidentally scratching his car, he sees it as irredeemably damaged.

Such a person tends to magnify his weaknesses and to see his minor mistakes as disasters; he dwells on his failures and dismisses his achievements.

The first step in therapy is to identify the automatic thoughts that make up the faulty thinking patterns. This is done by keeping a diary of anxiety-related events together with a description of the thoughts and fantasies and levels of emotion which accompany them. These thoughts are then tested against reality by asking what evidence there is to justify them. Are they plausible? Should they be challenged? Does it matter if what the person fears happens? If the automatic thoughts do not stand up to reality testing, he will need to modify them. Another common error is that of over-estimating danger and underestimating coping abilities. Recognizing when stress is caused by habitual thinking errors and not by a specific event immediately reduces the impact of the event or situation. Some thought patterns may need to become more positive and less negative, but the principal aim of therapy is to help the individual adopt a more realistic view of himself, his world and his future (Beck 1976).

Recognition of the value of Beck's cognitive therapy is increasing. Over the last 30 years its effects on a variety of major mental health problems have been compared with those of pharmacological treatments, behaviour therapy and interpersonal psychotherapy, and found to be either superior or of equal efficacy (Butler et al 2006, Elkin et al 1989, Gloaguen et al 1998, Hollon et al 2005).

Both Ellis and Beck see the individual as having the ability to control his thoughts, and thus having the power to modify his feelings and his behaviour if he wants to. Their models are respectively concerned with challenging irrational thoughts and questioning faulty thinking patterns. Such approaches belong to the area of cognitive restructuring, i.e. the combatting of 'self-defeating thought patterns by reordering the client's perceptions, values and attitudes' (Lichstein 1988). Although their theories are similar in many ways, their styles of therapy differ: Ellis adopts a confrontational approach while Beck is more collaborative (Neimeyer 1985).

While cognitive theory is referred to several times in this book, the theories of Beck and Ellis are particularly relevant to the chapters on stress (Ch. 2), cognitive-behavioural therapy (Ch. 16) and goal-directed visualization (Ch. 19).

A further researcher whose work has been influential in the cognitive field is Seligman (1975). He focused on the degree of control which a person perceives himself to have over his environment. People who lack this kind of control are subject to a state he termed 'learned helplessness' which predisposes them to depression. Seligman's recent work has been called 'positive psychology'. This work provides guidance on how to lead a meaningful and fulfilling life. Its principles are based on positive emotions, positive psychological traits and positive-minded institutions (Seligman & Csikszentmihalyi 2002).

Cognitive methods may be seen to include most approaches involving the mind. Thus, self-talk and mental diversion are cognitive, as are other techniques which aim to restructure the thoughts. Some of these, however, are less amenable to scientific investigation than the structured approach of Beck.

Behaviour theory

Behaviour theory, by contrast, is concerned with observable actions. Discounting what goes on in the mind, it sees behaviour as conditioned by environmental events. Such events are seen as leading the individual to act in predictable ways. In the case of classical conditioning, behaviour is governed by associations; for example, Pavlov's dog learned to salivate at the sound of a bell because the bell was linked with the smell of food. This automatic association has helped to explain how fear responses can develop. Any stimulus that regularly occurs within a situation where fear is elicited will itself come to trigger a fear response.

In the case of operant conditioning, behaviour is governed by a system of reinforcement (Skinner 1938). Positive reinforcement refers to a response which is strengthened by adding something to the situation; for example, giving an employee a bonus every time she makes a profit for the firm. This results in the employee continuing to work hard. Negative reinforcement refers to the strengthening of a response by removing something from the situation; for example, when a headache is relieved by taking an aspirin, the likelihood of taking an aspirin to relieve the next headache is increased. Together, these two concepts can be used to shape behaviour.

Since these theories were first propounded, behaviour theory has developed in ways which take it away from its original reductionist models. However, it still retains its central principle, that observable behaviour is more worthy of investigation than behaviour which is only inferred, i.e. mental processes.

Behavioural approaches include muscular relaxation, distraction, graded exposure and social skills training. Muscular relaxation is described in the early chapters of this book; distraction consists of activity which diverts the attention; graded exposure offers a step-by-step approach towards mastery over a feared object or situation; and social skills training concerns interpersonal communication and covers verbal and non-verbal behaviour. Assertiveness techniques, developed in the 1970s by Alberti & Emmons, are a central component of social skills training. These writers define the concept as behaviour where people are acting in their best interests without experiencing undue anxiety and without denying the rights of others (Alberti & Emmons 1982). Topics included in assertiveness training are:

- exercising personal rights
- setting personal priorities
- expressing views
- making requests
- refusing requests
- countering manipulative behaviour in others
- allowing oneself to make mistakes.

Behaviour styles can range from aggressive to submissive, but the style of choice in most situations is the assertive one. Knowing when and how to use it is one of the social skills.

Initially it was considered by behavioural therapists that thoughts and emotions were unnecessary to the understanding of behaviour. However, over time it became evident that such matters could not be fully considered in isolation and that a certain overlap between cognitive and behavioural methods existed (Homme 1965). It can be seen from the above items, for example, that assertiveness training contains a strong cognitive element. This has led some researchers to combine the two approaches.

Cognitive–behaviour theory

This theory brings together the ideas from both philosophies. The combined approach was referred to as cognitive–behavioural training. Both Beck and Ellis acknowledged the value of this new development and included behavioural exercises in their cognitive therapies (Davidson 2008). Research has shown it to be at least as effective as medication in a wide range of anxiety disorders (Blackburn & Twaddle 1996, Davis et al 2000). As a component of cognitive–behavioural interventions, relaxation training plays a key part in the treatment of the physiological symptoms in anxiety and other clinical disorders (Donaghy et al 2008).

Cognitive–behavioural principles are described in Chapter 16. They also underlie some of the stress-relieving strategies in Chapter 2 and feature in the goal-directed visualizations in Chapter 19.

From theory into practice

Stress can express itself in any of three modes: the somatic (physiological), the cognitive (psychological) and the behavioural (observable actions). It has been proposed that the pattern of changes produced by cognitive relaxation techniques will be different from those produced by physiological ones, and that benefit can be derived from matching the treatment to the problem. For example, tension headache may be more likely to respond to a somatic approach such as releasing muscle tension than to a cognitive one such as correcting faulty thinking patterns (Lehrer 1996, Yung et al 2004).

Current thinking in cognitive–behavioural theories, however, favours a model in which interactions occur between somatic, cognitive and behavioural processes; for example, a painful joint is not simply a physical symptom but one which also involves psychological factors such as worry, and behaviours such as avoidance of certain activities which are associated with pain (Vlaeyen & Morley 2005). While different techniques may be used to influence the various aspects of anxiety, the aim of any therapeutic intervention will be the seamless integration of its different elements (Ralston 2008).

Relaxation and emotion

Therapeutic interventions should consider the role of our emotions within this seamless integration. What, however, is an emotion? We all know what it feels like to experience love, joy, anger and jea-lousy and we also know that changes are occurring in the body alongside these emotions, for example, the experience of fear is accompanied by a fast-beating heart. The conditions of stress and relaxa-tion have both cognitive and somatic aspects. In the case of relaxation, the cognitive aspect refers to the experience of mental calmness while the somatic aspect refers to such physiological matters as diminished nerve and muscle activity.

Like the emotions, relaxation is linked, on the one hand, to thinking processes and on the other, to physiological ones. Connecting them is the area of our feelings. These are relayed to the mind which makes sense of them; it processes the mate-rial, in a way which is based on the information it receives. This leads to physiological changes. However, thoughts can spontaneously arise in the mind, triggering our feelings, which themselves lead to physiological changes in the body. Thus our thoughts can trigger our emotions as our emotions can trigger our thoughts (Donaghy 2007).

Deeply involved in this process is the hypo-thalamus, a key organ within the limbic system where emotions are thought to originate. The hypothalamus carries impulses in both directions and initiates the chemical changes which accom-pany emotional activity. A system of feedback thus underlies the integrated actions of emotion, cogni-tion and physiology.

Figure 1.7 shows this two-way flow between the cortex and the limbic system and on to the physiological structures which produce the body's response. In the cerebral cortex there is a complex interplay among the many neuronal connections. The result is that links involving thought, emotion and neurophysiological responses run throughout the brain, allowing it to make constant refinements to our behaviour (Gill 2008).

How does relaxation therapy work?

Some techniques, such as Benson's relaxation response, work by activating the parasympathetic division of the autonomic nervous system (Benson 1976). This is thought to decrease physiological arousal. Some techniques, such as progressive rela-xation, reduce muscle tension. Others work by creating a distracting effect which draws attention

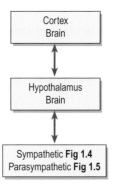

Figure 1.7 • Two-way flow of impulses between the brain and the physiological organs.

away from the source of the stress, as in imagery, or by focusing attention on a specified emotionally neutral object, such as the breath in meditation. In all these, the relaxation acts as a mediator, dimi-nishing the impact of the stressor.

Most techniques, however, have several effects, the principal one tending to generalize across the entire organism since the mind cannot be separa-ted from the body nor the body from the mind.

Practising relaxation skills is essential

All relaxation training involves the learning of new skills or the facilitation of already established ones. Practice is essential for the development of these skills and, for greatest benefit, should be under-taken daily. The length and quality of training and the dedication to home practice are vitally impor-tant to the outcome.

Borkovec & Matthews (1988) compared the anxiety levels of individuals trained in progressive relaxation with the levels of those untrained and found that the reduction in anxiety demonstrated in the trained group became considerably more pronounced as practice of the technique increased.

The learning process is aided by demonstration and feedback. Clients are also given information (printed as well as verbal) and this helps them to feel more in control of the procedure, provided the information is in a form which is meaningful to them. Feeling in control is thought to increase the client's motivation (Pomeroy 2007, Wulf 2007). Motivation can also be stimulated by record keeping on the part of the client; for example, a diary could record times of practice and changes in anxiety levels.

For those who wish to teach the technique, some kind of training is necessary. However, where this is not available the principles which underlie some of the methods can be woven into the skills already possessed by the health care professional. For example, attention to posture is a valuable and universal concept outside the domain of the Alexander technique, and images of warmth and heaviness can be induced without autogenic training.

The health care professional may sometimes feel inadequately equipped to deal with certain stress-induced conditions. Such a situation calls for consultation with a specialist in the area.

How to choose a technique

In selecting a technique for a particular disorder, the health care professional will be guided by the research. Chapter 26 contains research findings on a wide range of disorders for which relaxation training has been used, and Appendix 1 itemizes suggested applications for the different methods. It may be useful to consider the evidence alongside personal choice since a technique which gives the client a positive experience will probably have a relaxing effect.

Another guiding principle is the nature of the disorder and how it matches up with the technique. For example, a sports injury may respond best to a physical method such as progressive relaxation

Case study 1 Tension headache

Matthew works in an office where he spends most of his time seated at a computor. He likes his job and sets high standards for himself – sometimes impossibly high. He has been there for 15 years and has received promotion at regular intervals. He is married to Deborah who works in the local supermarket and they have two children. Matthew's hobbies are building model aircraft and growing orchids; he and Deborah are also enthusiastic ballroom dancers. In the last year or two, however, he has increasingly suffered from discomfort in his neck and from headaches which make his job difficult and interfere with his ballroom dancing events. The headaches seem to get worse as the day progresses. At first, he thought they were brought on by cigarette smoke but a ban on smoking has been imposed and the headaches have persisted. Sometimes things go wrong in the office, such as people taking advantage of his dedication to the work, and this makes the headaches worse. Also, the newly commissioned seating arrangements at work are not as comfortable as the old ones and seem to aggravate the pain in his neck which spreads to his shoulders. He has been arriving home exhausted and has to lie down. He worries about the cause; he also worries about his future in the job.

His friends tell him he should consult his GP, so eventually he does but the GP can find nothing organically wrong. Matthew is advised to start a course of relaxation training as the headaches might be associated with stress. He accepts this diagnosis – after all, many people suffer from stress, nothing to be ashamed of. He finds a therapist and arranges to meet at weekly intervals. His treatment begins with an investigation into his thoughts on the matter: what does he think causes the headaches? Does he have any thoughts which might help to find an explanation

for his own particular headaches? It is explained to him that such a dialogue approach has been found to be an effective way of tackling the problem. He is asked to keep a diary to record headache occurrences, rating the severity of each one, the circumstances in which it occurred and his feelings and thoughts about it.

In this way, the therapist gently prepares the ground for Matthew to make his own contribution to the diagnosis. He begins to feel he has been expecting too much of himself; it doesn't work to be a perfectionist; it leads to unnecessary anguish when things go wrong. Instead, he learns to be more assertive. Matthew is also introduced to posture exercises and stretchings to reverse the effects of the work posture. Perhaps his chair could be modified to make it more comfortable. Progressive relaxation is a further way of relaxing the tension, being a technique which has a direct effect on the muscles.

He responds favourably to all these procedures and is encouraged to integrate them into his work situation. He particularly likes the Jacobson technique which he finds easy to learn, effective and something he can do without attracting the attention of other people. Gradually, after a lot of daily practice, he begins to feel more at ease with himself and with his life. He stops worrying about the headaches which grow less frequent and less intense until after a few weeks they stop altogether. He is delighted. Things start to improve at work too. He seems to be getting on better with his colleagues; only yesterday he made a joke which made them all laugh. He feels happier; however, he realizes that the headaches could easily start again, so he decides to continue with daily exercise practice to ensure that he remains free of pain.

Case study 2 Panic disorder and agoraphobia

Angela is a professional carer who has looked after a succession of disabled people in the 20 years she has been in the job. She has enjoyed her work most of the time. It took her out and about and she always managed to find herself with people who appreciated her visits. She found the job emotionally rewarding. Bill, her husband, an insurance agent, would pick her up after work in his car and they would drive home together. Bill would settle down to read his paper while she prepared the evening meal. Eighteen months ago, however, Bill died. Angela was devastated. Her life crumbled. No Bill at home. No lifts after work. The whole structure of her life collapsed. At 52 she was left high and dry with apparently nothing to live for.

Everything seemed to be going wrong. Her job evaporated. Her mortgage payments fell behind. Things rose to crisis pitch one day when, selecting fruit in her supermarket she accidentally knocked over a tall stand of tomatoes. She abandoned her trolley and rushed out of the shop.

Since that occasion she has not been back and has become increasingly tied to the house. Not eating properly, she began to feel physically ill. Pressure from friends, neighbours and relatives drove her to look for treatment and she was given antidepressants. The medication made her feel better but only for as long as she took it. If she stopped, her symptoms returned. But she didn't want to take antidepressants for ever.

Then one day she saw advertised a class for people suffering from agoraphobia. This could be for me, she hesitatingly thought. It was not easy getting there but she steeled herself to do so, arriving in a cold sweat with palpitations, hard breathing and butterflies in her stomach. It was a talking group whose members were all experiencing what she was going through. She began to relax. Talking was good. As well as being able to talk to people with the same problem, she learned what she could do about it. Change your thoughts, they said. But how? Why worry about a tomato stand? It's probably been knocked over before. the shop is used

to it, we are sure nobody turned a hair. It's unlikely to happen to you again and, even if it does, it's not the end of the world. Get a diary, they say. Write down your fears as they occur and ask yourself what triggers them off. Are they justified? What is your way of dealing with them? We all have our particular solutions.

This was magical talk to her. She felt soothed by this new way of thinking. The group facilitator also taught a range of relaxation exercises: autogenics, passive muscular routines, imagery and visualizations. At first she was afraid to surrender herself to the relaxation experience as she feared losing consciousness. But she was reassured that could not happen. The visualizations entailed picturing herself returning to the supermarket and successfully making purchases without the least trace of panic. Angela liked the visualizations; they showed her coming out on top. But it was made clear to her that in order to benefit from this teaching she would have to practise three times a day.

She went home after the first visit in a mood she did not recognize in herself and resolved to carry out the instructions.

Over the next couple of months, with weekly visits, she found things were beginning to improve. She practised hard and was delighted with her new skills. In time she felt ready to start putting them to the test. Gingerly at first, just walking up to the shop. Nothing terrible happened. Nobody took any notice of her. Gradually over the next few days she began to feel confident enough to enter the shop and still nothing terrible happened. Her confidence grew over the next couple of weeks. She still had palpitations and butterflies but she could control them, and as her confidence grew her physical health improved.

She knew she hadn't fully thrown off the panic feelings, but now she had a way of dealing with them. And she was being invited to do some voluntary work which made her feel herself again.

whereas a cognitive disorder such as agoraphobia may benefit more from a psychological approach such as visualization. However, it is principally the evidence which should guide the practitioner in her choice of method to ensure that the best technique is selected for the particular situation.

Two examples will serve to illustrate how theory can inform practice. The first concerns a 55-year-old male office worker with tension headaches associated with pain in his neck and shoulders. The

second relates to a 35-year-old housewife with agoraphobia. They would each benefit from a course of relaxation training but whereas the first is a relatively straightforward problem, the second has more complex requirements.

Evidence of effectiveness

Techniques described in this book are known as mind–body approaches and include methods such as muscle relaxation, meditation and imagery. Measurement in this field has only developed in the last few decades, accounting for a relatively small research base, its development having possibly been delayed by the centuries-old dominance of the medical model. However, in recent years this research base has been growing and the evidence points to a variety of physical and psychological health benefits.

Reviewing the literature in 2003, Astin and colleagues found evidence to support the use of mind–body interventions. These included relaxation therapy in a variety of conditions such as cardiac rehabilitation, headache, insomnia, postsurgical pain, incontinence, chronic low back pain, cancer and the symptoms related to its treatment in the form of nausea and vomiting. For these conditions the evidence was considerable. Less robust evidence was found to support the use of mind–body techniques for hypertension and arthritis. The review excluded psychological disorders. On the basis of these results, Astin et al suggested that mind–body interventions be employed as adjuncts to conventional treatment.

A subsequent review in 2005 looked at the effects of relaxation techniques in a broader range of conditions that included psychological difficulties and disorders. It identified benefit in hypertension, cardiac arrhythmias, chronic pain, insomnia, anxiety, mild and moderate depression, premenstrual syndrome and infertility (Stefano & Esch 2005).

Evidence of the effect of relaxation training in reducing anxiety is shown in the systematic review of Manzoni et al (2008) in which relaxation techniques were found to be of consistent and significant benefit. State anxiety was shown to be more responsive to treatment than trait anxiety (see Ch. 15, p129 for definitions of state and trait anxiety) but equal benefit was derived from both group and individual sessions. Anxiolytic effects were markedly greater in participants who practised relaxation skills and a gradient of benefit related to the intensity of training could be seen.

With regard to depression, relaxation training can be seen as a potentially effective treatment. This is the conclusion drawn in a Cochrane review of 15 trials where relaxation techniques were found to be more effective than no treatment or minimal treatment, although less effective than cognitive–behavioural therapy. However, this latter treatment is not always available in which case relaxation techniques may be a useful first-line psychological treatment (Jorm et al 2008). Thus, important research developments are taking place.

In many cases, the relaxation method has been evaluated as a component of a larger scheme of stress management. Consequently it is not known what proportion of the success is due to the relaxation component. Another problem concerns inconsistency in the research findings; it reflects limitations in the methodology such as inadequate allocation, concealment and non-blinded outcome assessment including self-report. Other factors relate to procedural variability, for example different interpretations of the method.

Not all techniques have been through the systematic review process and this limits the drawing of conclusions in the field. At this moment, there is insufficient evidence to state that one method of relaxation is better than another.

KEY MESSAGES

- Relaxation is a state of low physiological arousal accompanied by a calm state of mind.
- It is possible to induce a state of relaxation in different ways, some focusing on the body and others on the thoughts in the head. The state induced, however, will involve both mind and body.
- Current evidence of effectiveness is presented but the research base is too small to declare one method superior to another.
- Practising the technique is essential. Greater practice leads to more effective results.

Further reading

Physiological background

Waugh, A., Grant, A., 2006. Ross & Wilson's Anatomy and Physiology in Health and Illness, Tenth ed. Churchill Livingstone Elsevier, Edinburgh (Chapter 9).

Cognitive background

Donaghy, M., Nicol, M., Davidson, K., 2008. Cognitive-Behavioural Interventions in Physiotherapy and Occupational Therapy. Butterworth Heinemann Elsevier, Oxford.

Stress: what is it?

CHAPTER CONTENTS

Stress is a commonly experienced emotion that is closely associated with physical symptoms such as increased heart rate, increased rate of breathing, and sweating. When we are stressed we are likely to experience feelings of anxiety, worry and fear. These are normal emotions. However, when stress in our everyday lives becomes unrelenting, it can cause ill health and absenteeism from work. In Europe, stress is now the most common cause of absenteeism, with 20 billion euros a year lost to job-related anxiety or stress (Ralston 2008).

Theories of stress

The concept of stress in the living organism was studied by Selye (1956). His work showed that when a body is subjected to a challenging stimulus, a characteristic response occurs. Selye identified three stages (Fig. 2.1):

- alarm
- resistance
- exhaustion.

Exposure to the stimulus results in the release of hormones and chemicals whose purpose is to create appropriate physiological changes. This is the alarm reaction. It is cancelled as soon as the stressor is

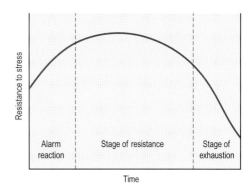

Figure 2.1 • The general adaptation syndrome.

withdrawn. If exposure to the stressor persists, the body will adapt by developing a resistance which serves it well at the time. Such resistance, however, takes a toll of the organism's resources and this stage will not last indefinitely. As body resources become depleted, a stage of exhaustion takes over. Together, these stages make up the 'general adaptation syndrome' (Selye 1956).

Selye, whose concern was centred on physiological aspects, viewed stress as the non-specific response of the body to any demand made on it. (By non-specific, he meant that the same response would occur irrespective of the nature of the stimulus.) Twenty years later, the psychologists Cox & Mackay (1976) defined stress as 'a perceptual phenomenon arising from a comparison between the demand on the person and his ability to cope. An imbalance gives rise to the experience of stress and to the stress response'. The emphasis here is on the individual's perceptions, on the subjective nature of stress and on its psychological dimension. Selye, in 1956, had ignored the role of psychological processes (Cox 1978).

Cox & Mackay's model introduces the idea of perceived coping powers as a factor governing the resulting stress. If an individual perceives his ability to cope as weak, and sees environmental demands as heavy, the level of stress he experiences will be high. If his self-perceived coping powers are strong, then those same demands may be readily tolerated and the level of stress experienced will be comparatively low. The environmental demands may, however, be too low, so low that stress arises from boredom. When the individual's perception of environmental demand is matched by his perceived coping ability, a state of balance can be said to exist.

It is clearly desirable for the individual to operate in situations where demands and coping skills are balanced. Establishing and maintaining that balance may involve regulating his exposure to the stressor. Alternatively he could reduce his anxiety levels and increase his coping ability.

This is a model which allows for variation among individuals as well as for changing perceptions over time in the same person. The ideas enshrined in it have led to the concept of the 'human performance curve' which is based on the relationship between demands placed on the individual and his coping ability (Fig. 2.2). Moderate levels of demand are associated with efficient performance. When demands are perceived as too heavy,

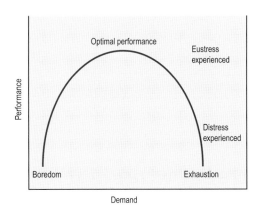

Figure 2.2●Human performance curve.

the overtaxed individual begins to experience fatigue; when they are too low, boredom results from understimulation. Distress is experienced in both events (Looker & Gregson 1989).

At the top of the curve is the zone of high performance. Here the individual is operating at levels of demand which match his coping skills. Daily variation may result in one slightly outweighing the other: for example, sometimes he feels that he has more capacity than he is being called upon to use, which gives him a feeling of confidence and control; at other times, he may feel that environmental demands are drawing on untapped inner resources, creating the rewarding experience of being pleasantly stretched. These feelings are collectively referred to as 'eustress' or 'good' stress.

Lower down the curve, on either side, the individual's performance gradually declines as the curve runs through transition zones of moderate stress and, ultimately, into zones of deep distress.

Thus, while distress erodes the person's quality of life, eustress enhances it. Working at levels of arousal that feel comfortable promotes not only the efficiency of the individual's output, but also his mental well-being.

The topic of stress has been developed further by Lazarus & Folkman (1984) who defined stress as an imbalance between the demands of the situation and the self-perceived resources of the individual. The imbalance gives him a subjective feeling of stress because he feels he does not have the capacity to control the demands made on him.

Most stress results from a sense of perceived harm or a sense of threat; however, if the individual feels confident to handle the situation, the conditions which give rise to it will appear more as a challenge than as a threat.

Symptoms of stress

Stress is associated with physiological symptoms characteristic of sympathetic nervous system activity. These symptoms relate to the fright/fight/flight response (p6) and are summarized below, together with the psychological symptoms of stress, both the subjective (how a person feels) and the behavioural (how a person acts), although there is considerable overlap in these areas.

The symptoms vary among individuals because of the differing sensitivities of organs to the experience of stress.

Physiological symptoms

As mentioned in Chapter 1, these comprise:
- raised heart rate
- increased blood pressure
- sweating
- raised blood coagulation rate
- increased ventilation
- raised blood glucose level.

Subjective symptoms

These include:
- tiredness and/or difficulty in sleeping
- muscle tension, particularly in neck and shoulder muscles
- indigestion, constipation, diarrhoea
- palpitations
- headache
- difficulty in concentrating and a tendency to worry
- impatience; feeling irritable and easily roused to anger.

Behavioural symptoms

Behavioural symptoms include:
- increased consumption of alcohol, tobacco, food, etc.
- loss of appetite or excessive eating
- restlessness
- loss of sexual interest
- a tendency to experience accidents.

Measuring stress

A physiological assessment of stress would include such measurements as heart rate, blood pressure, respiratory rate and skin conductance. Psychological as well as physiological methods have been devised to measure stress. One which has had some influence is the Social Readjustment Rating Scale (SRRS) of Holmes & Rahe (1967). These researchers compiled a table of life events ranging from minor violations of the law to the death of a spouse, rating each one in terms of the mental readjustment it demanded. A high score in any one year was associated with a high risk of developing a stress-related illness. But the SRRS has its critics: whereas Holmes & Rahe had proposed that any change in a person's circumstances, positive or negative, contributed to the risk, other researchers (Lazarus et al 1980) argued that positive experiences could moderate the effects of negative life events, making them less damaging to the immune system. For example, a broken bone is easier to tolerate if it coincides with the announcement of good exam results.

Another point of discussion raised by the SRRS is whether the stress caused by a series of minor adverse events is more harmful than one major adverse event. Lazarus believes it can be and has devised a tool for measuring small, day-to-day problems, calling it the Hassles Scale (Kanner et al 1981). Further research has supported the notion that a major crisis perceived to be solvable and of short-term duration is less harmful than a long-lasting succession of small hassles which the individual feels unable to control (Stevens & Price 1996).

The meaning that an event has for the individual also needs to be considered. Moving house, for example, can be a pleasant form of stress if you choose to move but a source of deep distress if you are forced to do so. Our interpretation of an event thus determines the nature and intensity of our response (Lazarus 1991).

In spite of these and other criticisms, the SRRS has been highly influential as a tool for measuring the effects of stress. Changing social values have, however, rendered some of the ratings out of date and created a need for additional items. As a result, the original scale was succeeded by a revised instrument, the Recent Life Changes Questionnaire (Rahe 1975), which has itself been rescaled (Miller & Rahe 1997) (Appendix 3). We acknowledge that there are other measures of life events which have been used in recent research (Picardi et al 2005). However, we have chosen to describe Miller & Rahe (1997) because of its historical relevance and its accessibility.

In the above measures, stress is represented in the form of life events. This is an objective way of viewing stress. Subjective measures also are in common use and consist of questionnaires which have been standardized for validity and reliability. Aspects of mood are itemized and the individual asked to tick the box which best reflects how he is feeling (see Chapter 25).

Sources of stress

Stress can arise from a multitude of sources. Broadly speaking, these sources can be categorized as those in the environment and those within the individual (Powell & Enright 1990).

Stress in the environment

The work environment

Conditions may be such that the levels of noise are excessively high; it may be too hot or too cold; the atmosphere may be polluted by tobacco smoke or exhaust fumes.

The individual may be suffering from work overload in the form of unrealistic deadlines, long hours or a feeling that the job is beyond his competence. On the other hand, the job may lack stimulation, causing him to feel bored, or it may lack opportunity for him to demonstrate his ability. There may be uncertainty as to the boundaries of his responsibility and the work objectives may be inadequately defined. Relationships with colleagues and superiors may be strained. He may be obliged to move to other departments or to other geographical locations. He may be declared redundant or be forced to retire before he wants to (Kovacs 2007).

The social environment

Social ties seem to play a large part in determining the way in which we cope with negative events. These ties include partners, relatives, friends and acquaintances and they act as a buffer between the event itself and the individual's reaction to it. Among the many researchers to demonstrate this association are Cohen & Wills (1985), who have shown that stress-related illnesses are less likely to occur among people with strong social support, and Pennebaker (1990), who shows the protective value of having a confidant. Social and cultural issues such as isolation, poverty and disability are considered to be major causes of mental stress (Goldberg & Huxley 1992).

Skelly (2003) highlights the importance of chemical stressors as a source of stress; these include additives in food and drink and pollutants in the air and water.

Stress in the individual

Personality types

Friedman & Rosenman (1974) described a personality type particularly associated with coronary heart disease. This type was characterized by a tendency for the individual to drive himself to achieve goals one after another, to create a programme filled with deadlines and to perform activities in a competitive manner with a constant need for recognition.

Individuals who displayed these tendencies were referred to as 'Type A' personalities, while those with the opposite characteristics were described as 'Type B'. Type B individuals were found to be almost immune to coronary heart disease. Type A characteristics are seen as negative insofar as they may lead to stress-related illness. However, they also lead to high achievement which is to be valued. Cooper (1981) suggests emphasizing the need to *manage* Type A behaviour rather than extinguish it. This may mean slowing down, resetting goals, regularly taking 5 minutes off and recording the occasions when this is performed. It may also mean seeking alternative ways of gaining rewards.

Kobasa (1982) described what he called the 'hardy' personality. Such a person was seen as being relatively resistant to stress by virtue of possessing three qualities: a sense of control over his life, a feeling of being committed to his work, hobby or family, and a sense of challenge in which change was viewed as an opportunity to develop himself rather than as a threat to his equilibrium. Individuals who do not possess these qualities are more likely to suffer from stress-related disease than those who do.

Personality traits are, however, not set in stone. The genetic predispositions we are born with are subject to external influences, particularly in early life, resulting in some traits being emphasized while others are diminished (Cassidy 1999). The findings from longitudinal research studies suggest that by early adulthood personality traits are more or less fixed (Matthews et al 2003). However, others would argue that since our actions are governed less by trait than by contingency (Dawes 1994), the genetic element is less influential than it appears. Stress levels and associated behaviour in the individual can vary which suggests a view of personality as a shifting entity (Apter 2003). The inability always to predict behaviour from personality traits has led to the development of theories around personal causation and self-confidence. These approaches include how effective we feel when predicting achievement in day-to-day activities and how much control we feel we have over our lives.

Self-efficacy

Self-efficacy is the term used to describe an individual's sense of his ability to deal with events and situations in his life. It is therefore concerned with confidence. Self-efficacy is the *belief* that a particular task can be successfully achieved. This leads into the area of expectation (Bandura 1977, 1986).

Bandura (1986) suggests that one's beliefs lead to expectations which can be classified in two ways: one is the expectation of efficacy and the other is the expectation of outcome. The first relates to the level of confidence a person has in being able to carry out a task successfully, i.e. whether he thinks he has the ability, and the second concerns beliefs which allow the prediction of results, i.e. whether he thinks his efforts will succeed. The theory is relevant to the self-management of chronic pain.

Self-efficacy is enhanced by the successful outcome of target behaviours. Increases in self-efficacy, in their turn, make it more likely that future outcomes will be successful since high levels of self-efficacy are related to self-perceptions of control and optimism. When we are successful

we build a sense of personal mastery which gives us a feeling of being in control of our lives. Being persuaded by other people that we can cope and succeed in difficult circumstances helps to intensify this feeling of mastery.

An individual who has low levels of confidence in predicting success can be helped to develop these qualities in several ways: by modelling himself on others who are successful, by the persuasive words of others and by emphasizing any success he may have had in the past.

In the context of the relaxation class, it may be helpful initially to invite such a person as an observer or provide him with a video to show the outcome of relaxation training, thereby allowing him to experience vicariously the success of others. The more strongly he believes in the benefits of the exercise, the more confident he will feel practising it and the greater will be the likelihood of success in managing the stress in his own life.

Self-efficacy, as a concept, originated in the clinical setting as a way of modifying the client's reactions to adverse events, such as those which lead to phobias (Bandura 1977, 1986, 1997). It has since proved to be a very powerful determinant of health-related behaviour (Schwartzer 1992).

Locus of control

Locus of control is a phrase which refers to the individual's perception of the degree of control he has over the environment (Rotter 1966). If he feels he has influence over most situations in his life, he is said to have an internal locus of control. If, on the other hand, he believes that his life is largely controlled by other factors such as fate or other people, his locus is said to be external.

Locus of control is a feature which has been studied in various contexts, one of which is stress where low vulnerability to stress seems to be related to internal locus and high vulnerability to external locus. Thus the more influence an individual believes he has over his environment, the less likely he will be to experience stress.

Other stressors of internal origin

Beck (1984) refers to stressors within the individual, such as the tendency to interpret events in a consistently negative way. Ellis (1962) points to the maladaptive effect of holding unrealistic belief systems, for instance believing one has to be right every time in order to be a worthwhile person (p10). Other maladaptive styles include:

- having unclear or unrealistic goals, leading to wasted effort and disappointment
- failing to make decisions: unmade decisions can so preoccupy the individual that he cannot get on with his life. The unresolved matter continues to claim his attention and eventually wears him out
- bottling up emotions: anxiety and anger are examples of emotions that people often keep to themselves, allowing the feelings to grow out of proportion
- having low self-esteem: a feeling that one lacks the rights that are accorded to others. Such a person may allow himself to be overruled on every side.

From theory into practice

As stress is an acknowledged component of many conditions, health care workers are increasingly being asked to help alleviate it. This does not mean that relaxation therapy should, in any sense, be seen as a substitute for medical help. Rather, it can be seen as a useful adjunct to other treatment. It also has a preventive role.

When offering relaxation training sessions to a group of people, the healthcare professional may wish to include certain topics and a discussion. This has been found to enhance outcomes (Payne 1989). The topics will relate to those conditions which group members are experiencing. for example anxiety, panic attack, depression and life changes. Coping is also a useful topic. For the purposes of this book, two of these topics, anxiety and coping, are considered.

Anxiety

Commonly experienced feelings of stress and anxiety are different from clinically recognized anxiety disorders where the anxiety is experienced at greater intensity and for longer duration. Unlike the fleeting periods of anxiety we experience in everyday life, clinical anxiety disorders may be profoundly disabling. If left undiagnosed and untreated, they tend to persist and may become chronic. While relaxation may be helpful in reducing stress,

it is likely that in the management of anxiety disorders, it will be used in conjunction with other interventions such as cognitive–behavioural therapy (CBT) or medication.

A number of anxiety disorders have been described by the American Psychiatric Association (1994).

- *Specific phobia*: significant and persistent anxiety in relation to a specific object or situation. Examples include spiders, storms, blood, injection, injury, tunnels and lifts. Contact leads to an immediate anxiety reaction. The person may rationalize that the fear is greater than it should be but feels powerless to avert the reaction. Situations are avoided for fear of further exposure.
- *Social phobia*: also known as social anxiety. The main feature is fear of one or more social situations where the individual worries that she will act in a way that is judged negatively by those around.
- *Generalized anxiety disorder*: main features here are significant worry and anxiety on most days, the worries covering a range of events and activities. The individual is likely to experience physical symptoms such as muscle tension, sleep disruption and poor concentration.
- *Panic disorder*: panic attacks involve an experience of intense fear which includes a range of symptoms including palpitations, sweating, trembling, chest pain, nausea and fear of losing control. Individuals with this condition experience these symptoms frequently and they worry about having further attacks. Panic disorder may also be associated with agoraphobia and a fear of enclosed spaces such as buses, trains and shops. Typically, these situations are avoided.
- *Obsessive compulsive disorder (OCD)*: this disorder consists of unwanted thoughts and images which intrude into a person's everyday life. The most commonly experienced obsessions revolve around fears of contamination with associated compulsions of frequent handwashing or bathing. Fears about personal safety are also common with associated compulsions of repeated checking of electrical appliances, door locking, etc. The compulsive behaviour reduces the anxiety for a short time but has to be repeated.
- *Post-traumatic stress disorder (PTSD)*: here the person has been exposed to a traumatic

event which may be relived over and over again. Intrusive images and upsetting dreams are features of the condition. In an attempt to protect herself, the individual will try and avoid any triggers such as places, thoughts, feelings and conversations relating to the event. Associated symptoms include feeling emotionally distant from others, disturbed sleep, irritability, difficulty concentrating, hypervigilance and heightened startle response.

One of the features of clinical anxiety disorders is co-morbidity with other conditions. Co-occurring depression (Brown et al 2001) affects as many as one in four, and substance abuse affects every second person with post-traumatic stress disorder (Kessler et al 1995). Reich et al (1987) have suggested that between 40% and 63% of people with panic disorder and agoraphobia have associated personality disorders. It is important, therefore, for health care professionals to recognize when anxiety symptoms reach the level of clinical disorder and to make the appropriate referral.

Coping

Coping has been defined as the way a person manages the demands of a situation when that situation is appraised as stressful. It refers to the thoughts he has about it as well as any particular behaviour it evokes (Lazarus & Folkman 1984). People who cope well may be employing one or more strategies to reduce the stress. For example, it is often possible to change the environment: if the monitor screen is too low and gives you a backache, it could be raised. This is problem-focused coping. Another way of coping is for the individual to change his response to the situation; instead of reacting angrily when things go wrong, he could practise one of the strategies in anger management. This is emotion-focused coping (Lazarus & Folkman 1984).

Higgins & Endler (1995) add a further category which describes the avoidance practised by some people; that is to say, by avoiding situations which are likely to create stress, they feel they are coping adequately. Developing these theories, other researchers have suggested an approach which protects against future stress. This is the proactive coping style (Aspinwall & Taylor 1997, Folkman & Moscovitz 2004). It searches out potential stressors and prepares a reserve of coping styles for handling them. For example, in situations of uncertainty it

is useful to have built up a store of information together with strategies to help retain one's control of the situation, in case it should develop in a negative way (Kovacs 2007).

Listed below are examples of coping skills which could feature as topics for discussion in group meetings.

1. Getting as much control over the stressor as circumstances allow. While accepting the restrictions of the situation, there may be areas of freedom which a person can develop.

2. If control is not possible or expedient, a person can change the way he thinks about the stressor: for example, instead of being irritated by traffic queues, he could see the time as an opportunity to play music tapes.

3. Training oneself to predict stressful situations in order to weaken their impact.

4. Being task oriented and not letting emotions take over. Emotions fuddle the mind and interfere with problem solving. If the emotion is strong, it can first be acknowledged then separated from the issue, which can then be judged dispassionately.

5. Avoidance of blaming; the latter tends to arouse anger. A more constructive attitude is to see mistakes as the result of a series of events which simply happened.

6. Dealing with anger. Some anger may serve a useful purpose; much anger, however, is purely destructive. The energy that goes into its arousal could often be more profitably spent in solving the problem. Ways in which anger can be controlled include:

    *   reinterpreting the stimulus in a more positive light; many situations contain ambiguities which allow reinterpretations to be made
    *   being realistic in one's expectations of other people
    *   modifying one's internal dialogue to include self-statements such as 'I am easygoing' or 'I keep my cool'
    *   focusing on the issue rather than the personality.

7. Giving oneself permission to make a mistake. It is part of being human to make mistakes occasionally.

8. Distancing oneself. If circumstances seem to be overwhelming, one can try stepping back mentally to get a more objective view (p19 and p20). It is sometimes useful to visualize another person coping with the same problem.

9. Introducing humour at suitable moments. When a person smiles and laughs, the relaxation response takes over.

10. Managing time efficiently. Priorities need to be established and time allotted to tasks proportionately. If time is short, inessentials can be cut out and tasks delegated. It is sometimes possible to say 'no' to demands when time is restricted.

11. Having someone to confide in.

12. Rewarding oneself for a job well done.

13. Living in the present. This means savouring the moment, enjoying the journey as well as the arrival. It is useful to remember that the future is to a large extent determined by the way we handle the present. A lot of stress arises from dwelling on the past with its regrets or on the future with its uncertainties.

14. Establishing good relationships. The support derived both from intimate relationships and the wider social network acts as a buffer to protect the individual from the full effects of stressful events (Ganster & Victor 1988). However, relationships, whether at work or at home, demand time and attention.

15. Taking exercise (see Ch. 15).

16. Learning to become more assertive.

Table 2.1 Stress-evoking factors and related coping strategies

Stress-evoking factor	Coping strategy
Faulty belief system	Cognitive restructuring
Unclear goals	Goal setting
Unmade decisions	Decision making
Low self-esteem	Building positive self-image
Bottling up feelings	Confiding, assertiveness
Deadlines and time constraints	Restructuring time
Deteriorating relationships	Enhancing personal interaction

Table 2.1 sets out some stress-evoking factors alongside appropriate coping strategies.

KEY MESSAGES

- Stress is an imbalance between the demands of the situation and the perceived resources of the individual.
- Stress can arise in the environment, in both work and social situations, or within the individual as a function of his personality or his behaviour.
- The force of the stressor can be ameliorated by social support which acts as a buffer.
- Relaxation can be used to ameliorate stress and feelings of anxiety. However, clinical anxiety may require additional interventions.
- Coping skills can strengthen the individual's perception of his abilities to handle stressful situations. This helps to turn a threat into a challenge.
- An important coping skill is knowing how to relax.

Chapter Three

Preparing for relaxation

This chapter provides a practical guide to generic aspects of relaxation training. The contents may be helpful for preparing people including students, self-help groups and practitioners, whether the training is delivered in one-to-one sessions, classes or through small group activity. Aspects of relaxation training which apply to all approaches are discussed here and include setting, confidentiality, position, introductory remarks, delivery, termination, debriefing, number of sessions, homework, the therapist, supervisory back-up and pitfalls (Payne 2004). Working with groups is then considered.

Aspects of procedure

Setting

Most authors advise a quiet, warm setting free from disturbance. However, others favour one that bears more resemblance to the normal environment, on the grounds that the relaxation skills learned will be more readily transferred to real life. Consequently, a background which includes faint external sounds may be deliberately sought since too heavy a silence can be artificial, even anxiety inducing.

Establishing confidentiality

In the case of group work, confidentiality must be established at the outset and re-established each time a new member joins. Confidentiality in this context means that nothing of a self-disclosing nature expressed by any member of the group is referred to outside the session. Topics can be discussed outside but only in a general sense.

Position

For deep relaxation lying is preferable to sitting, since a totally supported body will more readily lose its tension. However, some people, for different reasons, do not like lying. Another drawback of the lying position is a tendency on the part of the trainee to fall asleep (p30). In defence of sitting, however, it can be argued that the skill of relaxing transfers to everyday situations more effectively if it is taught in a position in which stress is more likely to occur, i.e. sitting rather than lying. Thus it can be seen that both positions have value and may be used on different occasions during tuition.

Various starting positions will be mentioned in later chapters. Mitchell (1987) lists three: lying supine, sitting and leaning forward with the arms and head supported on a high surface, and sitting with the back and head supported (p96). Jacobson (1938) mentions two: lying and sitting (p48). Bernstein & Borkovec (1973) favour a reclining chair or an easy chair with a footstool (p59), as does Poppen (1998) (p89). When lying on the floor, participants may find it comfortable to place a pillow under the knees as well as the head.

Many groups meet in public buildings, such as schools or church halls, where the floors are wooden or tiled. These are hard, but a length of foam or a beach mattress provides a suitably softer surface and can be supplied at very little cost by the participant himself. Women will find trousers more comfortable than a skirt for most of the exercises.

Whether the eyes are open or closed is determined by the nature of the approach and the preference of the trainee.

Introducing the method to participants

A short introduction will help to put the client at his ease.

Injury and illness can create stress, I think you'll agree. Stress is uncomfortable. It also interferes with the body's healing mechanisms because energy is diverted from the healing process in order to maintain a state of high alert. To reduce this state of high alert we need to promote a calm body and mind. Relaxation techniques can help to achieve this. There are different kinds of relaxation technique. Some involve the muscles and breathing pattern while others involve the thoughts in the head. Often both are involved.

When presenting any particular method it is believed that clients want to know two things above all others: that the approach is well established and that it works (Lichstein 1988). A short rationale addressed to the client is therefore appropriate. In addition, for the benefit of any trainees who fear that they are going to be hypnotized, Hendler & Redd (1986) suggest adding a disclaimer to reassure participants that such is not the purpose. It can also reduce the possibility of unintentional trance induction.

A sample introduction might be:

This relaxation procedure is one that has been practised for x [number of] years. It has been studied by researchers and found to be effective. You'll feel very relaxed and calm as a result. It is not the same as hypnosis and you will not lose consciousness at any point.

As some techniques involve the musculature, the concept of muscle action could be described, as in the paragraph below.

Muscle action

When a muscle contracts, its fibres shorten, making the muscle fat. On relaxing, the muscle returns to a resting state in which the fibres are by comparison long and thin. A contracting muscle feels hard to the touch. You can illustrate this by taking your thumb across the palm of your hand and, using the fingers of the other hand, feel the muscle below the thumb getting hard. Now, relax the thumb, and feel the muscle below it become soft.

This exercise demonstrates that the relaxation, as well as the contraction of skeletal muscles, is under the control of the will.

The introductory passages above need only be stated once; however, one of the two following passages may be used every time a session begins. These are used to help create the mood for relaxation by gently leading the trainee into a calm frame of mind. The first approach is called 'sinking' and the second 'imaginary bubble'. It is not necessary to use both.

Sinking

Make yourself as comfortable as you can ... become aware of the surface underneath you

*... let your body settle into it ... notice how
it supports you ... notice the points of contact
between you and the floor: your head ... shoulders ... spine ... ribs ... hips ... heels ... elbows
... forearms and hands ... feel your body
sinking into the surface you are lying on ... feel
the tension leaving it ... your body getting heavier as the tension ebbs away ... feel at peace
... Take one good breath and as you let it out,
feel it carrying all your tensions away ... then
let your breathing settle into a gentle rhythm ...*

Imaginary bubble

*As you lie or sit, reflect on the idea that you are
going to give the next half-hour to yourself. No
telephone can ring for you; no doorbell disturb
you; no-one will call your name. You may hear
sounds around you: voices, horns, sirens, bangs
and revs ... think of them as being outside your
world. With these thoughts in mind, draw an
imaginary circle around yourself, about 3 feet
from the centre. Create an imaginary bubble
... think of the interior as your space ... your
own private space. Feel how safe it is ... safe to
get in touch with yourself. Turn your thoughts
inwards.*

Delivery

Any relaxation procedure calls for a tone of voice
that is quiet and calm. That does not imply that it
should be hypnotic. Bernstein & Borkovec (1973)
suggest that the tone should be conversational to
begin with, but that the volume and pace of speech
should be gradually reduced as the session wears
on. They advise a tone which is 'smooth and quiet,
perhaps even monotonous, but not purposely
hypnotic'.

The pauses between instructions should always
be long to give the trainees time to carry out the
action or to evoke the image. Dots in the text indicate these pauses.

The 'live' voice is generally used for teaching.
Tapes also have value; for example, a trainee might
learn initially from the live voice, then continue
at home with a tape (preferably one containing
the trainer's voice) until he knows the technique.
A disadvantage of tapes is that the individual may
become dependent on them and unable to relax
without them. Any advantage that tapes have in

controlling the verbal aspect of the instruction is
more relevant to research than to therapy.

Termination

All deep relaxation procedures should be brought
to a gradual end, allowing the participant to make a
slow return to the alert state. A variety of methods
are described throughout this book. Some practitioners use a counting process, others a simple
sentence such as: 'When you feel ready, please
open your eyes and sit up'. Some teachers recommend bending and stretching the limbs, while
others advise sitting quietly for a few minutes.
Most of the relaxation approaches mentioned in
this book carry their own form of termination. The
following is a sample procedure.

*I am going to bring this relaxation session to an
end ... I'd like you gradually to become aware
of your surroundings ... feel the floor/chair
underneath you ... in your own time open your
eyes ... give your limbs a few gentle stretches
... make a few fists to stir up the circulation ...
have the feeling that you are alert and ready to
carry on with your life ...*

Termination is sometimes referred to as 'arousal' or
'return to everyday activity'. In autogenic training
it is called a cancellation.

Debriefing

At the end of a relaxation session there is a debriefing process, the object being twofold: to make
the experience more satisfying for the client and to
provide the therapist with feedback. The therapist
might open the discussion with questions such
as: 'How did you find that experience?', 'Did it
make you feel more relaxed?', 'Did you find the
technique easy to follow?', 'Was anything about it
confusing?', 'Were you able to relate to the different parts of the body?'. Plenty of time should be
allotted to the debriefing section to give clients the
opportunity to express their reactions or confide
their experiences, all of which helps the therapist
to understand her clients better. Trainers should
be prepared for feelings to be released during this
period since thoughts related to past trauma can
be unlocked by the relaxation experience.

Information gathered in this way is part of the ongoing assessment process and can help to increase the effectiveness of the following session.

Homework

Emphasis is placed on homework in every method of relaxation training as it leads to greater skill in using the technique. Skill is important because stress-related behaviour patterns tend to be resistant to change. Experienced use of the technique therefore increases its effectiveness.

Skill is built up by practice (see Ch. 1, p13). Only by regular and frequent practice will behavioural change take place. The need to practise, therefore, is paramount, a point that needs bringing out as trainees do not always appreciate its need. Investigating this topic in 1982, Hillenberg & Collins found significant levels of non-compliance in the home practice component of their study.

One way of increasing motivation is by introducing the record sheet or diary as a form of self-monitoring (see Ch. 1, p13). Regular, time-recorded entries of homework sessions and their outcomes are made on the sheet by the trainee and these provide feedback and encourage the trainee to continue. As it is important that these practice sessions fit in with the trainee's daily routine, convenient times can be discussed at the outset of treatment. Figure 9.3 (p82) offers a useful model.

The frequency and duration of homework are conventionally set at two periods a day, each lasting 15 minutes (Bernstein & Borkovec 1973). Whether or not this should be carried out soon after meals has been debated, the above researchers pointing to the benefits of postprandial low arousal. Others, however, favour avoidance of that time: Benson (1976) suggests that the process of digestion interferes with the physiological changes associated with meditation. Lichstein (1988), however, advises trainees to experiment and find the times that best suit them.

When the tuition course has come to an end, trainees are urged to continue practising, perhaps in some less frequent form, so that the benefits of training are not lost.

Number of sessions

It is possible to learn most methods in about six sessions, assuming that attention is given to home practice. Transcendental meditation can be taught in six, and progressive relaxation in 5–10 sessions (Lichstein 1988). Many relaxation courses, however, cover several methods and may do more than simply teach relaxation. They may include group discussion topics (see p23), mutual support and other concerns, thus extending the duration of the course beyond six sessions.

The trainer/instructor/therapist

On the thorny question of training, Luthe (1970), referring to autogenics, insists that only medically qualified practitioners are equipped to teach. Lichstein (1988) has viewed this position as untenable, believing that health care professionals have much to offer, provided they use their judgement and recognize the limits of their training. He feels that the interests of society are best served by allowing and even encouraging such individuals to teach relaxation methods.

The requirements for therapists who wish to teach relaxation methods include:

- basic training as a health care professional
- professional experience with the condition and type of group with whom they are working
- arrangements for supervision on a regular basis
- recognition that relaxation therapy is not a panacea, although it can be a powerful tool.

Today, there are validated courses on relaxation techniques which interested therapists are strongly advised to attend and, as relaxation training, in some form or other, has traditionally featured in the core training of many health care professionals, the therapy clinic becomes an appropriate setting for such work with clients (Potter & Grove 1999).

Supervisory back-up

Recommended to both group and individual relaxation therapy is the provision of supervisory back-up for the therapist. Its main purpose is to strengthen and maintain her skills, which in turn ensure the value of the treatment received by the client.

Supervision also helps to protect the therapist from emotional fatigue by providing an opportunity for her to release her own tensions, thereby guarding against the state of burn-out or exhausted empathy. Supervision performs another function, namely, in helping the therapist to handle her reactions if old wounds are re-opened during treatment, as they can be when past emotional experiences are stirred by listening to other people recounting theirs. Contact with a more experienced colleague is useful for resolving these and other problems which may arise in the course of work.

Finding a supervisor is the responsibility of the therapist.

Autonomy of the individual

A central feature of relaxation training is that the individual is seen as a self-determining being. Throughout all procedures he remains self-aware and free of control by outside forces. The state of relaxation he achieves is of his own making. In so doing, he assumes ownership of this state and responsibility for the progress he makes. Relaxation training is firmly rooted in this principle.

Measuring outcomes

Measurement of both physiological and psychological outcomes plays an important role in treatment and is discussed in Chapter 25.

Working with groups

The material in the succeeding chapters may be used with individuals or with groups of people. As group work is a subject on its own, a short summary will be relevant. Groups, in this context, may be of three kinds.

- *Led.* Here a leader offers a previously prepared programme. Although it is presented in a systematic way, the leader displays flexibility when appropriate.
- *Facilitated.* Responsibility for the group is taken by a particular individual who, at the same time, imposes no strict format. The facilitator helps to steer the group in the way the members have decided it shall go, but she avoids telling them what to do. Her role is to suggest possibilities. If problems arise, however, she is responsible for dealing with them.
- *Self-help.* There is no designated leader or facilitator. The style is informal but the members are usually highly committed, attending as they do for mutual help and

support. Relevant information is collected for circulation among them and their experiences are shared. A role of acting facilitator is often rotated.

Lichstein (1988) considers that the group format is an effective way of delivering relaxation. The led group particularly lends itself to this function since an entire course can be worked out in advance. Relaxation training also occurs in facilitated and self-help groups; however, since the facilitators may not have had relevant training and experience, extra care should be taken in avoiding the pitfalls.

Organization

Starting a group is one matter, but keeping it going can be more difficult. In order to build up and maintain group bonding, certain points need attention.

1. *Establishing and maintaining confidentiality.* The need for confidentiality was mentioned above. It is repeated here as it cannot be overstated.

2. *Course programme.* A knowledge of what to expect enables members to make plans. Dates should be supplied in advance together with, in the case of a formal course, a syllabus.

   Some classes offer relaxation alone; others begin each session with a topic related to the needs of the participants (p22), before moving into the area of relaxation itself.

3. *Client choice.* The sense of belonging to the group is enhanced if members are given some choice in the way it is run. How much choice depends on the nature of the group: in the formal led group, less choice may be appropriate than in the informal self-help group. However, choice can still be introduced into the formal group by finding out from the members at the outset why they joined and what they hope to get out of the meetings. This strategy helps the instructor to meet their needs and provides the participants with a more rewarding experience.

   A system of paper slips can be used to collect the written answers. The alternative is to ask members directly. However, many people find it threatening to have to voice their private thoughts in front of strangers; such an approach may also be non-productive if it draws false replies. In our experience, people prefer not to be asked such questions in front of a group, but respond more favourably to the paper slip system (Payne 1989).

4. *Ice-breakers*. These are strategies for relaxing the atmosphere. Their essential characteristic is that the members physically participate. Some are designed for use in pairs while others involve the whole group. An example of the first is seen when one member of each pair tells the other about something pleasant that happened in the previous week; then they switch over. Another example of working in pairs is when person A talks to person B for 2 minutes, telling him who she is and what she does. Then B talks to A.

   Whole-group activities are particularly useful for learning people's names. Remocker & Storch (1992) suggest a game in which each member wears a name tag. The aim is to collect everyone's name in the shortest time.

5. *Discussion*. Exchanging information and sharing experiences are features of the group debriefing period and give the session an extra dimension. The therapist now occupies the role of facilitator, maintaining the focus of the group and seeing that all members who wish to, get a chance to express their views. Clients tend to enjoy the discussion and normally display an eagerness to take part. There may, however, be a short period before clients have learned to trust each other when a natural reticence holds them back from disclosing personal information. This can cause the discussion to dry up. It can be revived by adopting the strategy of 'circular questions' (Powell & Enright 1990). This entails drawing one participant into conversation with another, for example: 'Peter, you've been in this situation. What would you say to Jenny who is going through the same experience?'. In most circumstances, however, the discussion period helps to hold the group together.

   Although the discussion period has value, participants should not feel under any obligation to take part. The voluntary principle, which states that pressure should never be exerted on individuals, must be upheld (Heron 1977).

6. *Handouts*. Printed material setting out the points made in the session acts as an aide-memoire for participants. Handouts should relate to the topic currently being discussed: the information loses its relevance if it is produced a week later.

7. *Sharing the time*. Inevitably, some people talk more than others. Trainers are glad to have 'talkers' in the group: they liven it up. At the same time, it is part of the trainer's responsibility to see that the quiet ones have an opportunity to speak. Thus, the trainer may feel that she sometimes has to intervene. A tactful way of doing it is the following: 'I don't want to dismiss what you are saying, but I wonder what X thinks about it?'.

8. *Friction-dispelling techniques*. Occasionally, friction arises; a member may consistently disagree with the way the group is run. Calmly facing such a person and asking how she would like things changed, then putting it to the rest of the group, often resolves the matter.

Falling asleep

There is a tendency in group work for some members to fall asleep during the session. This is discouraged by most therapists. Bernstein & Borkovec (1973) take the view that it interferes with the learning of a skill and suggest strategies for preventing or dealing with it:

- regularly asking for signals in the form of requests such as 'lift your index finger if you are beginning to feel relaxed'
- directing the voice towards any sleeping participant
- avoiding the early afternoon for teaching sessions.

Keable (1997) suggests informing participants at the outset that they will be awakened with a light tap if they fall asleep. Others suggest that people who are inclined to fall asleep should sit in a chair rather than lie down, since making people less comfortable reduces their tendency to fall asleep. Kokoszka (1992) refers to the effectiveness of focusing attention on a monotonous stimulus, e.g. counting breaths, for keeping people awake.

Thus, falling asleep tends to be seen in negative terms. Fanning (1988), however, takes the view that if people have come purely for respite from stress, they should be allowed to sleep.

 POTENTIAL PITFALLS

Relaxation training includes techniques which can have powerful effects. It therefore needs to be handled responsibly and with due regard to the attendant pitfalls. These are discussed in the relevant chapters. It is essential, before taking up any method, to become aware of its pitfalls.

KEY MESSAGES

- A simple explanation at every stage can help to reassure the client about the procedure.
- Debriefing the client after the session helps to make it more effective for him.
- Home practice is an important part of the learning process.
- Some training for the teacher is necessary.
- The methods described are suitable both for one-to-one sessions and for groups.

Section **Two**

Somatic approaches to relaxation

4

Breathing

CHAPTER CONTENTS

Introduction

A wide variety of breathing routines have been proposed to induce relaxation, such as slow breathing, deep breathing, breathing meditation and abdominal breathing. Using the breathing system as a means of gaining a relaxed state is clearly an accepted approach. Moreover, the techniques are easy to learn and can be carried out anywhere – a fact which makes them available in the stressful situation itself. Giving attention to the breathing is a feature of most relaxation techniques.

In this chapter the respiratory mechanism is first described; exercises which induce a relaxed breathing pattern are then presented; there is a section on hyperventilation, and also one on the pitfalls of breathing exercises.

The process of breathing

Breathing is an automatic process governed by centres in the brainstem (pons and medulla). These activate the diaphragm and costal muscles to open the rib cage which expands in three directions: vertically, laterally and anteroposteriorly. Negative pressure in the pleural cavity pulls the lungs out, causing air to be sucked in. Relaxation of the same muscles results in the recoil of the thoracic structures and the expulsion of air. The respiratory organs are illustrated in Figure 4.1.

Oxygenated blood leaves the lungs bound for the heart which pumps it round the body where its oxygen is exchanged for waste products, amongst them carbon dioxide. These are carried back to the heart. The spent blood is then returned to the lungs where it gives up its carbon dioxide and collects a fresh supply of oxygen. The interchange of blood gases takes place in the alveoli (air sacs) which contain surfaces richly supplied with hairlike blood vessels through which the gases diffuse (pass through membranes). The direction in which the gases pass is determined by their concentration, i.e. they move from a situation of high concentration to one of low concentration. Thus oxygen passes from the air in the bronchial tubes to the blood, and carbon dioxide passes from the blood to the air in the bronchial tubes. Each breath makes a contribution to the process. Figure 4.2 shows the structure of a terminal bronchiole with its air sacs.

Chemoreceptors in the walls of the aorta and the carotid arteries help to control breathing and are sensitive to changes in the amount of carbon dioxide circulating in the blood (Waugh & Grant 2006). The levels of carbon dioxide influence physiological activity, and are conventionally represented in terms of the partial pressure of carbon dioxide

(PCO_2). The arterial PCO_2 ($PaCO_2$) may range from 4.7 to 6.0 kPa in the healthy individual (Hough 2001). Carbon dioxide levels are measured using arterial blood gas samples or end-tidal airflow (air delivered at the end of exhalation and measured at the mouth or nostril); the results from either the blood or the airflow are very similar in normal lungs (Gardner & Bass 1989).

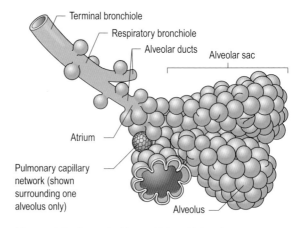

Figure 4.2 • A terminal bronchiole with its air sacs.

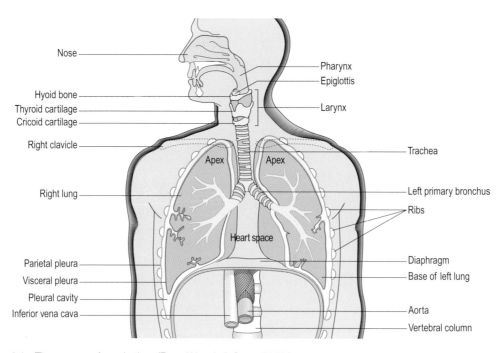

Figure 4.1 • The organs of respiration. (From Waugh & Grant 2006.)

Overbreathing and underbreathing

Overbreathing leads to excessive loss of carbon dioxide and a lowered $PaCO_2$ (hypocapnia); underbreathing leads to a build-up of carbon dioxide and a raised $PaCO_2$ (hypercapnia). A small rise (mild hypercapnia) is associated with lethargy and symptoms resembling those of parasympathetic dominance, i.e. relaxation (Slonim & Hamilton 1976).

Rationale of breathing control

Most relaxation methods such as imagery and muscle routines influence the autonomic nervous system by indirect routes. Breathing is different. It is directly linked to the system which controls physiological arousal. This adds to its potential as a means of inducing physiological relaxation.

The kind of breathing which accompanies sympathetic arousal is quite different from the kind of breathing characteristic of parasympathetic arousal; the first tends to be fast and staccato while the second tends to be slow and gentle. This connection between slow breathing and parasympathetic dominance has created a perception that slow breathing has stress-relieving properties and has led to its adoption as a relaxation technique (Sudsuang et al 1991). The approach is thus underpinned by physiological theory, but it also has cognitive elements in the form of the imagery which features in some of the exercises.

Its mechanism, however, is unclear. Lum (1981) proposed that slow breathing had a corrective effect on an abnormal pattern of breathing, while Garssen et al (1992) suggested that it may reduce stress for other reasons such as distraction.

Breathing awareness

This is a phrase which refers to the focusing of attention on the breathing pattern. It puts the individual in touch with the respiratory process and helps him to feel he has some control over it. As such, it forms a useful introduction to the topic. Breathing awareness begins with an exploration of the movements of the chest and abdomen which accompany respiration.

Exploring respiratory movements

During the inspiratory phase the chest expands through all dimensions. Participants can confirm this for themselves by the following exercises, for which plenty of time should be allowed.

1. **Lying or sitting**

    Place your hands on the lower edge of your ribs, fingertips a few centimetres apart. Feel your hands rise and separate as the air flows in and recoil as it flows out.

2. **Sitting with head and arms resting on a table**

    With movement in the front of the chest now restricted, you can feel the chest expanding backwards.

3. **Lying or sitting**

    Place your right hand over the solar plexus (the soft part between the ribs and the navel) and your left hand over the front of your chest below the clavicle (collar bone). Notice what happens under your hands when you breathe. As the air enters, feel the expansion growing, first under your right hand, then rising through the chest to reach the area under your left hand. Explore that idea for a minute or two.

The emotional state

Breathing is also subject to a person's emotional state.

Imagine for a few moments a situation that makes you feel uneasy ... Next, imagine one in which you feel at ease ... Did you notice any change in your breathing pattern from one to the other?

Breathing in a calm individual is associated with relaxed abdominal muscles and is characterized by visible movement of the upper abdomen; breathing in a stressed individual is associated with a predominantly upper costal movement and often involves contraction of the shoulder girdle muscles. Calm breathing tends to have a slow rate, stressful breathing a more rapid one.

Slow breathing

As mentioned above, relaxation is associated with a reduced rate of breathing. The natural pace of respiration in a resting individual is slow and since the oxygen requirement is low, breathing also tends to be rather shallow. The individual may occasionally take a deep breath and find it profoundly relaxing, but the natural tendency is for such a breath to be followed by the original pattern of slow and fairly shallow respiration. Certainly, the breathing of an unrelaxed individual is itself often shallow, but the difference between tense and relaxed shallow breathing is that the former occurs at a fast rate and is accompanied by tight shoulder muscles which restrict the natural movements of the thorax, whereas these factors are absent in a relaxed individual.

General points regarding breathing as a relaxation technique

1. Breathing should occur at the natural pace of the individual.
2. It should be seen in terms of 'letting the air in' rather than 'taking a breath'.
3. A smooth transfer should take place between inhalation and exhalation, and between exhalation and inhalation, unless the exercise indicates otherwise.
4. Breathing through the nose is preferable to breathing through the mouth since the nasal passages both filter and warm the incoming air.
5. Although some exercises may emphasize particular aspects of the breathing cycle, the respirations should always be gentle.
6. Artificially deep breaths should not be repeated in close succession because they can lead to hyperventilation.

The above principles are incorporated into the routines described here. When practising new forms of breathing control, it is helpful to adopt an attitude of quiet self-awareness rather than one which is intent on scrutinizing the performance (Van Dixhoorn & Duivenvoorden 1989).

Breathing routines for relaxation

1. Abdominal breathing
2. Breathing pouch
3. 'Out tension, in peace'
4. Breathing meditation (1)
5. Breathing meditation (2)
6. Breathing with cue words (cue-controlled relaxation)
7. A yoga exercise
8. Breathing 'chi'
9. Sighing

One breathing exercise is probably enough in one session. It can be repeated a few times, then dropped and taken up again later in the session. Allowing breaks between the exercises is a safeguard against overbreathing which may occur if the exercises are too enthusiastically carried out. Overbreathing or hyperventilation is discussed in a later section of this chapter.

Abdominal or diaphragmatic breathing

This refers to the kind of breathing which emphasizes the downward expansion of the chest cavity. It is useful at this point to inform or remind participants of the role of the diaphragm.

The diaphragm is a sheet of muscle whose edges are attached to the lower ribs, creating a floor to the chest. In the resting state it is dome-shaped. Contraction of the diaphragm flattens the dome, thereby lengthening the chest and drawing in air. Relaxation of the muscle causes it to reassume its dome shape which helps to push the air out. But the diaphragm also forms the roof of the abdomen and as such, its movements affect the position of the internal organs: as the contracting diaphragm presses down on the organs, it causes the abdomen to swell slightly. Similarly, as the relaxing diaphragm releases its pressure on the organs, the abdomen sinks back again.

To carry out an abdominal breathing exercise, the individual should first make himself as comfortable as possible, and spend a few minutes quietly resting. The following instructions may then be given.

Spend a few moments running through a sequence of pleasant imagery ... then, as your mind relaxes turn your attention to your breathing ... lay one hand lightly over the solar plexus. Focus your attention on this area. Start the exercise with a breath out ... a naturally occurring breath out. Notice a slight sinking of the area under your hand. Next, allow air to flow into the lungs, noticing the slight swelling which takes place under your hand. Then as the air is expelled, notice the area under the hand sinking back again. Allow the breathing to take place naturally.

Some writers teach abdominal breathing by urging pupils to 'think in and down' (Innocenti & Troup 2008). This helps to create a natural abdominal movement.

Breathing pouch

A variation of abdominal breathing, this exercise incorporates imagery. It is adapted from Everly & Rosenfeld (1981).

Concentrate on your breathing rhythm without trying to change it. Become aware of your upper abdomen swelling as you inhale and sinking as you exhale. Picture an imaginary, hollow pouch lying inside your abdomen ... as you breathe in, air travels down to fill the pouch, making the abdomen swell ... breathing out empties the pouch, causing the abdomen to sink back ... if you place your hand over your abdomen, you can feel gentle swelling and sinking taking place.

'Out tension, in peace'

Listen to your breathing without altering its pattern ... imagine your tensions being breathed out ... imagine them being carried away, a little at a time with each breath out ... and now, imagine that every time you inhale, you are breathing in peace, a little at a time with each breath ... breathe out tension ... breathe in

peace ... gently breathing ... feeling peace flowing through your body ... always keeping your breathing light ...

Breathing meditation (1)

Let your mind follow the path of the breath, taking care not to change its pace or its rhythm. Think of the air flowing in through your nostrils, along your nasal passages, down your windpipe and into your lungs ... then, gently and smoothly turning, it is carried out along the same route ... turning again as the air is drawn back in ... notice the feel of the air ... warm as it leaves, and cool as it enters ... continue on your own with this idea for a few minutes.

Breathing meditation (2)

This script illustrating 'breath mindfulness' is adapted from Lichstein (1988). It is particularly addressed to people with high blood pressure.

With your eyes closed, settle into your chair, couch or wherever you have chosen to be ... let your body lose its tension and let your mind gradually become calm by using some pleasant imagery ... allow your mind's eye to rest on the upper part of your abdomen ... be aware of it swelling and sinking as you breathe ... notice these breathing movements without trying to change them ... just observe them in the knowledge that your body takes full care of your breathing ... allow your breathing to continue on its own ... flowing gently and smoothly ... perhaps you can feel the rate getting slower ... this is because your resting body doesn't need as much oxygen as when you are active ... your heart rate also is lowered and your blood pressure falls, as a state of quiet settles on you ... allow yourself to enjoy this feeling of tranquillity ... let your mind continue to focus on your breathing for a few minutes longer.

Breathing with cue words

This exercise is described under the name of cue-controlled relaxation in Chapter 9 (p83).

A yoga exercise (quoted by Hough 2001)

Sit with your feet flat on the floor, and as you inhale, imagine the air being drawn in through the top of your head, travelling down through your body and passing out through your feet.

Breathing 'chi'

Breathe in the energy force, 'chi', and let it flow into the solar plexus ... then ... on the breath out ... let it flow to an area of your body that needs healing or soothing ...

Sighing

Enjoy the feeling of being relaxed and notice your slowed breathing. As the air leaves your body on the next breath, let it go with a sigh ... Aaaaah ... and then resume normal breathing ... two or three breaths later, repeat the sighing sound ...

Evidence of effectiveness of breathing retraining

In health, the breathing pattern reflects the metabolic needs of the organism. Sickness, on the other hand, can be associated with a disordered breathing pattern. Correcting this disordered breathing pattern might help to promote recovery from sickness. Gilbert (2003) reviewed evidence relating disordered breathing patterns to cardiorespiratory conditions such as angina, hypertension, chronic obstructive pulmonary disease and cardiac rehabilitation and found that normalizing the breathing pattern helped in some cases.

Matsumoto & Smith (2001) report that relatively little research has focused on breathing as a sole intervention. Breathing very often appears as a component of treatment but seldom on its own. Among the few published works on the topic is the comparison study of Bell & Saltikov (2000). These researchers compared the effectiveness of the Mitchell method inclusive of diaphragmatic breathing with diaphragmatic breathing alone in 45 normal male participants. Using heart rate as an outcome measure, significant reductions were found in both intervention groups relative to the control condition of supine lying. However, no significant difference in effectiveness was found between the two groups themselves. In other words, diaphragmatic breathing appears to be an effective relaxation technique on its own and becomes no more effective by being presented in conjunction with the Mitchell method. In their analysis these researchers suggest that physiological benefits of the Mitchell method may be largely due to the component of diaphragmatic breathing and that the technique of Mitchell may be only as effective as diaphragmatic breathing on its own (Bell & Saltikov 2000).

An earlier study looked at the effects of focused breathing on recovery after cardiac surgery. Twenty-nine patients were trained preoperatively in breathing routines. Investigating their reactions after surgery, Miller & Perry (1990) found significant decreases in both physiological responses and pain reports in the group who received the breathing instruction compared with those who did not receive it.

Some research has compared the effects of breathing retraining with those of drug therapy. The randomized trial of Kaushik et al (2005) compared biofeedback-assisted diaphragmatic breathing with propranolol in the long-term prophylaxis of migraine. Both approaches were found to be significantly effective but the breathing group had a significantly greater long-term prophylactic effect than the propranolol.

Treatment incorporating breathing components for a range of conditions may be found in Chapter 26.

Hyperventilation
(also known as dysfunctional breathing)

Exercises which succeed in slowing the breathing rate tend to reduce ventilation. This is a useful strategy to employ whenever a person is under stress, since stress tends to increase ventilation. However, ventilation in a person under stress can be increased to such an extent that it disturbs body systems. At this level it is called 'hyperventilation'.

In the state of hyperventilation, a person over-breathes: that is to say, he processes a greater volume of air than is required by his body at that moment (Innocenti & Troup 2008). Thus, a hyperventilating person is one who is breathing in excess of body needs: taking in too much oxygen and releasing too much carbon dioxide. This results in reduced levels of carbon dioxide in the arteries and body tissues. The $PaCO_2$, normally around 5.6 kPa, can fall to as low as 3.5 kPa (Innocenti 1983). Since carbon dioxide is acid, the pH value of the blood rises, creating alkalosis. This results in neuronal excitability, vasoconstriction and a widespread disturbance of the body chemistry.

Itself a symptom of stress, overbreathing thus creates symptoms on its own account, one of which is cerebral vasoconstriction (Gardner & Bass 1989). This is related to symptoms such as:

- dizziness
- headache
- visual disturbance.

Other symptoms listed by Hough 2001 include:

- paraesthesia (tingling) caused by alkalosis
- chest pain caused by coronary vasoconstriction
- palpitations caused by paroxysmal dysrhythmia
- anxiety and/or panic attack caused or aggravated by misattribution of physiological symptoms.

The breathing pattern of a hyperventilating person displays irregularities which may include any of the following (Hough 2001):

- rapid breathing, rising in some cases to 30 or more breaths a minute
- sighing, yawning, excessive sniffing and throat clearing
- halts in the breathing cycle
- marked movement in the upper region of the chest
- difficulty getting the breath.

These symptoms are collectively referred to as 'the hyperventilation syndrome'. Many of them resemble the symptoms of sympathetic nervous system activity. The apprehension they create can itself release catecholamines which reinforce the initial symptoms, setting up one vicious circle within another as shown in Figure 4.3.

Contrary to what might be supposed, the overbreathing does not lead to a greater availability of oxygen because the hypocapnia causes vascular changes which result in a decreased amount of oxygen being transferred to the tissues (Lum 1981).

The condition may be acute or chronic. Acute hyperventilation, which occurs in some people

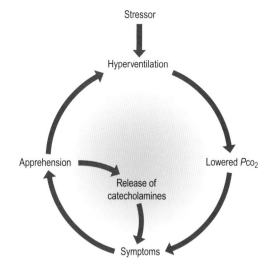

Figure 4.3 • The cyclic pattern of hyperventilation.

during moments of extreme stress, can give rise to marked symptoms. In chronic hyperventilation, however, there are often few visible symptoms; a process of adaptation appears to take place where the respiratory control mechanism undergoes 'resetting' to a lower level of $PaCO_2$ (Gardner 1992). However, in order to maintain this level, the respiratory drive must be increased, i.e. the individual must take deeper than normal breaths or suffer air hunger.

Although there is no conclusive way of testing for chronic hyperventilation, an indication of the state can be gained from simple tests. Four are described below.

- *Breathholding time*: the individual is asked to hold his breath. This is best done on an empty chest rather than a full one (CSP Interactive 2008). Difficulty in holding it for less than 20 seconds suggests that he may be hyperventilating. However, as people differ in the length of time they can hold their breath, the usefulness of the test lies in the repeated readings taken at regular intervals in the same individual. As the breathing pattern becomes more stable, the breath-holding time tends to increase (Innocenti & Troup 2008).
- *Provocation test*: the individual is asked to overbreathe rapidly for 3 minutes after which the expired CO_2 is measured at the mouth.

It is suggested that the end-tidal reading reflects the CO_2 level in the body (Bruton et al 2006). A fall in $PaCO_2$ of more than $1.33\,kPa$ and a slow recovery following the test are factors which suggest that the person may be hyperventilating (Innocenti & Troup 2008). The test is often used as a diagnostic tool by medical practitioners but it is not generally employed in therapy as patients tend to get distressed by the symptoms it creates (CSP Interactive 2008, Meuret et al 2005). It is inadvisable where cardiac irregularities exist, and Innocenti & Troup (2008) draw attention to its low accuracy rate.

- *The Nijmegen questionnaire (Van Doorn et al 1982)*: this contains a list of 16 subjective symptoms (Fig. 4.4). The individual marks the appropriate boxes and the values are added up to give a final score. This is expressed as a fraction of 64 which is the maximum score. If he scores above 23 he is considered to be experiencing the hyperventilation syndrome. Validity has been reported but is not conclusive. However, the scale is a useful component of the screening process and is widely used, particularly at the beginning and end of a course of treatment.

- *Observing the respiratory rate and pattern over 1 minute.*

Treatment

Breathing pattern re-education

The individual is first made aware of his existing breathing pattern which is then gradually replaced by a new one through a process of gentle re-education. Treatment is aimed at raising the levels of dissolved carbon dioxide in the arterial blood and reprogramming the respiratory centre to trigger inspiration at these higher levels (Innocenti & Troup 2008). This can be achieved by modifying the breathing pattern in different ways.

- Altering the rate and depth, making the breaths slower and/or shallower.
- Holding the breath for a few seconds.
- Changing the composition of inhaled air by rebreathing exhaled air.

Altering rate and depth

When people are asked to reduce their rate of breathing, they tend to take deeper breaths. This

	0 Never	1 Rarely	2 Sometimes	3 Often	4 Very often
Chest pain					
Feeling tense					
Blurred vision					
Dizzy spells					
Feeling confused					
Faster or deeper breathing					
Short of breath					
Tight feelings in chest					
Bloated feelings in stomach					
Tingling fingers					
Unable to breathe deeply					
Stiff fingers or arms					
Tight feelings around mouth					
Cold hands or feet					
Palpitations					
Feelings of anxiety					

Figure 4.4 • The Nijmegen questionnaire (Van Doorn et al 1982). (From Hough 2001, with kind permission from Stanley Thornes.)

will not change the $PaCO_2$ level. If it is to be changed, the interaction of rate and depth needs to be considered. When reducing one, the other has to be held constant if the $PaCO_2$ is to be raised. The individual can be reminded that slowing the rate means that the same volume of air is passing through, only travelling more slowly. A rate of 10–12 breaths a minute is a useful first target (Hough 2001). This can be reduced as the condition improves.

Breathing cycles which address rate and volume can be introduced (Innocenti & Troup 2008). For instance, a cycle for slowing the breath might consist of a gentle breath in followed by a slow breath out. Counting strategies can be incorporated, for example counting 'in … two … three' on the breath in and 'out … two … three … four …' on the breath out.

A regularity of breathing pattern is aimed at throughout the treatment and an abdominal form of breathing encouraged (Innocenti & Troup 2008).

In the early stages of re-education, controlled breathing may create air hunger because the brain continues to maintain a high respiratory drive. Later, however, following daily practice, the respiratory centre will begin to make the necessary adaptation (Rowbottom 1992).

Breath holding

If, during re-education, this feeling of air hunger becomes too great, the individual may sometimes find himself taking an excessively deep breath. This, of course, further lowers his $PaCO_2$ and temporarily worsens his condition. As a corrective measure, one breath hold is recommended lasting 5 or 6 counts (2 or 3 seconds), performed following the breath out. This compensates for the preceding unnaturally deep breath and helps to normalize the breathing pattern (Innocenti & Troup 2008). The same authors advocate the introduction of short gentle breath holds, performed at varying points in the breathing cycle, throughout the day (without altering the depth of the respiration). Otherwise, breath holds do not feature in most current treatment programmes (CSP Interactive 2008).

Changing the composition of inhaled air by rebreathing exhaled air

Air is made up of a variety of gases, of which oxygen contributes 21% and carbon dioxide 0.04% (Wilson 1990). However, this applies only to the air which enters the lungs. The air which leaves the lungs contains a lower proportion of oxygen and a higher proportion of carbon dioxide (exhaled air contains about 4% carbon dioxide). If a person in a hyperventilated state, i.e. with a low $PaCO_2$, rebreathes his own exhaled air, the condition will be temporarily corrected. A convenient way of doing this is to breathe into cupped hands placed over the nose and mouth and without releasing the hands, continue to breathe into them 4–5 times, taking a rest, then repeating the process if necessary. Hough (2001) emphasizes that the rebreathing should be gentle.

Rebreathing exhaled air is useful in acute hyperventilation and particularly if symptoms rise to panic level. Where symptoms are chronic, however, rebreathing will do little more than temporarily relieve them (Gardner & Bass 1989). Treatment for chronic hyperventilation should focus on the re-education of normal breathing patterns (as above).

People who habitually overbreathe need to understand that their symptoms are the result of a normal chemical reaction to stress. It occurs to some extent in everyone, particularly during crises. For certain individuals, however, it may become a habit, which they can be helped to overcome by correcting the breathing pattern and learning to identify the precipitating factors.

Relaxation

Because of the association between anxiety and hyperventilation, relaxation has a part to play, both as a preliminary to breathing re-education and as a component of stress management.

Home practice and self-management

Training the respiratory centres of chronically hyperventilating individuals to accept higher levels of PCO_2 takes time. Only practice can restore a normal breathing pattern. This practice consists of slow, smooth, shallow, abdominal breathing performed for about 15 minutes, three times a day (Hough 2001, Innocenti & Troup 2008). In addition to the therapeutic programme, there are other strategies which can help to slow the breathing rate, such as humming and reading aloud (Hough 2001).

People who hyperventilate may also need to examine environmental features which trigger or aggravate their condition, and deal with them in an appropriate way.

In their study of hyperventilating individuals, Pinney and colleagues (1987) demonstrated that a programme of education, relaxation and abdominal breathing helped to relieve the condition in 94% of participants.

Other approaches to treatment of hyperventilation

Hyperventilation has been associated with asthma. The theory underpinning the claim suggests that asthma is exacerbated by overbreathing with resulting hypocapnia and bronchoconstriction (Kellett & Mullan 2002). Two approaches are based on this assumption: the Buteyko and the Papworth methods. The principal feature of the Buteyko method is breath control and breath holding in order to reduce ventilation and reset normal CO_2 levels. Thomas (2004) found the condition responded favourably to the approach while Bowler et al (1998) found the approach resulted in a slightly decreased steroid use. Other researchers find the evidence lacking (Bruton & Lewith 2005). However, a randomized controlled trial carried out in Canada comparing the Buteyko breathing technique with physiotherapeutic breathing exercises showed significant reductions in asthma symptoms in both groups, with no difference between them. Benefit was maintained at 6 months (Cowie et al 2008).

The technique bears some resemblance to the Papworth method which employs diaphragmatic breathing, relaxation training and education to reduce hyperventilation A randomized controlled trial of the Papworth method found that asthma symptoms were reduced by one-third in participants who practised the technique. The method appeared to ease respiratory symptoms and dysfunctional breathing. These benefits were maintained at follow-up 1 year later. Accompanying depression and anxiety were also reduced (Holloway & West 2007).

Discussion

Cowley (1987) has shown that 50% of those who experience the hyperventilation syndrome also

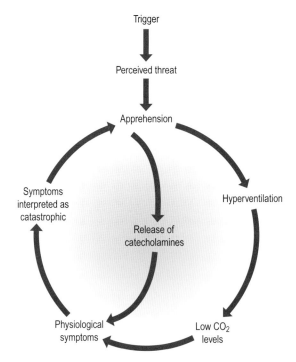

Figure 4.5•How hyperventilation might interact with cognitive factors to create a panic attack. (Adapted from Clark 1986.)

suffer from panic attacks. It is, however, often difficult to distinguish between hyperventilation in the acute form and panic attack. Similar symptoms occur in both conditions, being a result either of overbreathing or of stimulation of the sympathetic nervous system. Some researchers discuss the likelihood of an interaction between the two conditions, a possibility which is supported by the tendency for panic attacks to decline following treatment that focuses on respiratory control (Clark et al 1985). To cognitive researchers such as these, however, hyperventilation alone is not the cause of panic attacks. Cognitive factors predominate in their model in which it is suggested that resulting bodily sensations must be both perceived as unpleasant and interpreted in a catastrophic way for panic to develop. Figure 4.5 illustrates this idea.

However, respiratory retraining is important as it has been shown to result in a slower breathing rate, a decrease in anxiety and a reduction in the frequency and intensity of panic attacks (Han et al 1996). These are factors which make cognitive therapists reluctant to reject the benefits of breathing retraining (Meuret et al 2003).

Case study Continuation of the case study of panic and agoraphobia in Chapter One

Whenever Angela allowed her thoughts to dwell on the supermarket incident, she could feel her mouth getting dry, her throat constricting and the butterflies returning. Sometimes her hand would shake. But most of all she noticed a change in her breathing. It became halting, shallow and so high it was almost in her neck. She felt she might collapse. These panicky feelings accompanied every journey she made to the self-help class. The facilitator suggested she was hyperventilating – overbreathing, she said – and went on to explain how it caused loss of carbon dioxide and made her symptoms worse. She emphasized the need to breathe gently, slowly, smoothly and low down

in her chest – so low in fact that Angela could feel her stomach rising and sinking.

It certainly helped to calm her down. Angela decided to practise this breathing routine regularly. After a few days she found she was able to calm herself down without help and as the days went by, in an ever shorter time as she became more skilled at the routine. The panic she felt as she made her way to the class was losing its intensity. What particularly pleased her was that, besides calming her physical symptoms, the breathing sequences also seemed to settle her fears. Her head became clearer and she felt more able to choose her thoughts.

POTENTIAL PITFALLS

1. Breathing exercises for inducing relaxation should not be seen as a substitute for medical treatment where a disorder exists. They may, however, be used as a complement if the physician or physiotherapist agrees.

2. The individual should never feel he is straining or forcing the breaths; they must always feel comfortable.

3. Dizziness during the exercises is probably a symptom of hyperventilation, i.e. the exercises are being performed too deeply or too quickly. Remedies may be found in the section on hyperventilation. Alternatively, the individual could take a rest from the exercise. It is useful if the instructor describes the condition of hyperventilation at the outset.

4. Since individuals vary in their breathing rates, routines imposed by the instructor are not recommended in a group situation. The instructions can be phrased in such a way that participants individually decide on a pace that suits them.

5. Although slow, abdominal breathing can be an effective way of inducing relaxation, it may not suit everyone. In particular, people who suffer from air hunger, for whatever reason, may not find it helpful to manipulate their breathing rate.

6. Although people who suffer from panic disorder have been shown to derive benefit from

relaxation, a few individuals occasionally report the occurrence of panic attacks during periods of relaxation. Two possible explanations are offered here. One comes from Hough (2001), who points out that relaxation weakens the psychological defences and may allow disturbing feelings to rise to the surface. An alternative explanation is put forward by Ley (1988) who suggests that if a person who is currently hyperventilating begins to relax, he lowers his metabolic rate. This reduces his production of carbon dioxide. If he does not make a corresponding reduction in ventilation, his hypocapnia will increase and his symptoms become more marked.

KEY MESSAGES

- The respiratory system is strongly influenced by the emotional state.
- Unlike other body systems, the respiratory system is directly linked to that which controls physiological arousal.
- Breathing routines accompany most relaxation approaches.
- Abdominal breathing plays an important role in the promotion of relaxation.
- Hyperventilation can be corrected by breathing pattern re-education.

Chapter Five

Progressive relaxation

5

CHAPTER CONTENTS

History and description

To many people, relaxation training means learning techniques such as 'tense-release', i.e. the tightening and letting go of specific muscle groups. Tense–release is an active process in the sense that the individual is working his muscles. Some muscle relaxation methods, however, are concerned only with the 'release' part of the sequence, and these could be described as passive muscular approaches.

This chapter introduces the work of Edmund Jacobson, a pioneer in this field. His work lays the foundation of both the tense–release and the passive approaches, which are described here and developed in Chapters 6–9.

Working as a physiologist-physician in the 1930s, Jacobson was investigating the startle reaction that follows a sudden loud noise. He noticed that people who were able to fully relax their muscles made no start. Thus, the state of the muscle influenced the magnitude of the reflex. He invented a technique for measuring the electrical activity in muscles and nerves which became known as electromyography (EMG), and which allowed him to study hitherto unexplored aspects of physiology. Arising out of this new technology, he was able to demonstrate that thinking was related to muscle state and that mental images, particularly those associated with movement, were accompanied by small but detectable levels of activity in the muscles concerned (Jacobson 1938).

This integrated activity between the mind and the muscles led him to view the brain centres and the voluntary muscles as working together 'in one effort circuit' (Jacobson 1970); a neuromuscular circuit, since it was composed of both neural and muscular tissue. Just as a calm mind would be reflected in a tension-free body, so, Jacobson proposed, a relaxed musculature would be accompanied by the quietening of thoughts and the reduction of sympathetic activity, notions that would have relevance in the treatment of anxiety and associated conditions. The task facing Jacobson, therefore, was to find a way of inducing the skeletal muscles to lose their tension.

Muscle activity is accompanied by sensations so faint that we do not normally notice them. To promote awareness of tension, Jacobson emphasized the need to concentrate on those sensations, cultivating what he called 'learned awareness'. Once tension had been recognized, it would be easier to release it. If relaxation were then achieved, however, how deep would it be?

It is traditionally held that, in the waking state, healthy muscle, even during rest, is in a state of sustained, slight contraction. This is called muscle tone. Jacobson's EMG studies (1938) did not, however, support this notion. He found that voluntary muscle could achieve a state of complete relaxation during rest. He consequently formed the view that the aim of relaxation training should be to eliminate *all* tension, and relaxation could only be called complete if it proceeded 'to the zero point of tonus for the part or parts involved' (Jacobson 1938). Any tension that remained while resting a muscle was called 'residual' and it was this residual tension that Jacobson sought to eliminate in deep relaxation. 'Doing away with residual tension is … the essential feature of the present method' (Jacobson 1976).

Defining relaxation as the cessation of activity in the skeletal (voluntary) muscles, Jacobson devised a technique which he called progressive relaxation. It consisted of systematically working through the major skeletal muscle groups, creating and releasing tension. As a result, the trainee learned how to recognize muscle tension. Only one muscle action was carried out in each session and it was repeated twice. The rest of the time was spent releasing tension.

Jacobson (1938) insisted that his method be regarded as a skill to be learned. Unlike most other approaches, the use of suggestion was discouraged. Trainers were urged to avoid planting ideas of the kind: 'Your limbs are heavy/limp/ relaxed' or even 'Notice how your limbs are feeling heavy/limp/ relaxed'. Jacobson wanted the learner to make his own discoveries.

Rationale

Progressive relaxation (PR) is based on the idea that people think more clearly when they are relaxed and this helps them to solve their emotional problems (Lehrer 1982). Jacobson proposed that relaxation of the musculature offered a means to that end, since he further proposed that a relaxed musculature exerted a calming influence on the whole organism, including the mind. The effect was non-specific. The approach is a physiologically oriented one since its procedures are concerned with physical organs, i.e. muscles and nerves, although the act of focusing on muscular sensations gives it also a cognitive slant.

Presenting progressive relaxation

Conditions

Ideal conditions for presenting progressive relaxation include the following.

- A room that is quiet.
- Somewhere to lie down. A large room with a carpeted floor is suitable for a group. Trainees may be asked to bring a beach mattress or the equivalent to lie on, and a small pillow for the head. Lying is the position of choice; however, it is possible to learn progressive relaxation in the sitting position.

Introducing the method

Before starting the training proper, the basis of the method must be introduced. With the trainees seated, the trainer describes the rationale of progressive relaxation on the following lines.

Knowing how to rest the body enables body energy to be used more efficiently. It can also help to protect us from illness. This is a method of relaxing that involves the muscles. By creating and releasing tension, you will learn to tune into subtle feelings in the muscles, to recognize different levels of tension and to release that tension.

Muscle tension is believed to be closely associated with your state of mind: it is believed that muscles which are unnecessarily tense reflect their tension in the mind. If that muscle tension can be released, you will feel mentally calmer.

Your internal organs will also benefit in that pulse rate and blood pressure will be lowered while you are relaxing.

The method we are using is called progressive relaxation. It is not possible to learn it in one lesson. However, every bit as important as the lessons is the practice that you put in between them. Like any skill, the more you practise it, the more proficient you will become, and the more you will benefit from its effects, in this case relaxation.

The muscle action to be taught is then demonstrated, after which trainees are asked to lie down, face upwards, with arms resting on either side of the body, legs uncrossed. The eyes are open to begin with, but after 3 or 4 minutes trainees are asked to close them and to spend a few minutes quietly unwinding.

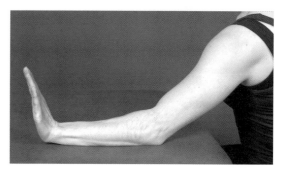

Figure 5.1 • Wrist bending backwards.

Procedure

First session: wrist bending backwards

A first session would take the following form. The trainee is asked to extend the left wrist (bend it back) and to hold it in that position for one minute (Fig. 5.1). He then releases the tension, letting go all at once, and continues to relax the part for 3 minutes during which any residual tension is also released. This action is then repeated twice. The instruction might run as follows.

Would you please bend the left hand back at the wrist. Do this steadily without seesawing ... and avoid raising the forearm ... continue to hold the hand back for a full minute, noticing the different sensations you get from doing it.

Using Jacobson's technique, it is not suggested to the trainee what these sensations might be; the idea is that the trainee should discover them for himself. However, in this case they would include tension in the working muscles situated along the top of the forearm and across the back of the hand, together with some sensations of strain in the wrist joint and skin stretching in the palm. Of these, it is the muscle sensations that the trainee should learn to focus on.

As you continue to bend your wrist back, distinguish between the various feelings you are experiencing ... pick out particularly those related to the muscles ... concentrate on the sensation of tenseness ... keeping the action sustained until the minute is up ...

And now, discontinue the action ... allow the hand to fall by its own weight. Let it flop

down. Avoid lowering it slowly or in any way controlling its descent.

Although you have let go as completely as you could, there may still be some tension there. Give it plenty of time to disappear ... give it at least 3 minutes as you focus on the sensation in the muscles ...

Now, bend the wrist back a second time ... feel the effort ... if you are finding difficulty in sorting out the feelings in the arm, allow the hand to fall down and try the following: with your right hand, pick up the left hand and gently press it back as if it didn't belong to you ... continue to press for about half a minute. Make sure the right hand does all the work. The feelings you're getting are coming from the wrist and from the palm. With your left hand still bent back, take away your right hand and as you do, transfer the power to your left arm. You are now using muscles in the left forearm to hold the left wrist back. Notice the new feelings you are getting ... these are the feelings you are asked to concentrate on ... continue to hold the wrist back for about a minute ...

Now, cease the action and allow the hand to fall down, letting all the tension go ... letting the muscle go negative ... concentrating on the feelings you are getting from it ... continue in that direction for the next 3 minutes ...

The trainee is not asked to 'relax', which Jacobson felt might create tensions on its own account, but to 'discontinue', 'cease to bend' or 'go negative'. Relaxation occurs on its own as the learner releases tension.

One further repetition is carried out before the trainee adopts a state of continuous rest for the remainder of the hour when the session comes to an end.

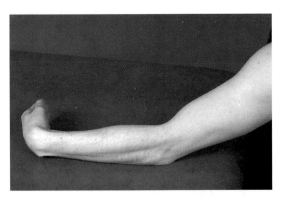

Figure 5.2 • Wrist bending forwards.

Second session: wrist bending forwards

At the following session a new action is introduced: wrist flexion (bending forwards). This action follows the same pattern as the previous one except that the wrist is bent forwards instead of backwards (Fig. 5.2).

> I'd like you to bend the left hand forward at the wrist ... hold the position steadily ... locate the feeling of tenseness (the underside of the forearm) ... and (when the minute is up) ... discontinue the action ... let the hand fall back ... continue letting go any remaining tension over the next few minutes ... tuning in to the feelings in the muscle in the forearm ...

Two repetitions are carried out, after which the trainee rests. That marks the end of session number two.

Third and subsequent sessions

The third session does not contain any tensing component. Instead, the time is entirely devoted to releasing tension. Subsequent sessions are spent addressing other actions and may cover many weeks. The protocol is outlined below and laid out in full in Table 5.1.

- *Arms:* five items for each arm; tensing and releasing of arm and hand muscles.
- *Legs:* seven items for each leg; tensing and releasing of thigh, leg and foot muscles.
- *Trunk:* seven items; tensing and releasing of back, abdomen and shoulder muscles.
- *Neck:* four items; tensing and relaxing of muscles around the neck.

- *Eye area:* eight items; tensing and relaxing the muscles of the forehead and the eyes.
- *Visualization:* six items; imagining different objects, moving and stationary.
- *Speech area:* 15 items; tensing and relaxing muscles associated with speech; counting and reciting, first in a normal voice, then gradually getting fainter.

Only one or two new actions are introduced at each period of tuition, and the whole programme takes about 50 sessions. In addition, an hour a day is devoted to home practice.

'Diminishing tensions'

Jacobson avoided using the word 'exercise' to describe the actions, since exercise, designed as it is to strengthen muscles, implies increasing effort. The wrist bending and other actions in progressive relaxation are introduced simply to teach awareness of the different sensations that arise in activated muscle tissue. Learning to recognize these sensations requires differing levels of muscle tension. Of these, the lower levels are the most useful for picking up residual tension as it is here that sensitivity to small fluctuations is greatest (Jacobson 1970, Lehrer et al 1988). Thus, the actions require an ever-*decreasing* intensity of contraction to fulfil their purpose.

To help the trainee become sensitized to low levels of tension, Jacobson devised a technique called 'diminishing tensions'. It is introduced as the learner becomes proficient in recognizing the sensation of tension. Returning to the action of wrist bending, the trainee would be instructed in the following way.

> Bend your wrist back but this time using only half as much effort as you did the first time. Hold it back for about a minute, noticing the sensations you're getting from the muscle ... and at the end of the minute ... cease holding it back. Go negative ... feel the tension leaving ... allow plenty of time for the remaining tension to disappear ... allow 3 minutes ... then bend the wrist back again, this time tensing the muscle half as much as last time ... hold it for about a minute, tuning in to the sensations ... then release the tension ... release it further ... and further still ... allow 3 minutes ... now, raise the wrist the smallest amount possible ...

Table 5.1 Progressive relaxation: schedule of items (adapted from Jacobson 1964)

Arms	Extend wrist (bend hand back)
	Flex wrist (bend hand forward)
	Relax only
	Flex (bend) elbow
	Extend elbow (straighten arm)
	Relax only
	Stiffen whole arm
Legs	Dorsiflex foot (bend foot up at ankle joint)
	Plantarflex foot (bend foot down at ankle joint)
	Relax only
	Extend (straighten) knee from a bent position
	Flex (bend) knee, dragging foot along floor
	Relax only
	Flex hip (raise bent knee towards chest)
	Extend hip (press thigh down into the supporting surface)
	Relax only
	Stiffen entire leg
Trunk	Contract (pull in) abdomen
	Extend spine (arch back slightly)
	Relax only
	Observe the action of breathing
	Brace shoulders back
	Relax only
	Flex shoulder joint (bring bent arm across chest)
	Repeat with other arm
	Relax only
	Raise (hunch) shoulders
Neck	Press head back into pillow/headrest
	Raise head off pillow
	Relax only
	Bend head to right
	Bend head to left
	Relax only
Upper face area	Raise eyebrows
	Frown
	Relax only
Eye area	Close eyes tightly
	Look left with eyes closed
	Relax only
	Look right with eyes closed
	Look up with eyes closed
	Relax only
	Look down with eyes closed
	Look forward with eyes closed
	Relax only
Visual imagination	Imagine a pen moving slowly, then fast
	Imagine a train passing, a person walking by
	Relax eyes

(Continued)

Table 5.1 Continued

	Imagine a bird flying and stationary
	Imagine a ball rolling, the Houses of Parliament
	Relax eyes
	Imagine a horse grazing, a reel of cotton
	Imagine the Prime Minister
	Relax eyes
Jaw, voice and auditory imagination	Close jaws firmly
	Open jaws
	Relax only
	Bare teeth
	Pout
	Relax only
	Press tongue against teeth
	Pull tongue backwards
	Relax only
	Count aloud up to 10
	Count half as loudly up to 10
	Relax only
	Count softly up to 10
	Count under your breath up to 10
	Relax only
	Imagine you are counting
	Imagine you are reciting the alphabet
	Relax only
	Imagine saying: your name three times, your address three times, the Prime Minister's name three times

hold it there … for 1 minute … discontinue … allow 3 minutes … and finally, make the action just a thought … hold the thought for 1 minute … go negative … spend 3 minutes continuing to go negative…

These progressively diminishing tensions train the individual to recognize differing levels, thus increasing his control over the voluntary musculature.

Jacobson's assigning of every third session exclusively to passive relaxation is evidence of the high value he placed on the relaxation phase and the relatively low value he gave to the contraction phase, using it simply as a means of cultivating sensitivity to the tension sensation. Many of his successors have, by contrast, attached great importance to the contraction, claiming that it leads to a deepening of the subsequent relaxation. Jacobson argued that the reverse may be the case, namely, that tensions which build up during the contraction phase would continue to persist for some time, thus hindering relaxation. In untrained participants

he showed that muscle tension continues to remain elevated for up to several minutes following a contraction, even when the participant is co-operating with appeals to 'go negative' (Jacobson 1934). Thus, deliberate muscle tensing may, in the short term at least, actually obstruct the relaxation process.

The issue of tense-release versus a release-only approach has not been satisfactorily resolved. It has been common in clinical practice to favour tense–release. However, the results of a study in 1991 (Lucic et al) support the view that initial tensing is detrimental to relaxation, and this finding may have strengthened interest in passive approaches.

Eye movements

The procedures for the eye and forehead and for the area of the speech muscles differ somewhat from those of the trunk and limbs. Consequently they are presented in more detail.

Although Jacobson (1938) indicated that only one or two actions should be carried out in each session, it is customary today to work through all the eye actions in a single session. Plenty of time should still be allowed for 'going negative'.

Jacobson's studies had demonstrated the effectiveness of progressive relaxation in reducing muscle tension. He had also been able to show that a relaxed musculature had a calming effect on the mind (Jacobson 1938). Muscle relaxation could thus be seen as a mental relaxant. But Jacobson went further: he claimed that in deep relaxation, thought itself disappeared. In the totally relaxed body, the mind would be a blank.

The eye muscles were considered by him to be particularly closely related to thought, since thinking created mental images which were accompanied by a sense of tension around the eyes. Releasing tension from the eyes, Jacobson believed, had the effect of cancelling those images. The following sequences are adapted from Jacobson (1970). Time should be allowed between the items for the trainee to absorb the message.

With your eyes open, raise your eyebrows … feel the tension … and release it … frown … feel the tension … and discontinue … shut your eyes tightly … feel the tension … and let it go … with your eyes still closed, spend a few minutes releasing tension in this part of your face …

Moving on to the eyes themselves (they are still closed) … without moving your head, turn your eyes upwards as if you were looking at the ceiling. As you do so, notice the sensation you get in the eye region … next, turn your eyes downwards as if you were looking at your feet, again taking note of the feelings around the eyes … repeat that several times, until you become familiar with the sensation in the eye muscles … then discontinue, going negative for a minute or so … still with your eyes closed, turn your eyes to the left for a few moments … now to the right … repeat this a few times to experience the transient sensations in the muscles … then, cease the action … do nothing for a few minutes …

Would you now, still with your eyes closed, imagine you are looking at the ceiling and the floor; do not actively look up and down, but simply think of looking up and down … notice the feelings (that is, the same sensations as when you deliberately turned your eyes up and down, although to a much lesser degree) … when you have identified the feeling, let your eye muscles go negative … notice what happens to the images … rest for a few minutes …

Now, imagine that you see the wall on your left … and the wall on your right … imagine seeing one after the other, noticing that slight tensions accompany the images … now, let your eyes go … and notice what happens to the images …

Similar effects can be created by imagining objects from everyday life: imagine a car passing … or a ball bouncing up and down … notice the sensation that accompanies the image … then let the eye muscles go negative and notice what happens to the images …

Multiply 16 by 80 in your head … when you have got the answer, notice how the eyes felt during the task … then, rest the eyes and notice what happens to the figures …

If the eyes are completely relaxed, the image disappears and the thought dies (Jacobson 1964). The individual, however, has made no effort to stop the thought process. He is asked only to release tension, 'letting other effects come as they may' (Jacobson 1976). Whether thought does in fact disappear in a totally relaxed body has not been scientifically established. Jacobson (1938) was, however, able to produce clinical evidence of the success of ocular relaxation in overcoming insomnia.

Speech movements

The speech muscles are also closely related to thought. Thinking with the use of words causes minute flickers of tension in the muscles of the tongue and jaw. Conversely, when these muscles are relaxed, thinking with the use of words is no longer possible (Jacobson 1970).

The following script begins with tensing of the speech muscles and ends with sequences of counting using 'diminishing tensions'. As with the eye actions, it is customary today to present the whole group in one session. As a rough guide, 5–10 seconds can be allowed for each action and 30–40 seconds for 'going negative'. Each action is repeated once.

Close the jaws firmly, noticing the sensations you get from the action … hold it … and … discontinue … let your jaw drop … feel the tension leaving you … and continuing to leave you … then repeat the sequence…

Next, bare your teeth ... feel the tension in the cheeks ... hold it for a few seconds ... and cease the action ...

Make a tight 'O' with your lips ... hold it, while you register tension in the lips ... and ... go negative ...

Press your tongue against your teeth ... feel the pressure ... and discontinue ...

Now, pull the tongue back towards the throat. Feel the muscles drawing it back and note the sensations you get from this action ... and ... let it go negative ...

Tune in to the presence of residual tension in any of the muscles associated with speech and let that tension recede ... and go on receding ...

(Allow several minutes for the last phase.)

A counting sequence follows, using diminishing tensions.

Count aloud slowly from one to ten, picking up the sensations you get from the muscles in the mouth, throat, face and chest. Repeat it a few times ... then stop counting ... allow time for the full release of tension ...

Now, count again, half as loudly ... noticing the reduced amount of tension in the speech muscles ... discontinue ... next time, count softly ... notice the tension ... and let it go ... and now, under your breath ... still concentrating on the feelings you get in the mouth, jaw and throat ... rest a moment ... and now, simply imagine the counting ... here perhaps you can detect a flickering in the speech muscles ... finally, cease to count altogether ...

When the speech muscles ceased to be involved, Jacobson (1938, 1964, 1976) claimed that it was no longer possible to think in verbal terms. The notion that thought disappears in states of deep muscle relaxation is consistent with a theory which sees mental processes being influenced by the state of the skeletal musculature (Lehrer 1982).

Further work of Jacobson's

Differential relaxation

Jacobson (1938) also investigated the degree of tension necessary for carrying out a particular activity. He drew a distinction between those muscles actually performing the activity and those muscles not involved in it. The first group needed the minimum level of tension consistent with performing the task; the second group could be totally relaxed or as relaxed as possible. This differential in the degree of tension required was studied by Jacobson for the purpose of reducing both the excessive effort often used by the first group and the unnecessary effort often used by the second. Differential relaxation is discussed in more detail in Chapter 13.

Self-operations control

In addition to progressive relaxation, Jacobson (1964) developed a method of instruction which he called 'self-operations control'. The principles of recognizing and eliminating tension are the same as those of progressive relaxation. The emphasis, however, is placed on self-direction: the individual controlling his muscle tension throughout the events of daily life, learning 'to go on and off ... as different occasions may require' (Jacobson 1964). He learns to monitor all sensations of tension, simultaneously and automatically, and to release those tensions which are not desired, in a continuing process (McGuigan 1984). The result is a decreased consumption of energy, which effect extends to other body systems such as the autonomic nervous system, where sympathetic activity is reduced. Thought processes are also believed to benefit from the tension-decreasing effect (McGuigan 1981).

This method, however, takes as long to learn as Jacobson's original technique.

Evidence of effectiveness

Progressive relaxation in one form or another is widely used in the clinical field and its effectiveness has been tested in many conditions. Kwekkeboom & Gretarsdottir (2006) investigated its effectiveness alongside that of a range of other mind–body methods in the treatment of pain in adults. Eight of the 15 trials reviewed contained evidence supporting their use. The intervention most frequently cited was PR where arthritis pain was singled out as deriving particular benefit. Postoperative pain responded best to jaw relaxation and systematic relaxation. There was little evidence in favour of autogenic training and still less for rhythmic breathing or other techniques. These conclusions are, however, tentative; strong conclusions cannot be drawn because of weaknesses in the methodology of some of the studies.

Another systematic review looked at the effects of PR on patients experiencing generalized anxiety disorder and panic disorder but the authors were unable to find evidence to support the use of muscle relaxation in those conditions. Better designed studies are needed before firm conclusions can be drawn (Conrad & Roth 2007).

Hui et al (2006) compared the effects of PR with qigong to determine their relative properties when applied to the quality of life among cardiac patients. Sixty-five patients with cardiac diseases ranging through myocardial infarct, valve replacement, postcoronary intervention and ischaemic heart disease took part in a study consisting of eight 20-minute sessions. Both interventions were effective in reducing blood pressure but PR provided greater benefit. PR was also found to be more effective in somatic domains while qigong seemed more effective in psychological ones.

In her review of relaxation techniques, Kerr (2000) cites studies which have shown reductions in both physiological and psychological indicators of stress following a course of PR. These results suggest that PR has the potential to promote relaxation (Kerr 2000). When PR has been compared with other stress-reducing approaches, PR often appears equally effective, as in Salt & Kerr's (1997) study where PR was compared with the Mitchell method in 24 normotensive participants. Whereas significant reductions in heart rate, respiratory rate and blood pressure were found in both methods, the study did not show any significant difference in effectiveness between the two interventions. Similarly, Crist & Rickard (1993) found no difference in outcome between muscular and imaginal relaxation in 100 healthy students although both experimental conditions showed significant training effects.

Progressive relaxation is widely used in the clinical field for reducing mental tension. In its early form, however, it is seldom practised; its great length, accompanied by problems of time and money, constitute a major disadvantage. It has in many instances been replaced by modifications, one of which is described in the following chapter.

POTENTIAL PITFALLS

The pitfalls described cover Chapters 5, 6, 7 and 9.

It would seem that progressive relaxation is appropriate in any circumstances where rest is prescribed (McGuigan 1984). The method is unlikely to create negative effects and Jacobson did not refer to any. Some points, however, need to be considered.

1. Training in relaxation should never be viewed as a substitute for medical treatment; wherever a disorder is present or suspected, medical help should be sought.

2. Variations in the blood pressure may occur in the course of relaxation training: it can rise when limbs are being tensed and fall during deep relaxation. The fall in blood pressure which accompanies deep relaxation is only that which occurs under any resting condition. Following a session of relaxation, it is important to allow time for the individual to adjust before becoming active to avoid the risk of fainting.

3. For people whose blood pressure is already high and cardiac patients, a release-only method (see Ch. 8) is preferable to one which consists of muscle tensings.

4. Antenatal and labouring mothers are no longer given tense–release exercises because of the possibility of interference with uterine contractions. Release-only forms (i.e. passive relaxation) would, however, be appropriate.

5. Tense–release procedures performed with excessive tightening may lead to cramp. In order to avoid this, trainees can be advised to shorten the tension period (Bernstein et al 2000). Recurrent cramp would indicate the unsuitability of the technique for that individual. Overtensing the spine and the neck should also be avoided since it can lead to spinal damage.

6. Some individuals find that focusing on the body intensifies their perception of pain (Snyder 1985), and for them, muscular approaches may be less useful than cognitive ones such as imagery or meditation.

7. Trainees who, because of disability or disorder, are in doubt as to the suitability of any exercise should begin by performing it very gently. This applies, for example, to individuals with back or neck problems.

8. Some tense–release scripts make use of imagery. They will therefore, in addition, be subject to the pitfalls listed in Chapter 18 (p159).

KEY MESSAGES

- Jacobson formulated his progressive relaxation programme as a result of his experiments on the startle reaction.
- The programme is based on the notion that a relaxed musculature exerts a calming influence on the mind.
- The progressive relaxation programme itself consists of the alternative tensing and releasing of skeletal muscle groups during which the trainee is asked to take note of the sensations in the working muscle groups.
- In particular, Jacobson asks the client to recognize and release residual tension.
- As the trainee becomes more proficient, the tension component is dropped and attention is focused exclusively on release.
- Progressive relaxation is a skill, the mastery of which depends on daily practice.

Chapter Six

6

Progressive relaxation training

History and description

Although Jacobson's method (see Ch. 5) was found to reduce both pulse rate and blood pressure, it was time-consuming and unlikely to have wide appeal as it stood. Some form of abbreviation was needed. The first major attempt at shortening the format was made by Wolpe (1958), who reduced the training to six sessions and later reduced it further to one. Countless other modifications have followed, of which Bernstein & Borkovec's (1973) is one of the best known.

Named progressive relaxation training (PRT) by its authors, the approach is defined as learning to relax specific muscle groups while paying attention to the feelings associated with both the tensed and relaxed states. Its aims are (Bernstein & Given 1984):

- to achieve a state of deep relaxation in increasingly shorter periods
- to control excess tension in stress-inducing situations.

The trainee works through the sequential tensing and releasing of 16 muscle groups. These are reduced to seven in the next stage and to four in a subsequent stage. The tension component is then withdrawn, in what is called 'relaxation through recall', and the final stage consists of a mental summary of the previously learned techniques. Proficiency at each level depends on the skill obtained in the previous stage. The tense-release element of PRT is described in this chapter (p59). Relaxation through recall is presented in Chapter 8 (p72). Two additional components are described in later chapters: 'conditioned relaxation' in Chapter 9 (p83) and 'differential relaxation' in Chapter 13 (p113).

Differences between progressive relaxation and progressive relaxation training

Although PRT is founded on Jacobson's principles of recognizing and eliminating tension, there are important differences between the two approaches (Table 6.1).

Table 6.1 Differences between Jacobson's progressive relaxation method and Bernstein & Borkovec's progressive relaxation training

	Progressive relaxation	Progressive relaxation training
Position of relaxation	Lying or sitting	Reclining
Total number of muscle groups worked	40+	16
Number of new muscle groups worked in one session	1 or 2	All groups
Emphasis of technique	Releasing tension	'Producing' relaxation through tense–release cycles
Perceived value of the contraction	To alert the individual to the tension sensation	To deepen each relaxation component by providing a 'running start'; a strong contraction leads to a deep relaxation
Part played by suggestion	None: the technique is purely a muscular skill	Indirect suggestion is used to enhance the effect
Use of tapes	Not used	Advised against
Number of sessions needed	50+	8–12

The contraction phase

One of these differences is the prominence given to the tensing component in the modified version. Bernstein & Borkovec (1973) describe an effect whereby the strength of the contraction determines the depth of the relaxation which follows it, in the manner of a pendulum which, when lifted high on one side, swings back to the same height on the other side. Thus, the stronger the initial contraction, the deeper the subsequent relaxation. Jacobson (1938, 1970) does not share this view. He sees the contraction phase simply as a means of cultivating the individual's sensitivity to the presence of muscle tension. He never intended it as a means of 'producing' relaxation (Lehrer et al 1988).

The strength of the contraction is not specified by Jacobson, except in such terms as 'Do not stiffen your arm to the point of extreme effort, but only in moderation' (Jacobson 1964), and the command to 'tense', even at greatest magnitude, is taken to convey only a comfortable level, since the object is merely to enable the individual to identify the sensation of tension. To Jacobson, the lower the level of the contraction, the more useful it was. Bernstein & Borkovec, in contrast, use phrases such as 'tight fist' and refer to 'trembling neck muscles', suggesting a high level of tension. Wolpe & Lazarus (1966), similarly, in their version, urge clients to clench the fist 'tighter and tighter'.

Use of suggestion

Both Jacobson (1938) and Bernstein & Borkovec (1973) discuss suggestion. The argument in favour of using suggestion is that it increases cognitive awareness of the affective component which is believed to enhance the overall effect (Fig. 6.1).

Addressing trainees who fear they might be put into a trance state, Bernstein & Borkovec point out the difference between hypnosis and relaxation. In hypnosis, maximum use is made of direct suggestion such as 'Now your arm is limp'. Direct suggestion, so crucial in hypnosis, is not appropriate in relaxation.

PRT does, however, use indirect suggestion, such as 'Notice how your muscles are feeling more and more relaxed' and 'Let a feeling of relaxation flow through your limbs', in order to deepen the sense of relaxation. Voice modulations to reinforce the distinction between tension and relaxation are also encouraged: crisp tones during the tensing component and soothing tones during the relaxation component.

To Jacobson, however, even indirect suggestion is unacceptable. He sees progressive relaxation exclusively as a muscular skill, the mastery of which is impeded by any kind of suggestion.

Relevant to this discussion is the work of Paul (1969) who has shown relaxation training to be more effective than hypnosis at reducing muscle tension.

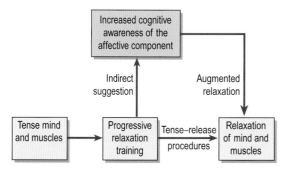

Figure 6.1 • How the inclusion of suggestion may increase the effect of a muscular procedure.

Rationale

As with progressive relaxation, it is proposed that relaxing the musculature exerts a calming effect on the whole organism, including the mind. The contraction phase in PRT, however, is given greater prominence since it is believed that initial tensing actually produces relaxation (Bernstein & Borkovec 1973).

The PRT procedure

The first session

In Bernstein & Borkovec's approach, training is governed by a fixed procedure.

1. The rationale of the technique is presented to the trainee, and the items involving the 16 muscle groups are then described and demonstrated. (See *Introductory remarks* section below.)

2. For the procedure itself the trainee is seated in a reclining chair. If this is not available, the trainee can sit in a chair with a high, sloping back and arm rests.

3. The procedure starts with the trainee being asked to focus attention on a given muscle group. (See *Item one* section below.)

4. A signal, such as the word 'Now', indicates that the muscle group is to be tensed.

5. The contraction is carried out all at once, not gradually.

6. Tension is maintained for 5–7 seconds during which the instructor asks the trainee to focus on the sensations of muscle contraction.

7. On a predetermined cue such as the word 'Release', 'Relax' or 'Let go', the muscle group is relaxed (again, all at once).

8. As the muscle group relaxes, the trainee is asked to notice the feelings that accompany the relaxation while the trainer maintains a patter which is indirectly suggestive of relaxation.

9. This continues for the duration of the relaxation period which is 30–40 seconds.

10. All 16 muscle groups are worked in the first training session.

Introductory remarks to trainees

The method you are going to learn is called 'progressive relaxation training' and it consists of tensing and releasing muscle groups throughout the body. The object is to produce relaxation and this occurs after the tension is released. A firm contraction can lead to a deep relaxation, rather like a pendulum swinging high on both sides. You will be asked to concentrate on the feelings that accompany the tension and the relaxation; feelings that up to now, you may have taken for granted. There are 16 muscle groups to be tensed and released and it takes about 40 minutes to complete the whole schedule. First, I'll run through the items, demonstrating them and giving you a chance to try them out.

The trainer demonstrates the following items.

1. Making a fist with the dominant hand without involving the upper arm.

2. Pushing the elbow of the same arm down against the arm of the chair (activating the biceps), while keeping the hand relaxed.

3/4. The non-dominant arm is worked separately.

5. Raising the eyebrows.

6. Screwing up the eyes and wrinkling the nose.

7. Clenching the teeth and pulling back the corners of the mouth.

8. Pulling the chin in and pressing the head back against a support, tensing the neck muscles.

9. Drawing the shoulders back.

10. Tightening the abdominal muscles (making the stomach hard).

11. Tensing the thigh of the dominant leg by attempting to contract the knee flexors and extensors together.

12. Pointing the dominant foot down (plantarflexion).

13. Pulling the dominant foot up towards the face (dorsiflexion).

14/15.16. The non-dominant leg is worked separately.

The trainer continues:

> *When we begin, I'll first describe each item but please do not tense the part until I give you the cue word 'Now'. Similarly, let it go only when I give you the cue word 'Relax'. Then let it go completely. Would you please close your eyes?*

Item one

The first item involves the muscles of the right hand and forearm; the hand is drawn into a fist (Fig. 6.2).

> *We'll start with the right hand and forearm. I'm going to ask you to tense the muscles in the right hand and lower arm, by drawing up your hand into a tight fist ... Now ... clench the hand ... keep it tight ... feel the tension in the muscles as you pull hard ... and ... Relax ... let go immediately and as the fingers uncurl, notice the feelings you now have in the muscles of the hand ... focus on the sensations you are getting in the muscles of the forearm also, as they lose their tension ... feel relaxation flowing into the area as the muscles get more and more deeply relaxed ... completely relaxed ... notice the way your muscles feel at this moment, compared to how they felt when tensed.*

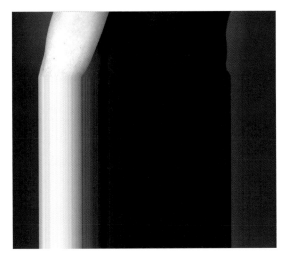

Figure 6.2 • Making a fist.

All items are performed a second time, after which there is an extended relaxation phase lasting a full minute. Trainees can be asked to raise the little finger of the right hand to indicate that they are fully relaxed before the next item is introduced.

Item two and subsequent items

Item two involves the muscles of the right upper arm: the bent elbow is pressed down into the arm of the chair (Fig. 6.3). A wooden arm rest can be softened with a cushion.

> *Let the hand and forearm go on relaxing while you transfer your attention to the muscles in the right upper arm. I'd like you this time to press your elbow down against the arm of the chair. Do this without involving the muscles of the hand and forearm ... Now ... feel the tension in your upper arm as the elbow presses down ... and ... Relax ... let it go completely ... focus your attention on the relaxing muscles ... feel the tension flowing out ... enjoy the pleasant feelings of the muscles unwinding ... experience the feeling of deep relaxation and of comfort ... then notice if the upper arm feels as relaxed as the lower arm ... if it does, then signal with your little finger.*

The above items give an idea of the nature of PRT, and in the first session the remaining 14 items are also worked through. Bernstein et al (2000) have introduced a slight change in procedure from the original schedule. It requires the trainee to take a

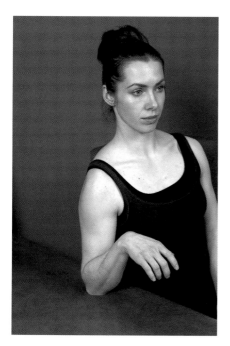

Figure 6.3 • Pressing the elbow down onto the arm of a chair.

deep breath and hold it before carrying out each of the items which involve the trunk and legs. The breath is released as the muscle group relaxes.

Ending the session

At the end, the trainer terminates.

I am going to bring the session to an end by counting backwards from four to one ... four ... start to move your legs and feet ... three ... bend and stretch your arms and hands ... two ... move your head slowly ... and ... one ... open your eyes, noticing how peaceful and relaxed you feel ... as if you'd just woken from a short sleep.

Practice

Two daily practice sessions of 15–20 minutes each are considered essential, the trainee picking moments when he is not under any pressure.

Summarized versions

When the trainee has learned the above procedure, it can be regrouped in a summarized form, enabling him to cover the process in a shorter time.

1. Right arm items combined.
2. Left arm items combined.
3. Face and head movements worked together.
4. Neck and shoulder region combined.
5. Torso items worked together.
6. Right leg items combined.
7. Left leg items combined.

A further summary cuts the process down to four items.

1. Both arms are worked together.
2. Face, head and neck items worked together.
3. Shoulder and torso movements combined.
4. Both legs are tensed together. (People who find this difficult should work the legs separately.)

Relaxation through recall

PRT continues with relaxation through recall. This is described in Chapter 8 (p72).

Evidence of effectiveness

PRT has produced favourable results in many conditions such as anxiety (Rasid & Parish 1998), hypertension (Yung et al 2001), insomnia (Bootzin & Perlis 1992), asthma (Vazquez & Buceta 1993), epilepsy (Puskarich et al 1992), dyspnoea and anxiety in chronic obstructive pulmonary disease (Gift et al 1992) and rheumatic pain (Stenstrom et al 1996).

The study by Stenstrom and colleagues compared the effects of dynamic muscle training with those of PRT in 54 patients with inflammatory rheumatic disease. Participants in both interventions trained for half an hour, 5 days a week for 3 months. At the end of that time the relaxation group exhibited marked improvements in muscle function which were significantly greater than those recorded in the dynamic exercise group.

Comparison studies in general, however, often show equal efficacy as in the study of Crist & Rickard (1993) where muscular relaxation was compared with imaginal relaxation in 100 healthy college students.

A randomized controlled trial was mounted by Cheung et al (2003) to evaluate the effect of a course of PRT on anxiety and quality of life among patients with colorectal cancer following surgery. Results showed a significant reduction in state anxiety and an improved quality of life in patients practising the relaxation technique.

Carlson & Hoyle (1993) reviewed studies featuring abbreviated progressive relaxation techniques such as PRT. The studies covered a wide range of conditions but the largest effect sizes were found in tension headache. Other conditions such as cancer chemotherapy and hypertension showed smaller effect sizes. Overall, the intervention was found to be moderately effective.

The debate about the value of the initial contraction continues. While some authors, such as Bernstein & Borkovec, see the contraction as a means of promoting relaxation, others claim that it obstructs the process and point to an increased muscle–nerve sympathetic activity resulting from the isometric contractions which feature in methods such as PRT (Farrell et al 1991). Ritz (2001) has suggested that tensing might provide benefit in the treatment of some respiratory conditions, since the tension component is associated with sympathetic activity and dilation of the pulmonary air passages; the release component, on the other hand, is associated with parasympathetic activity and constriction of the air passages. This has application in the treatment of asthma (see Ch. 26, p220).

Shortened and standardized versions of progressive relaxation, such as Bernstein & Borkovec's, are, in general, favoured by researchers and clinicians alike, although Lehrer, re-evaluating Jacobson's work in 1982, argued for the superior benefit of the lengthy original. Lichstein (1988), reviewing studies comparing the two approaches, found the evidence inconclusive.

Because of its various advantages, PRT has been widely practised. With regard to the evidence, however, the picture is far from clear since some of the research suffers from methodological problems.

In recent years, Bernstein et al (2000) have restated their approach and published their revised directions in a guidebook for the healthcare professional Their work in the field of anxiety continues. Borkovec has carried PRT into the cognitive–behaviour field where he has integrated it with other components of that approach (Borkovec et al 2002, Newman & Borkovec 2002).

 ## POTENTIAL PITFALLS

The pitfalls of muscular approaches are listed in Chapter 5.

KEY MESSAGES

- PRT is one of the many modifications of progressive relaxation.
- This particular modification places emphasis on the supposed value of the tensing component which precedes the release.
- PRT also promotes the use of suggestion which its authors believe augments the effect of the tense-release sequence.
- The programme is also presented over a much shorter time than progressive relaxation, i.e. 8–12 sessions instead of 50.
- As a skill, PRT requires regular practice.

Further reading

Bernstein, D.A., Borkovec, T.D., Hazlett-Stevens, H., 2000. New directions in progressive relxaxtion training: a guidebook for helping professionals. Praeger, Connecticut.

A tense–release script

CHAPTER CONTENTS

The script set out below lies in the tradition of progressive relaxation. In procedure, however, it more closely resembles progressive relaxation training, except that reduced effort is put into the repeats in the manner of Jacobson's diminishing tensions. The exercises themselves are drawn from a variety of sources. Trainees may be lying or sitting in a high-backed chair to perform them, although while the procedure is being introduced a sitting position is more suitable.

Introduction to the method

I am going to lead you through some of the major muscle groups of the body, asking you to contract and relax them, one by one. Tensing and releasing muscles can help to induce a feeling of physical relaxation. You may also feel mentally relaxed. As you carry out the items, you'll experience sensations in the muscles. These sensations indicate tension which you will learn to identify and to release. This is a skill which enables you to relax yourself any time you want to and the more you practise it, the easier it will become.

The following exercises should first be demonstrated by the trainer in order to familiarize participants with the procedure. Participants are then invited to try them out. It is worth spending time on the demonstration so that group members feel they know the exercises before the instruction begins.

The exercises

- Breathing (1)
- Arm: spider hand, rod-like arm
- Leg: plantar- and dorsiflexion (foot bending down and up), toe flexion (bending down) and extension (bending up)
- Breathing (2)
- Abdominal muscle tensing
- Shoulder bracing
- Shoulder hunching
- Head pressing back

- Upper face: brow raising, frowning, eye exercises
- Lower face: jaw, lips, tongue

Authors hold varying opinions as to the optimal duration of the tension and relaxation periods. Based on their collective judgements, we suggest 5 seconds for tensing and 30–40 seconds for relaxing.

It is explained to participants that each tension phase is carried out on the command 'Now'. The signal for the release of tension is the word 'Relax'. When calling the items, the tone of voice can be varied from slightly crisp during the tension phase to soothing during the relaxation phase.

Participants may have their eyes open or closed. When they have taken up their lying positions, the instructor begins.

Breathing (1)

The section on hyperventilation in Chapter 4 p40 is relevant to this exercise.

Please make yourself as comfortable as you can. Let your breathing settle down and observe its natural rhythm. After a minute or two, follow a natural breath out, making it a little bit longer than usual … then let the air in … let it gently fill your lungs … and … breathe out slowly, releasing your tensions with the air … and now let your breathing take care of itself … do not immediately repeat this deep breath …

You will recognize the exercises which follow. Please wait for the word 'Now' to perform the action.

Arm

Spider hand

This is adapted from Wallace (1980) (Fig. 7.1).

I'd like you to focus attention on your right arm, whether it's lying alongside you or resting on the arm of your chair. With the hand placed palm downwards, slowly press the fingertips into the surface, drawing them towards your palm so that your hand gradually takes on the shape of a spider … don't force the movement, just put a moderate amount of effort into it … Now … as you hold the position, notice the

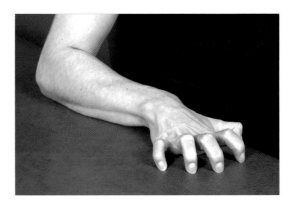

Figure 7.1• Spider hand.

tensions in the hand and the underside of the forearm … feel them build up … then … Relax … let the tension go … relax the muscles … let the tension disappear and go on disappearing as you give the hand time to get more and more relaxed … notice how it feels when it's fully relaxed …

The 'spider' exercise is repeated once using less effort.

Rod-like arm (Fig. 7.2)

If you are seated, start with your right arm in your lap. Lying participants will have their right arm alongside them. I want you slowly to tense up all the muscles so that the arm becomes rigid. Begin with a little tension in the fingertips … let it grow until the fingers are drawn into the palm, making a fist shape. Then stretch out the arm, creating tension in the forearm and upper arm until the arm gets rigid like a rod … Now … feel the tension throughout the arm, but don't overdo it … and … Relax … let it flop down … feel the muscles going slack and the arm becoming limp … notice the relief, the pleasant tingling and the sense of warmth … let the arm go on relaxing … and relaxing a bit more … imagine the last remnant of tension flowing out through your fingertips … notice how the arm muscles feel when they are fully relaxed.

The exercise is performed again, using less effort the second time.

'Spider' and 'rod' are then carried out with the left arm.

Figure 7.2 • Rod-like arm.

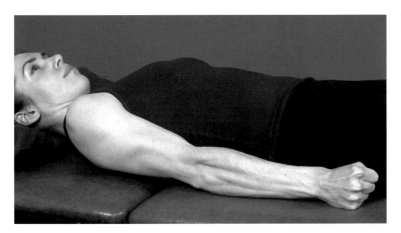

Leg

Next is a group of leg exercises. The first two are for those lying down and the second two are for those who are seated.

Feet pointing away from face

In this exercise the supine participant is asked to point his feet away from his face (Fig. 7.3).

Turning your attention to your legs which are lying flat on the ground, I'd like you to point your feet down, as if you were using them to indicate something. Don't overdo it, especially if you are prone to develop cramp … Now … as you hold the position, study the tensions in your calves … and then … Relax … let go … let all the tension dissolve … feel comfort returning to your lower legs … notice the sensations you get from relaxing the muscles … continue letting go until you feel they won't relax any further …

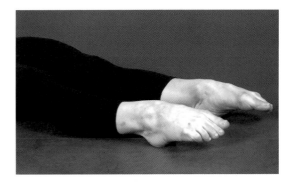

Figure 7.3 • Feet pointing away from face.

Feet pointing towards face

The feet are now pointed towards the face (Fig. 7.4).

This time, point your feet up towards your face, keeping the backs of your knees on the ground … Now … hold the position and notice the sensations you are getting in the working muscles around the shin bones … and then … Relax … as you let go your leg muscles, feel the tension leaving them … feel it draining out as your legs and feet become more and more relaxed …

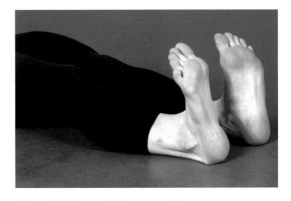

Figure 7.4 • Feet pointing towards face.

These two exercises are repeated once with reduced tension.

The following two leg exercises are addressed to seated participants.

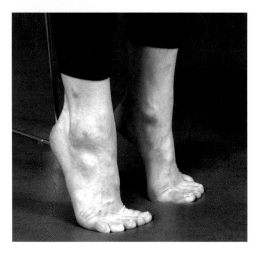

Figure 7.5•Heel raising.

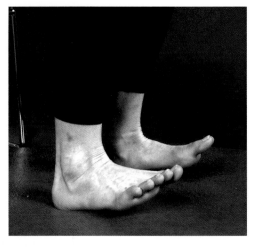

Figure 7.6•Toe raising.

Heel raising

Here, the seated participant is asked to raise her heels off the ground (Fig. 7.5).

Begin by making sure your feet are flat on the floor ... then, keeping your toes firmly in contact with the floor, raise your heels up in the air ... Now ... feel the tension in your calf muscles ... hold the action ... then ... Relax ... drop your heels to the ground ... notice the relief ... the comfort ... the warm, tingling sensation in your calves ... the enjoyable feeling of relaxing your feet ... go on letting those feelings continue until your feet and calves are completely relaxed ... then, a little bit further ...

Toe raising

In this exercise, the front part of the foot is raised off the ground (Fig. 7.6).

This time, keep your heels on the ground, and raise the front part of your feet as if you were about to tap a rhythm ... Now ... keep your toes up in the air while you take notice of the tension sensation in the muscles around the shinbones ... and ... Relax ... let the feet fall down ... notice the relief in the shin area ... feel the tension leaving you ... draining out through your feet and toes ... and continuing to drain out a bit longer ...

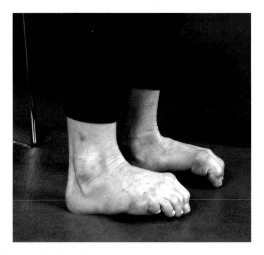

Figure 7.7•Toe flexion.

These two exercises are repeated with diminished tension.

The next exercise is addressed to both lying and seated participants.

Toe flexion and extension (Fig. 7.7)

Let your attention focus on your toes. Whether you are lying or sitting, curl your toes down, restricting the action to the toes themselves. Some people can do it more easily than others, but just do what you can ... Now ... feel the tension in the sole of the foot and the calf of the leg ... then ... Relax ... let it go ... feel the muscles going slack ... feel them going slacker as the tension disappears ... notice how the muscles feel when they are relaxed.

The exercise is repeated once using less tension.

It is followed by a similar exercise in which the toes are bent upwards. Here, muscle tension is felt along the top part of the foot and the shin.

Breathing (2)

At least a minute can be allotted to this item.

Turn your attention to your breathing again … notice its rhythm … place one hand over your upper abdomen and notice the gentle swell and recoil of the area underneath it … avoid any inclination to alter the rhythm … just let the breathing take care of itself …

Abdominal muscle tensing

Focus next on the abdominal muscles … make the area over your internal organs go flat and hard as you pull the muscles in … Now … feel the tension under your ribs, over your organs and around the back of your pelvis … then … Relax … let go … allow your muscles to spread themselves … feel a sense of deep relaxation … and let that relaxation become deeper as the moments pass …

One repeat is carried out using less tension.

Shoulder bracing (Fig. 7.8)

Moving to the region of the back, bring your attention to the bladebones behind your shoulders. Draw them back so that they get nearer to each other (without putting too much effort into it) … Now … feel them being gently squeezed together … notice also how your chest is lifted away from the supporting surface … and then … Relax … release the tension … let the muscles soften … feel your back lying once again in contact with the supporting surface … notice the feeling of relaxation and let that feeling continue on and on …

The exercise is repeated once with less tension.

Shoulder hunching (Fig. 7.9)

Moving to the neck region, I'd like you to lift your shoulders … hunch them up as if to touch your ears … Now … feel the tension in the lower neck … register the sensation … and …

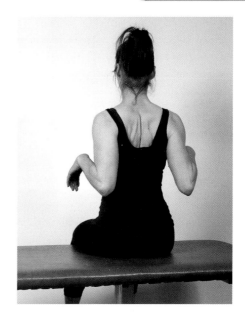

Figure 7.8 • Shoulder bracing.

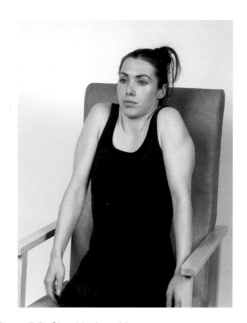

Figure 7.9 • Shoulder hunching.

Relax … let the shoulders drop … and go on dropping … further and further as the tension ebbs away … feel your shoulders completely relaxed …

The exercise is performed once more using diminished tension.

Head back

And the head: keeping your chin in, press your head back against the support (against the floor or back of the chair) … press it back, making double chins in the front … stop short of discomfort … Now … notice the feelings you get from the working muscles … tension in the back of the neck … and … Relax … let go … feel the area relax … notice the sense of ease that floods into the area … allow the relaxation to deepen until all the tension has left your neck …

One repeat is carried out using less tension.

Upper face

Eyebrow raising (Fig. 7.10)

Moving to the face, to the many muscles which control your facial expressions: would you now raise your eyebrows … raise them high, creating horizontal furrows … Now … feel the tension in the muscle that stretches across the brow … and … Relax … let the tension flow out … feel the furrows being smoothed … continue until there is no tension left in your brow … then a little bit further …

The repeat is carried out using less tension.

Frowning (Fig. 7.11)

Focus on your frowning muscle … bring the eyebrows closer together, buckling the skin between them into a deep frown … Now … hold it a few moments, taking note of the sensation you get from the action … then … Relax … release the tension … feel the eyebrows spread sideways … imagine the space between them getting wider and continuing to get wider … notice the comfortable feeling that accompanies this idea… continue until all the tension dies away …

The exercise is repeated once using diminished tension.

Eyes

We come to the eyes. First, I'd like you to screw them up and notice the sensation you get from the action … Now … spend a moment registering

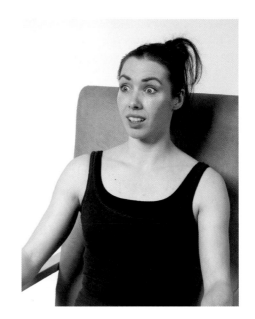

Figure 7.10 • Eyebrow raising.

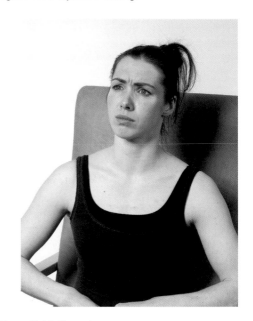

Figure 7.11 • Frowning.

it … then … Relax … let go … let the muscles loosen … notice the feeling you get from loosening them … feel the skin smoothing out …

The exercise is performed once more using diminished tension.

For the following exercise, the trainee's eyes should be closed. The format is slightly different in that, because there are so many eye movements, the relaxation is postponed until the end.

Next, without moving your head, turn your eyes upwards behind your closed lids …
Now … hold your gaze up for a few moments … notice the tension in the muscles … and … bring your eyes back to a central position … and, look down, as if towards your feet … Now … hold it a few moments … then return to the centre … look to the right … Now … keep a steady hold … and return to the front … and, to the left … Now … hold it … then bring your eyes back to the front … and … as they rest in a middle position, notice how they feel … compare this with how they felt when they were working … let them go on relaxing … continue relaxing for a full minute …
Finally, roll your eyes in a clockwise circle … Now … notice the sensations of tension … pause … roll them in an anticlockwise direction … Now … notice the feelings … and … Relax … let them fully relax … let them go on relaxing until all the tension has left them …

One repeat may be carried out using less tension.

A further exercise consists of focusing at different distances behind closed lids: first on a faraway object, then on an object placed close to the eyes (adapted from Madders 1981).

With your eyes still closed, imagine you are looking at an object on the distant horizon. You can't see it clearly but you are trying to make it out … Now … notice how it feels as you strain to identify it … then, releasing the tension, bring your eyes to focus on a piece of writing held very close … Now … notice the sensations as you make the effort to read the words … and … Relax … let your eyes settle on the middle distance … feel the relief as you let go of the tension in the muscles which control the focusing … enjoy the feeling of releasing that tension …

After a short rest, repeat the action with reduced tension.

Lower face

Jaw

Bring your back teeth together … do it firmly but without actually clenching them … Now

… feel a sensation in your jaw as if you'd been chewing tough meat … hold it … and … Relax … release the jaw muscles … feel the tension fading … continuing to fade … and then further still …

The exercise is repeated with diminished tension.

Lips

Press your lips tightly together as if you were rejecting some unpleasant medicine … Now … hold your lips pursed … then … Relax … let them go … and as they relax, notice feelings such as the warmth of the blood flowing back into your lips … tune in to the feelings of relaxation …

One repeat is carried out using less tension.

Tongue

Finally the tongue: press your tongue against the roof of your mouth and hold it there … Now … feel the tension in the tongue … and … Relax … notice how it feels when you relax it … and press it against the inside of your right cheek … Now … hold … and … Relax … and against your left cheek … Now … hold … and … Relax … and pull it back towards your throat (not too strongly) … Now … hold … and … Relax … and then let your tongue settle in the middle of your mouth, just touching the backs of your front teeth … feel it releasing tension … let it go on relaxing … enjoy the feeling of relaxation … let that feeling spread throughout your mouth and over your face, making them feel warm, glowing and relaxed … then, let it spread to cover your neck and shoulders … your arms … back … abdomen … and legs, so that your entire body experiences a feeling of complete relaxation … continue relaxing for several minutes …

Termination

And so, I'm going to bring this session to an end … gradually I'd like you to return to normal activity, but first I'll count from one to three to help you make the adjustment … when I get

to three, I'd like you to open your eyes, feeling
fresh and alert and ready to carry on with
your day ... one ... two ... three ... before
getting up, give a few gentle stretches to your
arms and legs.

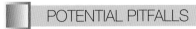

POTENTIAL PITFALLS

These can be found at the end of Chapter 5.

Chapter Eight

8

Passive muscular relaxation

Introduction and rationale

Muscular relaxation is a process by which contractile tension in voluntary muscles is reduced. The methods described in the previous three chapters are examples of the tense–release technique. Because of the contraction component, this is essentially an active procedure. When the contraction component is withdrawn, however, relaxation becomes a passive procedure. Jacobson's work covers both tense-release and passive relaxation.

Passive muscular relaxation consists of a systematic review of the skeletal muscle groups in the body. As attention is focused on each one in turn, the individual spots any tension and then releases it. Passive relaxation has certain practical advantages over active methods in that:

- the sequences can be carried out without drawing attention to the individual performing them. They are thus potentially useful in the workplace or other public locations where stress arises
- passive routines take less time to work through than tense–release ones
- the method is available to those with physical disabilities, the nature of which might preclude some of the tension routines.

Passive muscular relaxation, on the whole, requires previous knowledge of the tense–release approach. It is through tense–release that the individual learns to become aware of the sensations associated with muscle state, sensations that help him identify and release the tension.

Evidence of the value of passive relaxation comes from Lucic et al (1991), whose work supports the view that muscles relax more fully when the process is not preceded by a strong contraction. In other words, the tensing of muscle groups prior to relaxation may actually hinder their capacity to relax. These findings are thus in line with the view of Jacobson, whose work was essentially passive (though he did not use that word to describe it). Although his method has already been described in Chapter 5, reference must be made here to the position he holds as the pre-eminent exponent of the passive muscular approach. It is true that he used tensing procedures, but the emphasis of his work lay in the release of residual tension.

The authors whose work is described here are:

- Bernstein & Borkovec (1973)
- Everly & Rosenfeld (1981)
- Madders (1981), and
- Kermani (1990).

These authors have been included primarily because of the precise form of their presentations. Bernstein & Borkovec (1973) describe a release-only routine which they call 'relaxation through recall' in which muscle groups are relaxed by recalling the sensations associated with the release of tension.

Everly & Rosenfeld (1981) have developed a release-only approach which they call 'passive neuromuscular relaxation', defining it as a focusing of sensory awareness on particular muscle groups followed by their relaxation. These researchers see passive neuromuscular relaxation as a form of mental imagery which, together with its overtones of suggestion, departs from the strictly physical nature of Jacobson's progressive relaxation. On this account, the pitfalls of visualization (Ch. 18, p159) as well as those for muscular relaxation (Ch. 5, p55) should be read when adopting this approach.

The authors mentioned above are psychologists. Madders, a physiotherapist, includes passive relaxation in her book *Stress and Relaxation* (1981), while Kermani (1990), an autogenic training therapist, presents a scanning procedure.

Relaxation through recall

While giving prominence to tense–release sequences in progressive relaxation training (see Ch. 6), Bernstein & Borkovec (1973) also offer a release-only technique. 'Relaxation through recall' is the name given to this technique which is described here in an adapted form. It requires the trainee to have first learned the active form of progressive relaxation training, since the passive form is based on the memory of those routines.

The muscle groups involved are the final summarized groupings of arms, head and neck, trunk, and legs (p51). Two steps are involved.

1. The individual focuses on one of the groups, noticing any tension.

2. She recalls the sensation associated with releasing tension, and spends 30–45 seconds relaxing any tension that he finds.

Trainees are prepared by a short introduction.

Tensing and relaxing has made you highly sensitive to the feelings which accompany changes in the muscles, and now that you know the technique, I want to lead you to a more advanced version of it. I would like you to cast your mind back to the four-group tense-release procedure, but this time, to drop the tensing part. As we travel through these four groups, I'm going to ask you simply to look for any tension, and then, by recalling the sensations associated with its release, to let it go.

The trainee sits in a reclining chair or something that resembles it and the following script is presented.

Would you close your eyes please? I'd like you first to concentrate on the muscles of your hands and arms. See if you can identify any feeling of tension in them. If so, notice where it is 'notice how it feels ... and relax it away, remembering previous feelings of releasing tension in these muscles ... go on releasing tension as you recall those sensations ... go on until the muscles become more and more deeply relaxed ... until you feel relaxation flowing through all the muscles of your arms ... until they are totally free of tension ... signal with a lifted finger when the arms feel fully relaxed.

The trainer continues in this way for 30–45 seconds.

Next, bring your mind to focus on the muscles of your face and neck. Is there any tension there? If so, notice where it is and what it feels like ... then, recalling the feeling of letting the tension go, relax it ... feel the tension leaving the muscles ... note the pleasant feeling of relaxation ... allow the relaxation to deepen and go on deepening as you concentrate on the peaceful state of those muscles ...

Next, concentrate on the muscles of the trunk. Pick up any sensation of tension you may find ... notice where it is and what it feels like ... remember what it felt like when you previously relaxed tension in those muscles ... and relax them now ... relax any tension you find ... continue letting the tension go until your muscles feel quite loose. Go on relaxing them ... feel them getting looser and looser.

Finally, give your attention to your legs ... do you notice any tension there? ... notice exactly where it is ... notice how it feels ... and release it ... recalling the sensation of releasing it ... remembering that feeling ... letting all the tension dissolve ... further ... then further still ... until the muscles feel entirely relaxed ...

By practising relaxation through recall, the trainee will be able to reduce the time it takes to relax each muscle group from 45 to perhaps 15 seconds.

Relaxation through recall with counting

When the trainee feels skilled at relaxing through recall, the procedure can be still further shortened by introducing counting. Here, recited numbers correspond to the groups in the recall procedure as follows.

I'm going to count slowly from one to ten. As I count, I'd like you to focus on the same muscle groups as in the recall procedure, relaxing them as you did then.
One ... two, focusing on the arms and hands as they become more relaxed ... three ... four, relaxing the face and neck muscles ... five ... six, focusing on the muscles of the chest, back, shoulders and abdomen, feeling them becoming more and more relaxed ... seven ... eight, allowing relaxation to flow through the muscles of the legs and feet ... nine ... ten, relaxed all over ...

It is suggested that the counting be done at a pace which corresponds with the trainee's respirations. Once mastered, this technique can be used by the trainee when faced with challenging situations.

Passive neuromuscular relaxation

The technique described here is the work of Everly & Rosenfeld (1981). This method owes much to autogenic training (see Ch. 20) in its use of suggestion and its images of warmth and heaviness. It is, however, considered by its authors to be a muscular method and so belongs in this chapter.

Trainees are introduced to the approach with a short explanation on the following lines.

Tension in the muscles is associated with tension in the mind. If tension is eliminated from the muscles, then the subjective feeling of stress is reduced. In this method you will be asked to focus attention on one muscle group at a time, releasing any tension that exists. No activity is involved; the method is a passive one. It has been found that by concentrating on the muscles in this way, deep levels of relaxation can be achieved. Of course, the more you practise, the more effective it becomes.

The necessary conditions include a warm, quiet room where interruptions are unlikely to occur, and a comfortable chair to sit in or flat surface to lie on. The following script is adapted from Everly & Rosenfeld (1981).

Settle into the chair you're in or the surface you are lying on, letting your body weight sink into it. Close your eyes. To start with, I'd like you to turn your attention to your breathing ... follow the next breath out ... then, let the air in ... feel it gently filling your lungs ... pause for a moment ... and breathe out slowly ... then allow your breathing to follow its natural rhythm: gentle and slow ... getting gentler and slower ...
Now bring your attention to the muscles of your head. Begin to feel a slow warm wave of relaxation gathering at the top of your head and beginning to descend towards your forehead ... focusing on the muscles above your eyes ... feel those muscles becoming heavy and relaxed ... concentrate on the heavy feeling you are getting from them ... now shift your attention to the muscles of your eyes and cheeks and feel them also becoming heavy and relaxed ... now, focus on the muscles of your mouth and jaw ... allow them to grow heavy and relaxed ...

Pause for 10 seconds.

As your head and face continue to relax, let the wave of relaxation slowly descend into your neck ... focus your attention on the neck muscles and feel them becoming slacker and more relaxed with every moment that passes ...

73

Pause for 10 seconds.

The wave of relaxation continues to roll down, this time spreading warmth over your shoulder muscles ... focus on this area ... allow it to become heavy and relaxed as you concentrate your attention on it.

Pause for 10 seconds.

The head, neck and shoulders remain relaxed while you focus on your arms ... letting the wave of relaxation bring heaviness and warmth to them ... concentrate on the feelings in the arms ...

Pause for 10 seconds.

Now feel the wave of relaxation descending into your hands as you focus on them ... feel the muscles of your palms and fingers relaxing ... feel warmth flowing into them as they become more relaxed ...

Pause for 10 seconds.

Now, as the upper part of your body remains in deep relaxation, switch your attention to your abdomen and the wall of muscle covering your internal organs ... let those muscles loosen and spread ... then feel the wave of relaxation beginning to descend into your thigh muscles ... and as you concentrate on them, feel your thighs becoming heavy ... heavy as lead ...

Pause for 10 seconds.

The wave of relaxation continues to descend into your lower legs ... focus on your calf muscles ... feel the sense of heaviness and relaxation in your calves ...

Pause for 10 seconds.

Now, as the rest of your body remains relaxed, turn your attention to your feet ... feel the warm wave of relaxation descending into your foot muscles ... feel them becoming warm, heavy and relaxed ...

Pause for 10 seconds.

Then, as you feel all your muscles to be in a state of relaxation, start to recite the phrase, 'I am relaxed'; repeat it every time you breathe out.

After a 5-minute pause:

I'd like you now to bring your attention back to the room in which you are lying. I am going to count from one to five, and as I count, begin to feel more and more awake, more and more refreshed, with a clear head. When I reach five, I'd like you to open your eyes. One, begin to feel alert ... two ... three, more alert still ... four ... five ... open your eyes and gently stretch your arms and legs ...

The relaxation 'ripple'

Closely related to the above method is the relaxation 'ripple'. Adapted from Priest & Schott (1991), the technique consists of one continuous wave of relaxation which begins at the crown of the head and progresses down through the body to the toes. As the wave descends, the individual briefly scans the muscle groups, releasing tension. If she is lying down, all tension can be released; if she is standing, excess tension can be released. The effectiveness of the exercise is increased if it is timed to coincide with the outbreath. However, the participant should be discouraged from extending the outbreath for too long.

The exercise can be better understood if the first relaxation ripple is preceded by a tensing of the whole body (Schott & Priest 2002). Thereafter, it can be performed in a passive manner.

A passive relaxation approach

The script presented here is adapted from Madders (1981). It is addressed to trainees who are lying down. A supplementary section enables the instructor to adapt it for the seated participant.

Introductory remarks to trainees

This is a method which helps to relax your muscles and your thoughts. It consists of focusing on different parts of the body in turn and releasing any tension you find. There are no physical actions involved; relaxation occurs by virtue of a thought process. In spite of its length, the method is one which you can easily use to induce relaxation on your own.

Procedure for participants who are lying down

A firm support with a soft surface is needed, e.g. a length of foam spread out on the floor. The script could begin with the passage called 'Sinking' in Chapter 3, and continue as follows.

With your eyes closed, notice how slow and regular your breathing is becoming … easy, calm and even … leaving you more relaxed than you were before …

I'm going to ask you to take a trip round the body, checking that all the muscle groups are as relaxed as possible and letting go any tension that might still remain. If outside thoughts creep in, hold them in a bubble and let them float away. I'll begin with the feet.

Bring your attention to your toes … are they lying still? If they are curled or stretched out or in some way not entirely comfortable, waggle them gently. As they come to rest, feel the tension ebbing away … feel the tension leaving them as they lie motionless …

Let your feet roll out at the ankles. This is the most relaxed position for them. Let all the tension flow out of them … enjoy the sensation of just letting them go.

Moving on to the lower legs: feel the tension leaving the calf muscles and the shins. As the tension goes, so they feel heavier … so they feel warm and pleasantly tingling.

The thighs next: to be fully relaxed they need to be slightly rolling outwards … feel the relaxing effect of this position … make sure you have released all tension, and feel your thighs resting heavily on the floor.

Focus for a moment on the sensation of sagging heaviness throughout your legs … let the muscles shed their last remaining hint of tension and settle into a deep relaxation.

And now, think of your hips. Let them settle into the surface you are lying on … recognize any tension that lingers in the muscles … then

relax it away … let it go on relaxing a bit further than you thought possible.

Settle your spine into the rug or mattress … become aware of how it is resting on the floor. Let it sink down, making contact wherever it wants to … all tension draining out of it.

Let your abdominal muscles lose their tension. Let them go soft and loose. Feel them spreading as they give up their last vestige of tension … notice how your relaxed abdomen rises and falls with your breathing … rises as the air is drawn in and falls as the air is expelled … abdominal breathing is relaxed breathing.

Moving up to your shoulders, to muscles which are prone to carry tension … feel them letting go … feel them spreading … feel them easing into the floor, limp and heavy … feel them dropping down towards your feet … imagine them shedding their burdens … and as the space between your shoulders and your neck opens out, imagine your neck a bit longer than it was before.

Now, direct your thoughts to the muscles of your left arm. Check that it lies limply on the ground. Notice the feeling of relaxation and allow this feeling to sweep down to your wrist and hand. Think of the fingers, are they curved and still? … neither drawn up nor stretched out …in a hand that is neither open nor closed, but gently resting … totally relaxed. As you breathe out, let the arm relax a little bit more … let it lie heavy and loose … so heavy and loose that if someone were to pick it up, then let go, it would flop down again like the arm of a rag doll.

Repeat the last paragraph with the muscles of the right arm.

Your neck muscles have no need to work with your head supported, so let them go … enjoy the feeling of 'letting go' in muscles which work so hard the rest of the time to keep your head upright. If you find any tension in the neck, release it and let this process of releasing continue, even below the surface … feel how pleasant it is when you let go the tension in these muscles.

Bring your attention now to your face, to the many small muscles whose job it is to manage your expressions. At the moment there's no need to have any expression at all on your face, so allow your muscles to feel relaxed … imagine how your face is when you are asleep … calm and motionless …

Now, think about the jaw … and as you do, allow it to drop slightly so that your teeth are separated … feel it relaxing with your lips gently touching. Check that your tongue is still, and lying in the middle of your mouth, soft and shapeless. Relax your throat so that all tension leaves it and the muscles feel smooth and resting.

With no expression on your face, your cheeks are relaxed and soft. If you think of your nose, let it be just to register the passage of cool air travelling up your nostrils while warmer air passes down … breathe tension out with the warm air … breathe stillness in with the cool air.

Check that your forehead is smooth … not furrowed in any direction … and as you release its remaining tension, imagine it being a little higher and a little wider that it was before … let this feeling of relaxation extend through your scalp muscles, over the crown of your head and down behind your ears … feel a sense of calm as you do this.

Let your attention focus on your eyes as they lie behind gently closed lids. Think of them resting in their sockets, floating rather than fixed … and as they come to rest, so do your thoughts also.

Spend a few minutes continuing to relax, deepening the effect of the above sequences …

You have now relaxed all the major muscle groups in your body. Think about them now as a whole … a totally relaxed whole … and soothed by your gentle breathing rhythm, feel the peacefulness of this idea …

Images may drift in and out of your mind … see them as thoughts passing through. Feel yourself letting go of them. Say to yourself: 'I am feeling calm, I am feeling peaceful'. Let your mind conjure up a scene of contentment.

Trainees can relax quietly for a few minutes, before the session is brought to an end.

Termination

I am going to ask you to bring yourself slowly back to the room you are lying in. Gradually

become aware of it. Gently move your arms and legs … wriggle your spine, and in your own time, allow your eyes to open. Slowly sit up and take in your surroundings. Give your body plenty of time to adjust from the relaxed to the alert state.

Before the meeting breaks up, the value of practice should be emphasized. If carried out on a daily basis, the technique will help the trainee to relax herself more effectively.

Adapted procedure for seated trainees

The trainee picks the chair he finds most comfortable, although in a public building the choice may be limited. For deep relaxation the body needs to be well supported. The procedure begins in the following way.

Settle into your chair, sitting well back into the seat, your feet flat on the floor and your hands in your lap. Close your eyes. Become aware of the parts of your body that touch the chair and the floor. Feel the weight of your body passing through those points: hips, thighs, feet, back and arms, some of them carrying more weight than others. If the back of the chair is high enough, use it to support your head. If not, your head may be dropping forwards which is all right if you find it comfortable, but it tends to put a strain on the neck muscles if held for a long time. Try raising your head and seeing it as a weight supported by a pole. If you can balance it in this way, on your spine, you will be giving your neck muscles a rest.

The same script as for the lying position may be used, substituting the words 'sitting' for 'lying' and 'chair' for 'floor'. The paragraph about the neck muscles can be deleted, and also the one referring to the feet.

Kermani's scanning technique

To 'scan', in this sense, is to run the attention over all the voluntary muscles.

Scanning may be used for at least two purposes: as a means of checking to see if tension exists, and as a device to enable the individual to feel in touch with his body as a whole. Both purposes are relevant in the context of relaxation, and the method forms a quick and simple version of the passive relaxation approach.

Here is an example adapted from Kermani (1990).

I'll ask you to spend a moment getting in touch with the different parts of your body, acknowledging them as part of you and checking that they feel relaxed and comfortable. Begin by bringing your attention to your feet. First the toes ... working up through the ankles ... to the calves and shins ... over the knees ... along the thighs ... the abdomen ... then the chest. Think now of your shoulders ... of travelling down to the elbows ... through the forearms ... and into the wrists ... hands and fingers. Become aware even of your fingertips.

Next, move across to the lower spine and the pelvis. Give your attention to the lumbar region ... rising to the back of the chest and the bladebones ... continuing up into the neck and scalp ... to the crown of the head ... then slowly begin to descend to the forehead ... ending with the jaw ... feel that every part of your body is relaxed ...

You might like to think of a giant paint brush sweeping over your body, following the same route.

Another passive method

A release-only method is described in Chapter 9 (p83) as one component of Ost's applied relaxation.

POTENTIAL PITFALLS

Passive relaxation is subject to the pitfalls of other muscular approaches (Ch. 5, p55). Because passive methods often include imagery and suggestion, the pitfalls relating to visualizations should also be taken into account (Ch. 18, p159).

KEY MESSAGES

- Different authors have proposed variations of passive relaxation. Four are included in this chapter: Bernstein & Borkovec, Everly & Rosenfeld, Madders and Kermani.
- Passive muscular relaxation is derived from Jacobson's progressive relaxation but differs from it in its absence of tensing component.
- Summarized versions of these methods constitute scanning procedures.
- Passive forms of relaxation are useful for people who cannot tolerate tensing actions.
- Progressive muscular relaxation is a skill and as such requires regular practice.

Chapter Nine

Applied relaxation

9

CHAPTER CONTENTS

History

The methods described in previous chapters have, on the whole, been concerned with the induction of deep relaxation. Their purpose is to equip the individual with routines to be performed in the privacy of his own home. As such, these methods are useful for unwinding after a stressful day but may not provide strategies for coping with stress as it occurs. For this, some kind of shortened version that can be linked into life activities is required.

Jacobson's (1938) differential relaxation (p113) and Wolpe's (1958) systematic desensitization represent early attempts at applied formats. However, it was Goldfried (1971) who, recognizing the extent of the gulf between relaxation in the therapeutic environment and relaxation in the stressful situation, focused expressly on the issue of the application of the skills. He emphasized the need for a portable and shortened form of progressive relaxation; a form which could be used to defuse anxiety as it occurred, and one which the individual could use as a general coping skill in everyday life. In so doing, he gave the individual a new role, defining him as an active agent in his treatment rather than a passive client. The approach was called 'training in self-control' because it implied active mastery of anxiety by the individual himself.

Description

Öst's (1987) applied relaxation method is a more recent version of Goldfried's approach. Using progressive relaxation as a core technique, the method teaches the individual to relax in successively shorter periods and to transfer these relaxation effects to everyday situations. Thus the individual is equipped with a strategy to control his reactions to stressful events as they occur.

The method consists of six components, in each of which a particular aspect of relaxation is taught:

* tense–release technique
* release-only technique
* cue-controlled (conditioned) relaxation

- differential relaxation
- rapid relaxation
- application training.

It is estimated that by using the tense–release method taught here (Wolpe & Lazarus 1966), the trained individual can achieve a relaxed state in 15–20 minutes; by using the release-only technique he can achieve it in 5–7 minutes; using the cue-controlled, in 2–3 minutes; the differential technique, in 60–90 seconds; and using rapid relaxation, in 20–30 seconds. The final goal is to be able to apply relaxation skills to the experience of everyday stressful events.

The components must be taught in a precise order since progression to each depends largely on mastery of the preceding one. A total of 8–12 sessions of tuition is required, backed up by home practice which should be carried out twice a day, and is itself an important part of programme.

Rationale

As with all versions of progressive relaxation, applied relaxation is said to calm the thoughts as a result of relaxing the musculature. Thus, it can be used for coping with day-to-day stress. Öst's method, however, was designed principally for use with people who suffer from panic and other kinds of anxiety. In this context, an understanding of anxiety as a state is crucial to the success of the training and an explanation should be given to the participant at the outset.

Anxiety may be seen as having three aspects: the physiological, the cognitive and the behavioural. The physiological aspect is represented by such phenomena as raised heart rate and blood pressure, sweating and increased muscle tension; the cognitive aspect by negative thoughts such as 'This is too much for me to cope with' or 'I'm going to have a heart attack', and the behavioural aspect by tense posture and different kinds of unrelaxed activity. These effects can escalate with one inflaming the other. In particular, the physiological and cognitive aspects can create a vicious circle with negative thoughts leading to sympathetic changes which are themselves interpreted in a negative way. The result can be a spiralling of anxiety (Clark 1986) (Fig. 9.1).

One way of breaking the circle would be to reinterpret the bodily changes in a more positive light, i.e. instead of thinking he is about to collapse with a heart attack, the individual could reassure himself

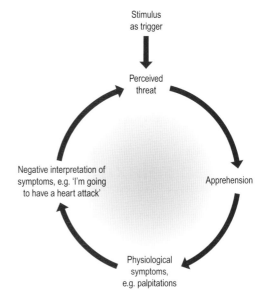

Figure 9.1 • A cognitive model of panic attacks. (Adapted from Clark 1986.)

that everyone gets palpitations sometimes. This constitutes a cognitive approach. Another way of breaking the circle would be to neutralize the anxiety with the use of a relaxation technique such as progressive relaxation. This draws on physiological theory. A third way would be to introduce graded exposure to the feared item which represents a behavioural approach. All three are incorporated in Öst's applied relaxation which can thus be seen as a cognitive-behavioural method (Heimberg 2002).

Because anxiety is easier to relieve when it is mild, it should be addressed before it reaches a peak. Early signals or signs of rising anxiety levels such as a pounding heart, sweating, fast breathing or tense muscles can be used as cues to employ the technique. Experiences of anxiety-provoking events can be recorded by means of 'self-monitoring', where the individual notes on a printed form the situations, the intensity of his anxiety and the remedial action taken by him (Fig. 9.2). This form, over time, reflects his progress in coping with such events.

Procedure

Conditions for training sessions

It is suggested that participants sit for the exercises since daily stress frequently occurs in this posture

Date	Situation	Reaction, i.e. anxiety signals	Intensity (0–10)	Action taken

Figure 9.2 • Form for recording self-observed early anxiety signals. (Adapted from Öst 1987.)

rather than in a lying one. The chair should be comfortable and have arm rests. The procedures are first demonstrated by the trainer and carried out by the trainee to ensure that they have been understood. The trainee then closes his eyes while the instructor runs through the programme. At the end, the trainee rates the degree of relaxation gained on a 0–100 scale.

Each component requires 1–2 weeks of practice for the trainee to become proficient in it.

Introductory remarks to participants

Before beginning the programme of relaxation, the rationale of the treatment is presented to participants.

As its name suggests, this method will show you how to apply relaxation skills in everyday life. This means the techniques have to be quick-acting and unobtrusive. The aim is to be able to relax in 20–30 seconds and to transfer this skill to situations of stress.

When people experience anxiety they tend to react in three different ways: a physiological way in which their blood pressure rises and they become breathless with a pounding heart and a cold sweat; a psychological way in which distressing thoughts go through their head; and a behavioural way whereby they find themselves trying to escape.

If the physiological symptoms are viewed as threatening, the body will respond by intensifying those symptoms, which in turn will make the thoughts more negative. This is the way a panic attack develops.

However, this vicious circle can be broken and one way of doing this is by learning not to react so strongly. This will reduce your feeling of distress and your symptoms will tend to subside.

I am going to lead you through a well-tested method which will help you to achieve this. You'll be learning a skill so it's important to practise it, but once you've mastered it, you'll find it useful in nearly all situations.

The approach starts by introducing you to progressive relaxation which consists of tensing and releasing the muscles throughout the body. When that is learned and practised daily, the tensing part of the exercise is dropped.

Next, you'll be asked to repeat the word 'relax' to yourself when you are in a state of relaxation. Attaching the word to the state has the effect of turning the word into a cue; a cue to invoke a state of relaxation. This only happens, of course, after repeated associations.

Learning how to use reduced amounts of muscle tension when carrying out specific tasks is the next procedure, followed by a rapid-acting technique for maintaining low levels of stress throughout the day. Finally, these skills are applied to particular situations of stress.

These exercises enable you to achieve relaxation in progressively shorter periods of time. Success depends on practice.

Tense-release

Two sessions of tuition are devoted to learning this version of progressive relaxation.

First session

The first session is spent working on the hands, arms, face, neck and shoulders. Each muscle group is taken through one tense-release cycle in which 5 seconds are allotted for the tension and 10–15 seconds for the release, as follows.

> *Begin by clenching the right hand … make a fist … make it tight … notice the sensation of tension in the hand and forearm while you hold it for five seconds … then let it go … feel the hand and forearm becoming relaxed and comfortable … warm and relaxed … relaxed and heavy …*

The release is continued for 10 seconds.

The other actions featuring in session one are:
- clenching the left hand
- bending the right elbow
- straightening the right elbow by pressing the wrist down on the arm of the chair
- bending the left elbow
- straightening the left elbow
- raising the eyebrows and wrinkling the forehead
- bringing the eyebrows together and frowning
- screwing the eyes up tight
- biting the teeth together
- pressing the tongue against the roof of the mouth
- pressing the lips together

- pressing the head against the back of the chair
- pressing the chin down on to the collarbone
- hunching the shoulders up to the ears
- bracing the shoulders back to bring the blades together.

Termination

When the above exercises have been worked through, the session is brought to an end.

> *The relaxation session is over now, and to help you return to activity, I'm going to count from one to five, and when I get to five, I want you to open your eyes, feeling calm and relaxed … one, feeling calm … two, feeling relaxed … three, very calm … four, very relaxed … five … open your eyes, feeling ready to carry on with your everyday life.*

A debriefing period follows (Ch 3, p27). Participants are instructed to practise for 15 minutes twice daily. They are asked to record the level of relaxation achieved, using a 0–100 scale where 0 = total relaxation, 100 = maximum tension, and 50 represents normal. They are also asked to keep a note of the length of practice time taken to reach the level achieved. The form shown in Figure 9.3 serves to

0 = totally relaxed
100 = maximum tension

Date	Time	Component	Degree of relaxation (0–100)		Time taken to achieve it
			Before	After	

Figure 9.3 • Form for recording relaxation training homework. (Adapted from Öst 1987.)

motivate the individual to practise as well as to record the details of the homework session.

Second session

Session two starts with a review of the work done in the first session followed by tense–release exercises for the chest, stomach, back, legs and feet. These are:

- tensing the muscles which pull the stomach in
- arching the back so that the spine leaves the back of the chair
- tensing the buttock muscles by pressing the feet down into the floor
- raising the heels with the toes remaining on the ground
- raising the front part of the foot, keeping the heels on the ground.

The second session is terminated in the same way as the first and trainees are reminded to practise.

Release-only

In this phase of instruction, the 'tension' part of the sequence is eliminated, leaving just the 'release' part. As a result, the relaxed state can be achieved in less time than when working with the full sequence; 5–7 minutes are suggested instead of the 15 of the tense–release session.

The training session begins with breathing instructions, followed by a scanning of all the voluntary muscles starting with the head and working down to the toes. The following instructions are adapted from Öst (1987).

In a moment I'm going to ask you to focus your attention on your breathing and, in particular, on the movement of your upper abdomen ... notice how it swells slightly as you breathe in, and sinks back as you breathe out ... do not change it in any way ... just tune in to its rhythmic pattern ... feel yourself relaxing more with each breath ... feel your muscles letting go from the top of your head ... your forehead ... eyebrows ... eyelids ... cheeks ... temples ... jaws ... throat ... tongue ... lips ... feel your entire face relaxed ... now ... your neck ... shoulders ... arms ... and down to the tips of your fingers ... and while you are doing this, let your breathing continue at its own pace, expanding the stomach region in particular ...

Now, relax your back ... now, the lower part of your body ... hips ... thighs ... knees ... calves ... shins ... . feet ... toes ... still breathing gently and noticing the relaxing effect of each breath ... feel yourself relaxing more and more ...

The sequence is terminated in the same way as for the first component.

Again, the homework assignment is a twice-daily practice, the trainee being asked to record afterwards the level of relaxation achieved and how long it took to reach it.

Cue-controlled or conditioned relaxation

This component of the training focuses on the breathing. It begins by asking the trainee to relax himself by employing the release-only method of progressive relaxation. Once relaxed, he is asked to begin silently to recite the word 'relax'; he recites it once each time he breathes out. Following many repetitions, an association is built up between the word and the relaxed state whereby the word alone becomes capable of inducing a measure of relaxation. The word has thus become a cue. The stronger the association, the greater the power of the cue word. Expressed in other terms, a conditioning process has been set up, as a result of which the trainee feels himself relaxed whenever he thinks the word 'relax'.

The trainer introduces the exercise in the following manner.

Spend a few moments with your eyes closed ... relax yourself by running through the release-only routine ... signal to me by raising your right index finger when you feel fully relaxed ... if you are ready, turn your attention now to your breathing ... tune in to its rhythm ... let it adopt its own pace ... do not be tempted to alter it ... and just before you breathe in, think the word 'inhale' ... just before you breathe out, think the word 'relax' ...

Leading with the instructions of 'inhale' and 'relax' for five breaths, the trainer then asks the participant to continue on his own for a further five breaths. After a few minutes' rest, the full sequence is repeated.

If there is more than one participant, the trainer will not attempt to synchronize their respirations but will let them conduct their own exercise. As proficiency increases, the command 'inhale' can be dropped, and the word 'relax' used on its own.

Homework consists of 20 pairings a day of the word 'relax' with the state of relaxation. Participants should be warned against overbreathing, i.e. allowing the breathing to become deeper or more rapid (Ch. 4, p40). The trainee keeps a record of the level of relaxation achieved and the time taken to reach it.

Once learned, it takes only 2–3 minutes to become fully relaxed by this method.

Differential relaxation

So far, the sessions have been concerned with teaching basic techniques. The application of those skills now begins. Differential relaxation focuses on controlling the levels of muscle tension while the individual is engaged in some activity. Although some tension is needed in order to carry out the task, the level is often greater than is necessary and may need to be reduced. Also there may be unnecessary tension in the muscles not directly engaged in the task. Different levels of tension (or relaxation) are required for each.

Since an ability to recognize muscle tension at its varying levels is essential for developing this skill, differential relaxation is presented after the individual has been trained in progressive relaxation.

Two sessions of tuition are indicated, one dealing with sitting and the other with standing activities. Both sessions begin with a revision of cue-controlled relaxation.

The first session: sitting

In the first session, the trainee, seated in an armchair, is instructed to make certain movements while maintaining a relaxed state in the rest of the body.

Please make yourself as comfortable as possible. Settle into the chair with your feet flat on the floor. With your eyes closed, relax yourself using your cue word with breathing … when you are ready, would you raise your right index finger … I'd like you now to open your eyes and look around the room without moving

your head … notice the tension in the eye muscles but keep the body relaxed …

Next, look around the room allowing your head to move in order to increase your range of vision. Keep a minimum of tension in the neck muscles while you do this, and check that the rest of your body is free from tension …

Would you now lift one arm, and as you do, remember to keep the other parts of your body relaxed … and, lower the arm. Continue to scan your body for signs of unnecessary tension.

Now, lift one leg off the ground, keeping the rest of your body as relaxed as possible … and, let it down.

If you had any difficulty with this exercise, perhaps we could discuss it before moving on.

The routine is then carried out on the other arm and leg, after which the trainee is moved from his armchair to an upright chair. He relaxes himself in this new sitting position before being led through the same procedure of eye, head and limb movements. Next, he is seated at a table and asked to write something short such as his name and address, using the minimum of muscle tension needed to accomplish the task. As an alternative, in practice sessions, he could make a short telephone call, adopting the same relaxed state.

The second session: standing

In the second session of differential relaxation, the trainee stands. His position should be near a wall or some form of support, in case he feels unsteady, but he should not be leaning on it. The session begins with cue-controlled relaxation, after which the same schedule of head, arm and leg movements is worked through.

Lastly, the trainee is asked to practise relaxation while walking. Emphasis is placed on finding an easy way of moving and on relaxing the muscles not used, such as those of the face and hands. Any initial awkwardness will disappear as the individual discovers more relaxed ways of holding his body.

With the skills he has learned and practised, the individual will be able to achieve a state of relaxation consistent with effective task performance within 60–90 seconds. Differential relaxation is expanded in Chapter 13.

Rapid relaxation

As its name implies, this component is designed to reduce still further the time it takes to become relaxed; it also gives the trainee the opportunity to practise in everyday situations. First, the trainee's environment is arranged so that a regularly used appliance acts as a cue to relax; for example, the wristwatch or the telephone are marked with a coloured dot which reminds the individual to relax whenever he sees it. Every time he looks at his watch or makes a telephone call he is reminded to release tension. This means that stress is in general held at low levels in the everyday setting. Rapid relaxation consists of the following routine performed each time the individual sees the coloured dot.

Take a slow breath ... think 'relax' ... then exhale. Repeat this twice ... scan the body for unnecessary tensions ... and release them.

Regular practice of this short sequence (15–20 times a day) makes the technique more effective and results in the trainee being able to relax in a still shorter space of time. It has been found that after 1 or 2 weeks' practice, he can relax himself by this method in as little as 20–30 seconds.

Application training

Applying relaxation skills to situations of potential stress is the subject of this phase. With the use of a system of graded exposure (Ch. 1, p11), the trainee is encouraged to face the situation of stress. Anxiety-provoking situations should, however, be presented at a level of challenge which the trainee can cope with, neither too high nor too low.

Take yourself to a situation that you know is likely to provoke stress for you. Relax yourself before entering the scene. Observe your reactions. If you feel anxiety levels beginning to rise, bring out your cue word 'relax'. Continue to apply it until you feel your anxiety levels falling.

It may not work the first time because, like any skill, practice is necessary to achieve success, but gradually you will find you are gaining more control over your anxiety levels.

As a preliminary, the individual could visualize himself successfully coping in the stress-provoking situation before exposing himself to the same event in real life (see Ch. 19).

Maintenance programme

However successful the treatment, Öst suggests keeping up the habit of scanning the body for unnecessary tension and using rapid relaxation to release it.

Evidence of effectiveness

Öst addresses three modes of anxiety with the applied relaxation approach: the physiological, the cognitive and the behavioural. The physiological aspect is addressed through muscle relaxation; the cognitive through the cue word; and the behavioural through differential relaxation and exposure to the stressor. A multivariate approach such as this has advantages in a condition such as anxiety where changes occur in different modes.

As a method, applied relaxation has been tested in a wide variety of conditions including phobia, panic disorder, headache, epilepsy and tinnitus. In all these it has been found significantly more effective than no treatment or placebo conditions. Follow-up at varying times from 5 to 19 months showed that effects were maintained and in some cases augmented (Öst 1988).

Studies comparing applied relaxation with psychological methods often find very little difference in effectiveness; for example, in a study comparing the method with cognitive therapy on a population of 33 people experiencing generalized anxiety disorder, it was not possible to declare one method superior to the other. Both, however, were found to be effective (Öst & Breitholtz 2000).

In an earlier study, Spence and colleagues (1995) tested the effect of applied relaxation on chronic upper extremity pain caused by cumulative trauma. Forty-eight patients were randomly allocated to four groups: applied relaxation, electromyographic feedback, a combination of both and a waiting list control. After treatment twice weekly for 4 weeks, significant reductions in pain, depression, distress and anxiety were found in all the relaxation groups while minimal change occurred in the waiting list control. The greatest benefit, in the short term at least, was reported in the group who received applied relaxation.

Although effective therapies for anxiety exist, many individuals refrain from seeking treatment owing to the embarrassment associated with help seeking. Internet-based self-help supplemented by weekly telephone calls can be an alternative. Exploring the benefits of this approach, Carlbring et al (2003) randomly divided 22 participants experiencing panic disorder into two self-help groups. One was trained in cognitive-behavioural therapy, the other in applied relaxation. Therapist contact was minimal. Both trainings were found to be effective, achieving significant medium-to-large effects, providing support for the use of Internet-administered self-help. A further study by Carlbring et al was mounted in 2007 to compare Internet-directed cognitive-behavioural therapy with a waiting list control in people experiencing social phobia. Results of this randomized controlled trial showed greater reductions in anxiety in the treatment group than in the control group. Moreover, there was 93% adherence to the Internet programme with benefit maintained 1 year later. These results strengthen support for the use of Internet self-help.

POTENTIAL PITFALLS

Since applied relaxation is based on progressive relaxation, it is subject to the same potential pitfalls. They may be found in Chapter 5 (p55).

KEY MESSAGES

- Öst was one of many researchers who sought to apply the work of Jacobson to everyday life.
- The method uses a multivariate approach which addresses the physiological aspect through muscle relaxation, the cognitive through the cue word and the behavioural through exposure to the stressor.
- Öst's approach was designed to be learned in 8–12 sessions compared with the 50 of Jacobson's.
- Applied relaxation is a skill which has to be learned and therefore home practice is essential.
- As the trainee becomes more proficient, the state of relaxation can be achieved in ever shorter periods.

Chapter Ten

10

Behavioural relaxation training

History and rationale

A person who is tense adopts a characteristic pattern of muscular activity in the form of frowning, clenching and general body tenseness. The muscles of a relaxed person, by contrast, are free from excessive muscle tension. As a result, people who are tense look different from people who are relaxed. Their feelings are associated with a different posture in each case. Don Schilling, a psychologist

working in the early 1980s, found the converse also occurred; that is, people adopting a relaxed posture reported feeling more relaxed.

Schilling, who was teaching progressive relaxation to adolescent boys, noticed they were better at tensing than relaxing; In fact, they found it difficult to respond to the request to relax. He suggested to his pupils that instead of trying to *become* relaxed, they should adopt the more concrete objective of trying to *look* relaxed: to take up postures they would expect to see in people who *were* relaxed. The result was that the pupils not only succeeded in looking relaxed but reported actually feeling more relaxed. Thus, by adopting postures characteristic of relaxation, they had induced a subjective feeling of relaxation.

The idea is reminiscent of the facial and postural feedback hypotheses which state that feedback from facial expression and posture induces feelings that match those expressions and postures. In other words, people feel the emotions that correspond with their poses.

Based on these ideas, Schilling & Poppen (1983) set up a method of relaxation which they called behavioural relaxation training (BRT). Liberal feedback from the trainer provided reinforcement or corrective adjustment. The method is thus underpinned by behaviourist principles.

Description

Behavioural relaxation training is a method in which tense postures are replaced by relaxed ones.

The trainee is required to take up specified relaxed postures based on the way people look when they are relaxed. He then registers the feeling engendered by the posture itself.

Protocol for behavioural relaxation training

Setting

The ideal setting is a warm, quiet room with dimmed lighting. A padded recliner is the chair of choice but, since this may not be available, any flat surface will serve. Pillows may be used under the knees, forearms and head, as required. Women will find it convenient to wear trousers.

Introduction of method to participants

Participants are introduced to the method in the following way.

We can all recognize signs of tension: tightly drawn face muscles, clenching of teeth and

fingers. These are typical postures that people adopt when under stress. When people are relaxed, muscle tensions are released and a new posture results. The central idea of behavioural relaxation training is that by adopting the posture of a relaxed person, we can make ourselves feel more relaxed.

In this method you will be asked to make different parts of your body look as relaxed as possible and then to notice the effect the new position has on you; to notice how the new position feels. I'll describe and demonstrate each item before we begin. Please try out the items on yourself.

The postures, as described in Table 10.1, are then demonstrated and the trainee asked to copy them. The unrelaxed postures are also demonstrated to emphasize the point. Feedback is provided by the trainer in the form of praise or corrective instructions. The trainee is asked particularly to take note of the proprioceptive events, i.e. the joint and muscle feelings which convey the sense of body position as each new posture is adopted.

Following the demonstration, the trainee rests quietly with his eyes closed. After a few minutes, the

Table 10.1 Relaxed and unrelaxed behaviours (adapted from Poppen 1998, with permission from the author)

Item	Relaxed	Unrelaxed
Breathing	Breaths regular and fewer in number than recorded on the baseline	Breaths irregular and greater in number than recorded on the baseline
Quiet	No audible sounds such as sighs, words or movements	Talking, whispering, sighing, coughing, snoring or other audible sounds
Body	Symmetrical and fully resting on supporting surface	Holding any part tense or twisted
Head	Motionless and supported with nose in midline	Head turning or other movements; head unsupported or tilted; nose outside midline
Eyes	Lids lightly closed with eyes still	Eyes open or, if closed, darting about under tense and fluttering lids
Mouth	Lips parted at centre of mouth with teeth separated	Lips firmly closed with teeth held together or mouth uncomfortably open
Throat	No activity	Swallowing, twitching or preparing to speak
Shoulders	Dropped and level with each other; resting against support	Both hunched or one higher than the other; not resting on support
Hands	Both resting at sides, on armrests or on lap; palms down, fingers gently curled	Clasped, clenched tight or gripping the armrest
Feet	Comfortably rolled out so that the toes point away from each other	Pointing vertically, crossed or excessively rolled out

instructor may make an initial assessment (see the section on the Behavioural Relaxation Scale, p90).

Training procedure

The training procedure is then presented in its entirety. Below is a slightly paraphrased version of the protocol laid out in Poppen (1998), where it is suggested that each relaxed posture be held for 30–60 seconds. Trainees are asked to close their eyes.

Feet

Starting with the feet: these are relaxed when you feel they are flopping, with the toes slightly pointing away from each other. No effort is involved; it is the posture of rest. If you are putting any effort into it, then your muscles will be working and your feet will be tensed. Notice how your feet feel in the relaxed position.

Body

The next item is called 'body'. Your body is relaxed when your hips and shoulders are in line with each other and resting on the supporting surface. If you are lying in a crooked fashion, your body is not relaxed. If there is any movement you are not relaxed. Make a note of the sensation of having a relaxed body.

Hands

This posture is called 'hands'. Your hands are relaxed when they are resting on a surface with the fingers gently curled, that is to say, neither clenched nor stretched out. Notice the sensations in your hands as you relax them.

Shoulders

And now the shoulders: these are relaxed when they are level and dropped. If you feel one is twisted or higher than the other, then they are not relaxed. Register the feeling of having relaxed shoulders.

Head

The next posture is called 'head'. Make sure your head is resting on its cushion and facing forwards. Feel it being supported. Any attempt to turn or twist it will cause your neck muscles

to work. Notice the feelings you get as you relax your neck muscles.

Mouth

The next posture is called 'mouth'. Your mouth will be relaxed if your teeth are parted and your lips gently touching. If you are smiling, grimacing, licking your lips or pressing them together, your mouth is not relaxed. Take note of the feelings you get as you relax your mouth.

Throat

Now the area called 'throat': this is relaxed when you can feel no movement there. If you are swallowing or if your tongue is twitching, then your throat is not relaxed. However, if you need to swallow, do so, then return to your relaxed state. Notice the sensations in your throat as you relax it.

Breathing

The next item is called 'breathing'. Relaxed breathing is slow and gentle. Unrelaxed breathing is rapid, jerky and may be interrupted by coughing, sighing and yawning. Register the effect of your relaxed breathing.

Quiet

And now we come to an item called 'quiet'. This means that you are not making any sounds such as sniffing, umm-ing or talking. If you feel you have to clear your throat, that's all right, but return to your state of quiet afterwards, noticing the sensation of stillness.

Eyes

The last relaxed area is called 'eyes'. These are relaxed when the lids rest over them in a lightly closed position and when the eye movements are brought to rest. Eyes are unrelaxed when they dart about and when the lids are twitching. Notice the feelings you are getting from your eyes as you relax them.

The order is not important but it is suggested that the eyes are left until the end, since the trainee needs to use them to mentally observe the other behaviours (Poppen 1998).

A training session will last about 15–20 minutes, after which the trainee is instructed to continue relaxing as he silently reviews the items for a further 10–15 minutes. At the end of this period, the trainer may carry out a post-treatment assessment (see p91).

Arousal

Arousal takes place in the following manner.

Very slowly, I would like you to prepare to end the session. To help you transfer from your deeply relaxed state, I am going to count slowly from one to five: one … two … three, open your eyes … four … five … begin to move your limbs … and in your own time, sit up.

Practice

Since behavioural relaxation training is a skill, practice is necessary. Trainees are urged to spend 20 minutes a day practising. Poppen suggests that benefit can be derived from combining BRT with cognitive relaxation methods such as autogenics or meditation. In this way, the one can augment the effects of the other.

Variations of the protocol

Variations of the above protocol exist for different situations: first, where the only available chair is an upright chair and second, where the need for relaxation occurs in the middle of a task (termed 'mini-relaxation' by Poppen (1998)).

Script for trainee sitting in an upright chair

Where the trainee is seated in an upright chair, the following four areas of legs, back, arms and head should be substituted for feet, body, hands and head in the protocol given above.

Legs

This area is called 'legs', and these are relaxed when you have both feet flat on the floor with a right angle at the knees. Allow the knees to fall outwards into a comfortable position. The legs are unrelaxed when crossed, extended or

tucked under the chair. Notice the sensations in your legs when they are in the relaxed position.

Back

The next area is called 'back'. It is relaxed when your shoulder blades and hips touch the chair symmetrically. It is unrelaxed when you are bending forwards, arching backwards or leaning to one side. Register the feelings you get from the relaxed posture.

Arms

Next is the area is called 'arms'. These are relaxed when the wrists are resting on the thighs; they are unrelaxed when hanging down, when crossed or when being leant on. Notice the sensations as you relax your arms.

Head

Now we come to the area called 'head', and this is relaxed when it is held upright and is looking forwards. The head is unrelaxed when it is tilted or turned in any direction. Notice the feelings you get from holding your head in the relaxed position.

'Mini-relaxation'

Tension can arise in the course of any task or situation. For example, while talking, the individual might develop tension in the hands; while typing, in the shoulders, and while focusing on a difficult job, in the mouth and throat. Breaking off to release these tensions is what Poppen means by mini-relaxation. He suggests that a person, when engaged in any task, should take mini-relaxation breaks periodically. Thus, mini-relaxation can be seen as a form of differential relaxation (see Ch. 13).

Mini-relaxation can be practised throughout the day and reminders to do so provided by placing coloured dots on the telephone, watch, steering wheel, typewriter, kettle handle or any other frequently used appliance.

The Behavioural Relaxation Scale

There are no universally accepted procedures of assessment in relaxation; a reliable and valid measuring device has yet to be found. Schilling & Poppen's

(1983) Behavioural Relaxation Scale (BRS) is an attempt to fill one aspect of this gap. It was designed as an easy method for measuring the motor element of relaxation, i.e. that relating to the voluntary muscles. Although it specifically measures the behaviours taught in BRT, it may be used to assess the motor aspect of any relaxation procedure.

The scale is based on the assumption that a person who feels relaxed also looks relaxed. As a result, some kind of judgement of the degree to which a person is relaxed can be made by an onlooker. Using the same items that feature in BRT, the scale allows an objective assessment to be made, without the need for expensive equipment such as electromyographic instruments. Each posture is checked for its degree of relaxation with reference to the table of relaxed and unrelaxed postures (see Table 10.1). The order of the items in Table 10.1 is suggested by Poppen (1998) as being the most convenient for assessment purposes.

Using the Behavioural Relaxation Scale

Establishing the baseline breathing rate

The first measure concerns the breathing rate. This is counted over a 30-second interval (each count representing a complete cycle of inhalation and exhalation). The process is repeated 15 times and the total sum of the respirations divided by 15 to give the mean or average number of respirations in 30 seconds. The mean is then entered in the box marked 'breathing baseline' on the score sheet (Fig. 10.1). A diaphragmatic form of breathing is recommended (see Ch. 4).

General assessment

A general assessment covers five 1-minute periods in which the individual is observed for outward signs of relaxation. Each minute begins with a further count of the breathing rate lasting 30 seconds; it is entered in the empty box in the column marked '1' in Figure 10.1. If the answer is less than the baseline rate, then the adjacent plus sign is ringed; if it is more, the minus sign is ringed. The following 15 seconds are spent scanning the trainee's key postures, picking out any unrelaxed ones and repeating the appropriate word label, for example 'shoulders' for a hunched arm. The succeeding 15 seconds are spent ringing the items; plus for relaxed postures, minus for any that continue to be unrelaxed.

After the first minute, the procedure is repeated and the answers recorded under the figure '2', and so on until five columns have been completed. The ringed plus signs are added up and entered under 'total'.

Name .... Date .... Time .... Session no. ....

Breathing baseline ☐

+ relaxed
− unrelaxed

INTERVALS

		1		2		3		4		5	Total
Breathing	−		+	−		+	−		+	−		+	−		+	
Quiet	−	+	−	+	−	+	−	+	−	+	
Body	−	+	−	+	−	+	−	+	−	+	
Head	−	+	−	+	−	+	−	+	−	+	
Eyes	−	+	−	+	−	+	−	+	−	+	
Mouth	−	+	−	+	−	+	−	+	−	+	
Throat	−	+	−	+	−	+	−	+	−	+	
Shoulders	−	+	−	+	−	+	−	+	−	+	
Hands	−	+	−	+	−	+	−	+	−	+	
Feet	−	+	−	+	−	+	−	+	−	+	

Self-ratings 1 2 3 4 5 6 7   Score ☐

Figure 10.1 • Behavioural Relaxation Scale score sheet. (Adapted from Poppen 1998, with permission from the author.)

Working out the score

Scoring is expressed as a percentage arrived at in the following way: the total number of ringed 'plus' signs is counted and the sum divided by the total number of observations (i.e. the 10 behaviours multiplied by the five testings). The resulting figure is then multiplied by 100. For example, if there were a total of 40 ringed plus signs, they would be divided by the 50 observations. After multiplying the resulting fraction by 100, a figure of 80% would be obtained.

The pretreatment baseline

At the beginning of the course one pretreatment assessment is carried out. It acts as a baseline against which to measure progress, but should itself be carried out after a short period of rest to avoid confusing the effects of training with those which occur naturally whenever a person enters a restful environment (Lichstein et al 1981). Thereafter, assessment follows each training session to monitor progress.

Reliability and validity of the Behavioural Relaxation Scale

The reliability of the scale, i.e. its ability to produce the same scores when used on different occasions, has been tested. It was found that higher levels of reliability were obtained with trained observers than with untrained ones. Thus the training of observers is important.

Two forms of validity have been demonstrated: one procedural, where participants receiving other accepted forms of relaxation training showed statistically significant changes in relaxation scores on the Behavioural Relaxation Scale while controls did not (Schilling & Poppen 1983), and the other concurrent. Here, significant correlations were found between electromyographic measures of frontalis muscle and BRS scores, i.e. low EMG readings were associated with scores which reflect relaxed postures as described in the BRS, while high readings were associated with scores which reflect unrelaxed postures (Poppen & Maurer 1982). Further work has tended to strengthen confidence in these results (Norton et al 1997) but more research is needed.

Other methods of assessment of behavioural relaxation training

Because relaxation involves responses in subjective, physiological and behavioural spheres, a full assessment would take account of all three modalities. Poppen indicates the need to view behavioural assessment as part of a broader system of measurement. One of its components is self-report.

Self-report

As relaxation and anxiety are subjective states, it is appropriate and customary to include a self-rating measure when assessing their levels. Self-report can take the form of free description, but since this is difficult to quantify, preset descriptive phrases with associated numbered ratings are often used. The individual rings the number corresponding with the phrase that most accurately reflects his state.

A behavioural relaxation self-rating scale, adapted from Poppen (1998), is shown below.

1. Feeling extremely tense and upset throughout my body.
2. Feeling generally tense throughout my body.
3. Feeling some tension in some parts of my body.
4. Feeling relaxed as in my normal resting state.
5. Feeling more relaxed than usual.
6. Feeling completely relaxed throughout my entire body.
7. Feeling more deeply and completely relaxed than I ever have.

Discrepancy between self-report and objective testing

There are often wide discrepancies between self-reports and objective measurements. One of the reasons is that self-report may be coloured by factors of social desirability, for instance where the trainee gives the answer he thinks is expected of him. These matters are discussed further in Chapter 25.

Evidence of effectiveness

Behavioural relaxation training offers both therapy and means of assessment. As a therapy, it provides a form of body scanning in which relaxed postures are adopted and feelings of relaxation experienced. As an assessment tool, it provides a numerical measure of the level of relaxation present in the musculature.

The approach does not ask participants to recognize subtle degrees of arousal or to be conscious of different levels of relaxation; the method is easily learned and readily applied. These attributes make it a convenient technique for reducing anxiety in people with learning disabilities.

In this context, Lindsay and colleagues have carried out a series of studies charting the effect of BRT on cognitive performance. Results showed that where the disability was severe, short-term memory and learning significantly improved following 12 sessions of BRT, compared with quiet reading where no significant differences were reported (Lindsay & Morrison 1996).

In a later study, Lindsay et al (1997) tested concentration and responsiveness in eight participants, this time with profound learning disabilities. Four stress-relieving procedures were compared: snoezelen, aromatherapy massage, BRT and active therapy. Following each therapy participants were set simple concentration tasks. The treatments which led to the most successful outcomes were snoezelen and BRT, in which significant effects were recorded. There was no improvement in the aromatherapy group and the active group even showed a deterioration.

Brain injury is another area where the approach has been applied. Guercio et al (2001) taught BRT skills to one adult with an ataxic tremor resulting from an acquired brain injury. Having learned the skills, the participant was then connected to a biofeedback facility. Results demonstrated a significant reduction in the severity of the tremor.

The benefits of behavioural relaxation training can be seen after very little teaching: Schilling & Poppen (1983) observed benefit within as few as two training sessions. They also reported that effects were retained at follow-up 4–6 weeks later.

 POTENTIAL PITFALLS

As with any relaxation approach, possible pitfalls should be considered before taking it up. Chapter 5 contains a discussion of potential hazards relating to muscular approaches.

KEY MESSAGES

- Behavioural relaxation training rests on the principle that a relaxed body displays a different posture from a stressed body. The trainee is asked to *look* as relaxed as possible.
- The training procedure focuses on each muscle group in turn, checking it for relaxed appearance.
- Trainees are asked to register the feel of the relaxed postures.
- As a therapy it provides a form of body scanning in which relaxed postures are adopted and feelings of relaxation experienced.
- As an assessment tool it provides a numerical measure of the level of relaxation present in the musculature.
- The approach can be used by anyone. However, on account of its simplicity it has particular application for people with learning disabilities.

11

The Mitchell method

CHAPTER CONTENTS

History and rationale

In 1963 a new method of relaxation was introduced. Its originator was Laura Mitchell, a physiotherapist with a wide experience of teaching and practice in the field of obstetrics. She argued that it was useless to ask a person to notice tension in his muscles since there are no nerve endings in muscle tissue capable of conveying such information to the conscious brain. The sensory apparatus in the muscle connects only with the lower brain and spinal cord. Consequently, exhortations to become aware of the presence or absence of muscle tension are inappropriate. However, proprioceptive structures in the joints, and skin pressure receptors do have links with the conscious brain. The first tell us where our limbs are in space and the second tell us where the skin is being stretched or compressed. It is only, she claims, by moving the joints and stretching the skin that information about muscle state is relayed to the higher centres. Thus, the joints and the skin are the organs on which we need to focus attention.

Mitchell's approach is based on the physiological principle of reciprocal inhibition, i.e. when one group of muscles acting on a joint is working, the opposing group is obliged to relax. As the fibres of one group contract, the fibres of the opposing group become slack. It is a built-in mechanism to allow the smooth performance of movement.

Mitchell exploits this principle and makes it the nub of her approach. Stress-related posture, or what she calls 'the punching position', is studied, the working muscle groups are identified, and then relaxed by activating the opposing groups. The resulting changes of joint position and the accompanying skin sensations are then mentally registered as the part settles into the posture of ease. Thus, her approach consists of moving the body out of the posture of defence or stress, and training the mind to recognize the posture of ease or relaxation.

The aim of the procedure is to reduce stress and relax the mind. Mitchell proposes that the

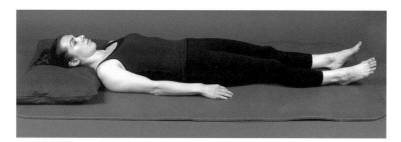

Figure 11.1 • Starting position: supine.

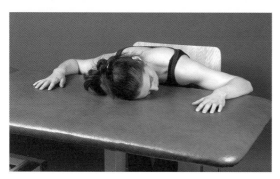

Figure 11.2 • Starting position: forward-lean sitting.

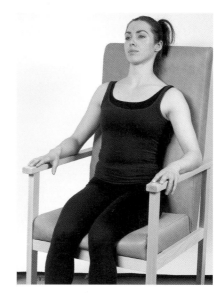

Figure 11.3 • Starting position: sitting.

relaxation induced by her method spreads throughout the organism to include the mind.

Description

Mitchell's method (Mitchell 1987) is composed of 13 items, referred to as joint changes (although they do not all involve joint activity). These changes reverse different aspects of the punching position, which is described below:

- shoulders hunched
- arms held close to sides
- fingers curled into the palms
- legs crossed
- feet dorsiflexed (drawn up towards face)
- torso bent forwards
- head held forwards
- breathing rapid with noticeable movement in the upper chest
- jaw clenched
- lips pursed
- tongue pressed into upper palate
- brow furrowed into a frown.

Mitchell does not suggest that the punching position is actually adopted under stress; rather, that the muscles responsible for it are contracting to a slight extent.

Procedure

Starting positions

Three starting positions are described.

1. Supine lying with a pillow under the head (Fig. 11.1). A pillow under the thighs is optional.
2. Forward-lean sitting, i.e. leaning forwards with head and arms resting on a table (Fig. 11.2).
3. Sitting in a high-backed chair with arm rests on which the hands are supported, palms downwards (Fig. 11.3).

Varying the starting position is useful in order to extend the range of application of the method. The eyes may be open or closed.

Instructions

The instructor begins by giving an order to direct a part of the body away from its posture of tension. The order is followed by the word 'Stop'. This means that the part is no longer being actively moved; it also means that the muscles responsible for the movement are no longer contracting. The part then falls naturally into the position of ease. This position is then mentally registered. Below is a list of the items to be worked.

Items of the Mitchell method of relaxation

1. Pull your shoulders towards your feet.
2. Slide your elbows away from your body.
3. Stretch your fingers and thumbs.
4. Turn your hips outwards.
5. Move your knees until they are comfortable.
6. Push your feet away from your face.
7. Breathing.
8. Push your body into the support.
9. Push your head into the support.
10. Drag your jaw downwards.
11. Press your tongue downwards in your mouth.
12. Close your eyes.
13. Think of a smoothing action which begins above your eyebrows, rises into your hairline, continues over the top of your head and down into the back of your neck.

Each item is modelled by the instructor who asks the trainee to copy it.

Introductory remarks to participants

Trainees are introduced to the method by a short description of the rationale and procedure.

I just want to say something about the Mitchell method before we begin. When people are under stress, there is a position which they tend to adopt. We could call this 'the punching position'. Although people don't actually present themselves in a punching posture, the muscles

which create it are tensing to a minute degree. This happens instinctively and helps to promote a feeling of being ready for anything.

If we move the body into the opposite of the punching position, we will be taking it into a position of ease or relaxation.

You might ask: 'How do we get the punching muscles to relax?'. This is where the physiological principle comes in: when one group of muscles acting on a joint is tensed, the opposing group automatically relaxes.

The trainer demonstrates.

When I bend my wrist forwards, the bending-back muscles relax, and vice versa. It's a reciprocal mechanism without which smooth action could not take place.

The method itself consists of a succession of changes of position. Each change moves a body part out of its position of defence and into its position of ease. As the part settles into the position of ease, you'll be asked to notice how it feels. The aim is to learn to recognize the relaxed position so that you can reproduce it more easily. I'll first demonstrate the items.

Working through the schedule

The schedule is then worked through in its entirety. It is presented here with the orders expressed in inverted commas.

1. Shoulders

'Pull your shoulders towards your feet.' Do this gently, but go on until you can't pull them down any more. Feel the space between your shoulders and your ears getting greater. 'Stop pulling.' Notice the feel of the new position. Take plenty of time to register the sensations you are getting from it.

2. Elbows (Figs 11.4–11.6)

'Elbows out and open.' For participants lying supine or sitting in a high-backed chair: slide your elbows sideways, carrying your arms away from your body until you reach a comfortable point (Figs 11.4, 11.6). For participants in forward-lean sitting: slide your

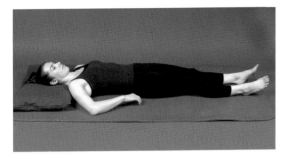

Figure 11.4 • 'Elbows out and open' in supine position.

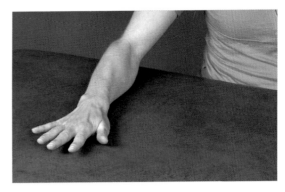

Figure 11.7 • 'Fingers and thumbs long.'

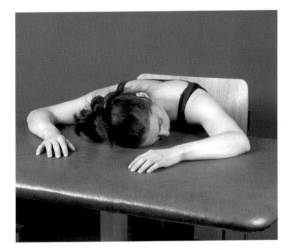

Figure 11.5 • 'Elbows out and open' in forward-lean sitting position.

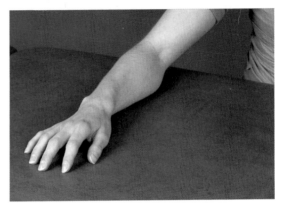

Figure 11.8 • Fingers recoiling.

arms away from your body, opening your arms at the elbow joint (Fig. 11.5). 'Stop moving.' Check that your arms are resting on the supporting surface and notice how it feels to have a space between your arms and your body. Feel this position.

3. Hands (Figs 11.7 and 11.8)

'Fingers and thumbs long.' Stretch and separate your fingers and thumbs while the heels of both hands remain in contact with the floor, the table or the arm of the chair. While the fingers and thumbs spread (Fig. 11.7), feel the palms getting taut. 'Stop.' As you stop, the fingers recoil and fall on to the supporting surface where they lie with the hand gently open, fingertips touching the surface underneath (Fig. 11.8). Notice how the hand feels; notice also, without disturbing your fingers, the texture of the surface under your fingertips. Spend a moment or two taking in these sensations.

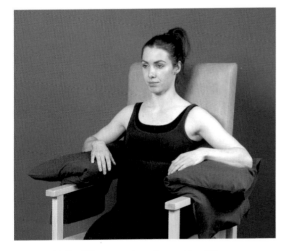

Figure 11.6 • 'Elbows out and open' in sitting position.

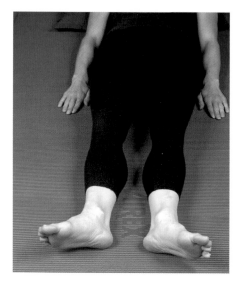

Figure 11.9 • 'Turn your hips outwards.'

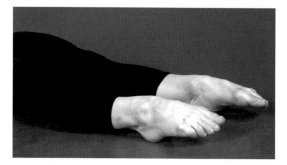

Figure 11.10 • 'Push your feet away from your face' in supine position.

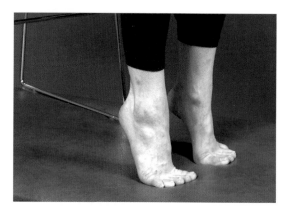

Figure 11.11 • 'Push your feet away from your face' in sitting position.

Extra time should be spent on the hand because of its disproportionately large sensory area in the brain.

4.   Hips (Fig. 11.9)

'Turn your hips outwards.' If you are lying, this means rolling your thighs outwards (Fig. 11.9). If you are sitting, it means swinging your knees apart. 'Stop.' Let your legs settle comfortably, noting how they feel in this position.

5.   Knees

'Move your knees until they are comfortable.' This simply means adjusting their position in whatever way enhances their comfort. 'Stop' and register that sense of ease.

6.   Feet and ankles (Figs 11.10 and 11.11)

'Push your feet away from your face.' If you are lying, point your feet and toes down, being careful not to induce cramp. If you are sitting with your feet on the floor, keep your toes in contact with it and raise your heels. You are working the calf muscles and reciprocally relaxing the muscles around the shin. 'Stop.' As you stop, your calf muscles stop working too. (If you are sitting, your heels drop down.) Take note of the feelings you are now getting from your feet and ankles. Spend a few minutes enjoying the sensation of ease in your legs.

7.   Breathing

There are no orders for this item because people have their own breathing rates. I'll describe the action first, then you can perform it in your own time.

I'd like you to think of the soft triangle between the front edge of your ribs and your waist. As you breathe in you can feel it swelling slightly; at the same time you can feel your ribs spreading outwards. As you breathe out, that soft area sinks back and your ribs recoil.

Allow your breathing to take place slowly and comfortably, without putting any effort into it and without attempting to alter its rhythm.

8.   Torso

'Push your body into the support.' Press against the support, whether it is underneath you or behind you. 'Stop.' Feel your body slumped into the floor, table or chair. Feel its weight being

supported. Notice the points where your body touches the support.

9.   Head

'Push your head into the support.' This will be the floor for those lying down, the table for those leaning forwards and the back of the chair for those seated. 'Stop.' As you stop pushing, notice that the support still carries the weight of your head. Feel your head being supported.

10.   Jaw

'Drag your jaw downwards.' Let your teeth come apart and your jaw hang down inside your mouth. 'Stop.' Feel the new position. Notice also the contact between your gently touching lips.

Spend a bit longer on this item because the lips, in common with the fingertips, are richly supplied with sensory nerve endings.

11.   Tongue

'Press your tongue downwards in your mouth.' Draw it away from the upper palate. 'Stop.' Feel your tongue lying loosely behind your teeth. Notice also your throat slackening.

12.   Eyes

'Close your eyes' (if they are not already closed). Simply lower your eyelids and gently keep them down. Let your eyes be as still as they can be. Feel the peace of the darkness.

13.   Forehead and scalp

'Think of a smoothing action which begins above your eyebrows, rises up into your hairline, continues over the crown of your head, and down to the back of your neck.' Savour the effect.

The above 13 items may be repeated.

Mind

Mitchell ends with a sequence for the thoughts.

Let your mind focus on a topic you find pleasant. Pick one that flows like a poem or a walk

in the country and let it hold your attention as it develops. Continue for a few minutes.

Termination

When you are ready, I'd like you to begin to make a gradual return to normal activity. Give your arms and legs a good stretch. Sit up slowly, giving your body plenty of time to adjust to an active state.

Practice

The Mitchell method of physiological relaxation is a skill which can be learned; the more it is practised, the greater will be the benefit gained from it. It is through practice that the individual can cultivate his awareness of the relaxed posture, thus enabling him to reproduce it at will.

Further aspects of the Mitchell method

'Keys' and 'triggers'

The items in Mitchell's schedule cover the whole body. Many individuals, however, have characteristic ways of displaying tension. This means that they will be likely to benefit more from some joint changes than from others. The joint change that an individual finds most effective in reducing tension is referred to by Mitchell as the 'key change', because it is instrumental in releasing tension in other parts of the body. The key change can be identified by asking the individual how he tends to react when experiencing anger, pain, anxiety or conflict. If he tends to make fists, his key change will be finger lengthening; if he tends to clench his teeth, it will be jaw dropping. Key changes, by their generalizing effects, can promote a sense of ease throughout the whole body.

Mitchell applies her technique to everyday activities, using the concept of 'triggers of tension', i.e. events which tend to provoke feelings of stress such as waiting at traffic lights or being interrupted by bells and alarms. She suggests sticking coloured tabs on potentially stressful appliances such as the steering wheel and the telephone as reminders to adopt the key change. Thus, to become more relaxed in daily life, there is first a need to recognize the triggers and second, a need to diminish their impact by using the key change to move the body into the ease position.

Benefit can also be gained from a partial use of the schedule. Mitchell suggests that selected joint changes be used during specific activities; for example, the face items can be carried out while driving or the leg items while reading. The idea is not far removed from differential relaxation (see Ch. 13).

The 'three-point pull'

This is a variation of the shoulder item where, in addition to pulling the shoulders down, the head gently reaches upwards. (It should be done without tilting the head backwards.) The action is useful for stretching the joints in the neck and may be practised in public situations without attracting attention.

Application of the method to specific conditions

The Mitchell method lends itself to a range of conditions including insomnia, psychiatric disorders, dyspnoea, osteoarthritis and cardiac rehabilitation, as well as everyday stress. It is widely used in the field of obstetrics where its advantage lies in its avoidance of tensing procedures. The required relaxation is achieved by simply moving the body part.

Mitchell's insistence that breathing should be slow and easy, and never include breath holding, is another reason for the method being favoured by those working in the obstetric field (Mantle et al 2004). For the same reasons the method is often adopted by those who work in the field of respiratory medicine (Hough 2001).

Comparison with other approaches

Both Jacobson (see Ch. 5) and Mitchell see their approaches as skills to be learned. Neither favours the use of tone of voice to influence the message. Instead, the participant is required simply to respond to the basic order. Again, like Jacobson, Mitchell avoids using the order 'Relax'. Her reason is that she finds it 'vague, generalized and ambiguous'. Jacobson avoided using it because he felt it provoked the trainee into making an effort

which was superfluous, when 'going negative' was the effect he wanted. On other points they are, of course, fundamentally opposed, Mitchell placing the highest value on joint and skin sensations and rejecting the idea of information coming from the muscles, while Jacobson is only interested in muscle feelings, dismissing any value that joint sensations might have.

Greater resemblance may be found between Mitchell and Alexander (see Ch. 12) in the value they both place on proprioceptive stimuli and awareness of posture. There is little difference between the 'three-point pull' of Mitchell and the 'neck lengthen' injunction of Alexander.

Evidence of effectiveness

Mitchell's method promotes awareness of relaxed postures. The method is simple and quick and many of the 'changes' can be carried out unobtrusively. It is widely practised as a stress-relieving strategy and clinical findings testify to its effectiveness. Scientific evaluation of the method, however, is limited. Jackson (1991) studied four rheumatoid arthritis sufferers trained in the Mitchell method, comparing them with controls who simply rested. Using electromyography to measure activity in the frontalis muscle (a sensitive indicator of general muscle state), she found a marked reduction of tension in the study group and very little change in the control group. No statistical analysis was reported.

An interesting comparison between the methods of Mitchell and Jacobson was made by Salt & Kerr (1997). With a sample of 14 men and 10 women, these authors measured the effects of both approaches on the cardiovascular and respiratory systems. The study was designed with a control condition of supine lying. Participants were randomly assigned to three groups in which they received the two trainings and the control condition, presented in different sequences to avoid order effects. Heart rate, systolic blood pressure, diastolic blood pressure and respiratory rate were recorded before and after every treatment.

Results showed significant reductions after treatment on all measures for both methods, with no significant differences between them. The control condition itself showed significant reductions in heart rate and respiratory rate; however, when compared to the control, both treatment methods were found to be significantly superior on measures of systolic blood pressure. On a subjective level, there was some evidence of participants finding the Mitchell method easier to follow and less demanding in concentration than progressive relaxation.

Thus, while each approach demonstrated greater effectiveness than supine lying on certain counts, the study has been unable to demonstrate a substantial difference in the separate capacities of the two approaches to induce physiological relaxation. This is the first study to investigate the Mitchell method using statistically analysed data. A later study compared the Mitchell method with diaphragmatic breathing (Bell & Saltikov 2000) and also found a lack of significant difference between the two. The study is reported in greater detail in Chapter 4.

 POTENTIAL PITFALLS

These are similar to the pitfalls of other muscular approaches (Ch. 5, p55).

KEY MESSAGES

- The Mitchell method is built around the physiological principle of reciprocal inhibition, i.e. when one group of muscles acting on a joint is working, the opposing group is obliged to relax. Thus, for example, in order to relax a flexor group of muscles, the client is asked to activate the extensor group.

- Each session takes the client through all the major voluntary muscle groups in the body.

- Practice is essential to obtain maximum benefit.

- 'Key changes' play an important role in the Mitchell method. These are particular items in the schedule which the client finds most effective, e.g. jaw dropping, finger lengthening or shoulders dropped down. In their effectiveness they act as a key to the whole body system.

- Triggers are another important concept. These are stress-provoking events such as traffic lights, bells and alarms. Mitchell urges the client to adopt stress-diffusing tactics in advance.

Chapter Twelve

The Alexander technique

CHAPTER CONTENTS

History and rationale

Posture refers to the way an individual habitually holds himself against the forces of gravity and is one of his recognizable features. A look round our acquaintances tells us that they all have characteristic ways of holding themselves; each one stands differently, walks differently and sits differently. Although a person's posture may be largely of genetic origin and thus beyond his control, we are inclined to think that it is also governed by the way he looks at and reacts to life.

Teachers of the Alexander technique point to the way young children use their bodies, describing the effect as 'poise'. They also indicate how this natural poise can become distorted by emotional and physical influences as the child grows towards maturity, resulting in the development of tension habits which interfere with healthy functioning.

This notion had earlier captured the attention of Matthias Alexander, at a time when he was experiencing a problem with his voice. An actor by profession, he noticed that he was developing hoarseness and a painful throat whenever he began to perform. Intuitively, he felt that posture lay at the root of it. Mirrors revealed that he was pulling his head back and tightening his neck muscles to the extent that he could not breathe properly. By freeing his neck and lengthening his spine he discovered he could regain control of his voice, and the manner in which he accomplished this forms the basis of the Alexander technique (Alexander 1932).

Principles of the Alexander technique

The Alexander technique is not underpinned by any established theory but it is based on principles of body positioning:

- primary control
- use and misuse

- faulty sensory perception
- inhibition
- 'end-gaining' and the 'means whereby'
- integration of mind and body.

Primary control

Alexander believed that the primary control of human posture lay in the relationships of the head to the neck and of the neck to the rest of the spine. So convinced was he of their crucial nature that an almost magical significance was attached to these relationships in his day. This status has, however, been modified over the years, and the Alexander teacher of today sees primary control less as an inviolable principle than as a useful starting point.

Primary control has three components:

- a neck that is free and whose muscles contain only enough tension to keep the head upright
- a head moving forward and up (Fig. 12.1), not back and down to crumple the spine (Fig. 12.2)
- a spine that feels lengthened, thus counteracting any tendency towards sagging.

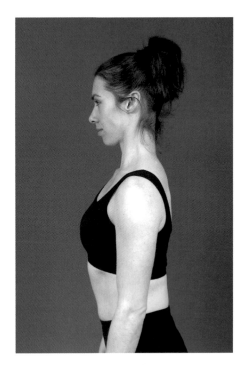

Figure 12.1 • Head held forward and up.

Use and misuse

'Use' refers to the characteristic way we have of holding our bodies. It is a neutral term. When there is harmony between the tension necessary to support the body and the relaxation necessary to allow it to move, the use is said to be 'balanced'. When, however, this is upset by too much or too little tension, a state of misuse is said to prevail (Barlow 1975). Examples of misuse are hunching of the shoulders, head sinking into the spine, chin thrusting out.

The regaining of 'balanced use' means the recovery of natural movement patterns, which can only occur if we review the messages we are getting about the position of the body in space.

Faulty sensory perceptions

All movement in the healthy organism is accompanied by sensory feedback in the form of proprioceptive impulses from the moving part. This gives us information about the position of body parts in space. In the young child these messages lead to responses which are natural, economic (in terms

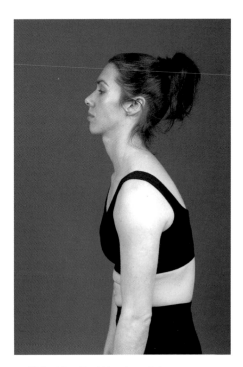

Figure 12.2 • Head held back and down.

of energy consumption) and uncontaminated by emotional factors, while those in the adult may be distorted by trauma (mental or physical).

Responses carried out repeatedly turn into habits which are then interpreted by the higher centres as normal, i.e. the way we habitually use our bodies will feel normal to us simply because we are used to it. Alexander's experience with the mirror showed him he was still pulling his head back even after he felt he had corrected it. This could only be because his body had got used to the 'bad' posture and had internalized it as normal, so that even the smallest degree of correction was interpreted by his conscious mind as overcorrection.

The phrase 'faulty sensory perception' refers to the way messages are interpreted in a misused body.

Inhibition

Many of our movements are automatic. If they show patterns of misuse which we want to change, it will be necessary to intercept them, that is, to examine them before they are automatically executed. A pause is required. This act of pausing constitutes what Alexander called 'inhibition'. It allows the individual to question the validity of his response. It gives him the chance to reconsider his action and to redirect his movement.

Inhibition, not to be confused with the Freudian meaning, is what happens when the individual ceases to react automatically to stimuli, thereby leaving him free to respond appropriately; to do nothing for a moment while the maladaptive, automatic response pattern is broken. 'When you stop doing the wrong thing, the right thing does itself' (Alexander 1932).

'End-gaining' and the 'means whereby'

Inhibition provides the opportunity to focus on the means whereby we achieve a certain end. It draws attention away from 'end-gaining', where action is performed too quickly and too energetically for one to give any thought as to the manner in which the end is gained. Alexander would say that if you pay attention to the means, the end will take care of itself (Maisel 1969).

Integration of mind and body

Central to the teachings of Alexander is a belief that the mind and the body are interdependent. Not only does the body posture reflect the individual's thoughts, but his mind responds to the way he uses his body. Such notions introduce a new dimension to the concept of body movement, and can be said to lie at the heart of the statement that 'we *are* our posture' (Barlow 1975).

The technique

The technique itself re-educates the body to perform in a balanced and energy-economical way (Gray 1990). Habits of misuse are identified and replaced by more appropriate ways of using the body. Assessment and correction are carried out in positions of lying, sitting, standing and walking. Gently using her hands, the teacher guides the pupil's body both in motion and at rest while the pupil mentally focuses on the message he is getting from the teacher's hands. For example, a supine pupil might be told to think of the words: 'shoulder release and widen', as the teacher is repositioning one of his shoulders. Thus, without actively performing the movement, the pupil directs his body to co-operate.

Some of the principal orders or directions are listed below, beginning with the three elements of primary control:

1. 'neck free'
2. 'head forward and up'
3. 'back lengthen'.

Other directions include:

4. 'keeping length'
5. 'back widen'
6. 'shoulder release and widen'.

The three elements of primary control

1. 'Neck free'

This means that the head is carried in such a way that no undue strain is put on the neck muscles.

The image of the nodding dog in the back of the car may help to convey the feeling of a free neck.

2. 'Head forward and up'

'Head forward and up' is the phrase for those who are sitting or standing. It means that the head is held with the chin pointing to the toes, not poking out. It also means that the head is lifted up and out of the vertebral column. The result is that the individual feels taller or longer, having 'grown' from a point at the back of the head. It is the opposite of a head which sinks into the shoulders with the chin thrust out. At the same time, no excessive effort should be made to extend the body. The effect described can often be achieved simply by 'thinking up'. Figures 12.1 and 12.2 illustrate the correct and incorrect ways of carrying the head.

3. 'Back lengthen'

An erect spine anteroposteriorly displays a succession of natural curves: concavities in the cervical and lumbar regions, convexity in the dorsal region. In urging 'back lengthen', it is not implied that efforts should be made to obliterate these natural curves, but rather that the curves should not be allowed to become overemphasized, since that would result in crumpling or shortening of the spine. Actions which particularly shorten the spine are:

- overextension of the cervical vertebrae (thrusting out the chin)
- overextension of the lumbar vertebrae (exaggerated lumbar concavity) (Fig. 12.3).

Similarly, slumping is to be avoided. Slumping occurs when the whole spine is rounded into a long C-shaped curve, with the neck hyperextended in order to allow the eyes to look forwards. Slumping also creates shortening of the spine (Fig. 12.4).

'Back lengthen' indicates that the spine should be allowed to reach its full length (or height) as opposed to being either crumpled (where spinal curves are exaggerated) or slumped (where the back is too rounded). An image that evokes the idea of lengthening the back is that of a jet of water springing up in the spine and lifting it gently. The head should feel lightly balanced on top.

Alexander's view of a balanced standing posture is one in which the body weight passes through the front of the heel, the knees are unbraced and the pelvis is in midposition, with the 'tail' neither thrown out nor forcibly tucked under. The direction

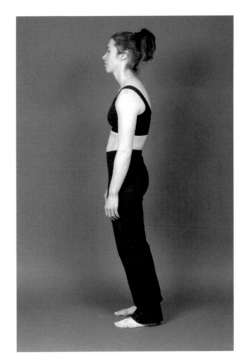

Figure 12.3 • Standing with exaggerated cervical and lumbar curves.

to 'think up' helps to convey the idea of standing straight but without making any forced effort to do so. Some teachers introduce the image of a helium-filled balloon lifting the head (Gray 1990). Figure 12.5 illustrates the correct standing position.

'Neck free', 'head forward and up' and 'back lengthen' are fundamental to the technique.

Other directions

4. 'Keeping length'

The order 'keeping length' is related to 'back lengthen'. Alexander applies it to the action of sitting down where he sees particular benefit to be gained from the avoidance of crumpling. His method of lowering the body is illustrated in the following passage (Leibowitz & Connington 1990).

Place your feet slightly apart and positioned so that the backs of your legs are lightly in contact with the chair seat. Let your arms hang loosely by your sides. Before lowering yourself, let your mind focus on the idea of 'keeping length', i.e. not crumpling the spine. Keep the head and neck in the same relation as they were in the

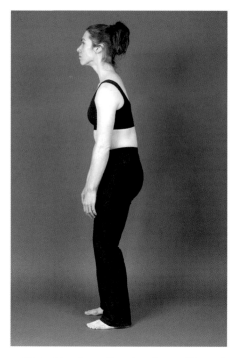

Figure 12.4 • Standing with spine slumped into a long C-shaped curve.

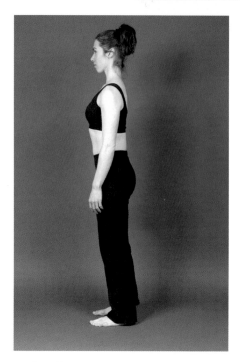

Figure 12.5 • Balanced standing posture.

standing position and as you lower yourself, flatten the lumbar curve. Although you are looking at the floor as you go down, make a point of thinking 'UP' to prevent any tendency of the spine to crumple.

Figure 12.6 demonstrates the correct way of lowering the body into a chair.

The wrong way of sitting down, according to Alexander, is to overextend both the neck and lumbar regions, i.e. to thrust the chin out and exaggerate the lumbar concavity. Their combined effect crumples and shortens the spine (Gray 1990). Figure 12.7 shows an incorrect way of lowering the body into a chair.

On rising from the chair, the head should start the movement and lead the body forwards. From that point the motions of sitting down are put into reverse.

What Alexander is saying is that the lumbar spine should be slightly flexed and the cervical spine prevented from extending itself in the actions of sitting down and rising. He urges applying the same ideas to other activities which carry the centre of gravity forwards, such as leaning over a basin to clean the teeth.

Alexander compared the action of tooth brushing in humans to the peeling of fruit by erect primates in the wild. Both actions take place anterior to the body itself. On noticing that primates adopted a particular stance to carry out their task, he concluded that mechanical advantage was being gained from it. The stance itself is characterized by bent knees and slightly flexed (flattened) lumbar and cervical spines; a posture which is referred to as the 'monkey stance' (Fig. 12.8).

The effect of the monkey stance is to keep the centre of gravity as close to the spine as possible, thereby relieving the strain on the lumbosacral junction. Where the monkey stance is not adopted for comparable tasks, a position of mechanical disadvantage is created. Figure 12.9 illustrates this idea: the arms and head reach forwards, pulling the centre of gravity with them, while the cervical and lumbar spines retain their concavities.

Common to both the monkey stance and the act of sitting (as recommended by Alexander) is a slight flexion of the lumbar spine. Alexander's insistence on the value of this posture has been supported by research (Adams & Hutton 1985, Adams et al 1994) which is discussed later in this chapter.

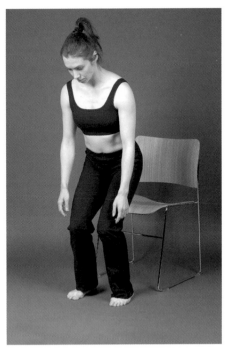

Figure 12.6 • Sitting down with the spine 'keeping length'.

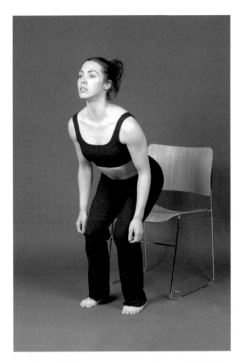

Figure 12.7 • Sitting down with a 'crumpled' spine.

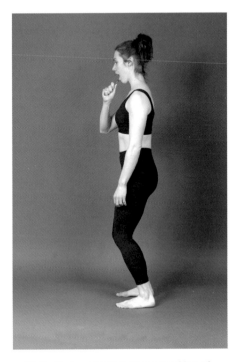

Figure 12.8 • Task performance in a position of mechanical advantage (the monkey stance).

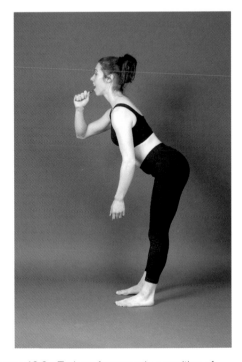

Figure 12.9 • Task performance in a position of mechanical disadvantage.

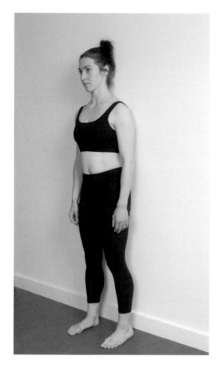

Figure 12.10 • Testing for body alignment 1: leaning against wall.

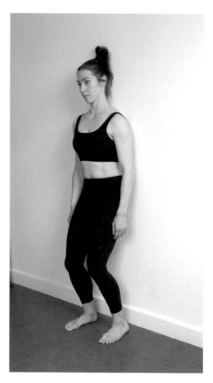

Figure 12.11 • Testing for body alignment 2: flattening the lumbar concavity as the body is lowered.

5.   'Back widen'

This phrase applies to the posterior part of the thorax which should be allowed to feel wide in order to permit full expansion of the ribs. To convey the idea of 'back widen', Gray (1990) promotes the image of the rib cage filling out into the back as the air enters the lungs.

6.   'Shoulder release and widen'

This is aimed at relaxing the muscles of the shoulder girdle which are often held more tensely than they need to be.

Recognizing and correcting misuse

Test for body alignment

As mentioned in the section on faulty sensory perception, a habitual posture, whether balanced or not, will feel 'right' to its owner. This makes it difficult for him to recognize misuse in himself. A procedure to solve this matter has been worked out by Barlow (1975).

Stand with your heels 5 centimetres (2 inches) from a wall, with your feet 46 centimetres (18 inches) apart. Let your body sway back until it touches the wall.

Figure 12.10 shows this position.

If your shoulders and hips touch simultaneously with each side level, your alignment is correct. However, you may find that one side touches the wall before the other or that your shoulders touch before your hips. Do what you can to realign yourself. Next, bend your knees slightly and notice that this action will tend to bring the lumbar vertebrae into contact with the wall (lumbar curve flattened).

Figure 12.11 demonstrates this effect.

If you can hold this position with relative comfort, then your body is not in a misused state. If you find it unduly tiring, then practice will make it easier and help to restore alignment.

Changing posture

Alexander sees misuse as resulting, largely, from stress and the demands of contemporary life; in its turn, misuse can be the cause of physical stress, leading to muscle and joint problems.

A person wishing to change his posture needs to consider three points. He should:

- be aware of the particular habit-governed movement that he wants to alter
- refuse to react automatically. This implies pausing to reassess the 'means whereby', i.e. being ready to say 'no' to the old method
- redirect his muscles by a thought process. In the early stages of re-education this signifies *thinking* about the corrected movement rather than driving the muscles to perform it. Such an approach allows the neuromuscular system to restructure its response. 'The mind gives the instruction, and little by little, the body absorbs the message' (Fontana 1992) until the corrected form of the movement becomes automatic.

Regularly practising new responses will result in a gradual weakening of the old ones and turn a pattern of misuse into one of more balanced use. There are no defined stages of progress nor specified goals of perfection. Individual problems call for individual remedies. Common to all remedies, however, is the cultivation of a sensitive approach to the movement of one's own body (Barlow 1975).

Relaxation effects

Although proponents speak of 'balanced use' rather than relaxation, the technique can nonetheless be seen as a method for promoting relaxation. Balanced use is associated with the elimination of excess muscular activity and is concerned with establishing minimum levels of muscle tension. These are concepts that are found in Jacobson's differential relaxation. For Alexander, however, they form the basis of his technique, whereas for Jacobson they are subsidiary to his main concern, which is the release of residual tension.

Alexander suggests a daily 15-minute session of rest, to be carried out in a crook lying position (knees bent up, feet flat on the ground) with a book under the head (where the height of the book is determined by the shape of the spine). The object is to allow the body to regain its natural symmetry; the procedure is also, however, a relaxing one (Fig. 12.12).

Teaching the Alexander technique

The purpose in writing this chapter is to give a general idea of the principles underlying the Alexander technique, rather than to show how to teach it; such training involves a 3-year course. The principles, however, may be woven into other approaches, particularly where posture is a key item.

Trained teachers of the Alexander method often work in the field of the performing arts in the belief that the approach can identify unwanted movement patterns which can interfere with performance (Batson 1996). However, the technique has universal relevance.

Evidence of effectiveness

Alexander's method is among the few approaches to focus systematically on relaxation of the body while it is in motion (Woolfolk & Lehrer 1984). As such, it is a form of kinesthetic re-education. The technique is based on the assumption that the way

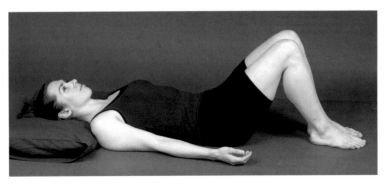

Figure 12.12 • Promoting body symmetry in a relaxed position.

we use our bodies affects our general functioning. However, there is no ideal; it is for each to explore his or her possibilities and find better ways of using the body. For this and other reasons, the technique does not readily lend itself to systematic investigation and has not until recently begun to receive scientifically rigorous assessment.

Little et al (2008) have suggested that one-to-one lessons in the Alexander technique are effective for people with chronic back pain. In their randomized controlled trial of 579 patients, these researchers found that 24 lessons provided significant benefit in 3 months. This was statistically significant. At 12 months, the benefit was even greater. The study also showed that it is possible to achieve a similar effect with fewer lessons: the researchers found that six lessons followed by prescribed exercise was almost as effective.

Wide use is made of the Alexander technique in the field of motor problems. Stallibrass et al (2002) tested its efficacy in people experiencing symptoms of Parkinson's disease. Ninety-three participants were randomly divided into three groups: one received 24 lessons in the Alexander technique, one received 24 sessions of massage and there was a control which received no treatment. Results showed that, from pre- to post-intervention, motor symptoms in the Alexander group improved significantly compared to the no treatment group and this improvement was maintained at 6-month follow-up. These benefits were not demonstrated in the massage group. Both intervention groups, however, recorded positive changes on the Beck Depression Inventory whereas the control group registered no such changes.

The work of the anatomist Adams (Adams & Hutton 1985, Adams et al 1994) is relevant with regard to some of the postural claims made by Alexander. Adams has studied the effect of actions which impose physical stress on the lumbar spine. He has found that a moderate degree of flexion (i.e. flattening of the lumbar curve) is mechanically advantageous, which supports Alexander's views about the action of sitting down and the value of the monkey stance.

In her critical review of relaxation techniques, Kerr (2000) finds that the available research suggests that the Alexander technique may offer benefit in states of stress; it may also have a positive effect in conditions such as anxiety and depression.

A systematic review of controlled clinical trials concluded that the evidence in favour of the Alexander technique is 'encouraging' rather than 'convincing' (Ernst & Canter 2003). However, the research base is small and not all studies meet the requirements of being methodologically sound and clinically relevant. More research, both psychological and physiological, is needed to help clarify the position. Until that has been carried out and conclusions drawn, the technique must, in Barlow's words, continue to be regarded as a hypothesis (Barlow 1975).

KEY MESSAGES

- Alexander's technique is a process of psychophysical re-education.
- The re-education includes the unlearning of disadvantageous postural habits and the learning of alternative ones so that the muscles work in a more energy-economical way.
- Posture plays a central role in this approach. Phrases such as 'spine lengthening' and 'head held forward and up' illustrate the basic principles of Alexander's technique.
- His message is: if the posture is right, the body will be relaxed and the mind also.
- By its emphasis on balance, the technique helps to defuse body stress and this has application in the area of the performing arts.
- There is some evidence that the technique can help to reduce disability in Parkinson's disease. Different forms of paralysis such as stroke and multiple sclerosis may also respond favourably to the approach.

Chapter Thirteen

13

Differential relaxation

CHAPTER CONTENTS

Definition and rationale

Differential relaxation, a phrase introduced by Jacobson (1938), means, in his own words: 'the minimum of tensions in the muscles requisite for an act, along with the relaxation of other muscles' (Jacobson 1976). This is to say that the muscles engaged in performing any activity, for instance typing, should exhibit a minimum level of tension consistent with task efficiency, while those not directly engaged in the task are relaxed. This leaves the body as relaxed as it can be while achieving the objective, i.e. typing the page. Thus, differential relaxation is progressive relaxation applied to everyday tasks.

We need muscle tension in order to live our lives. It is essential for carrying out purposeful activity, of the type that Jacobson calls 'primary'. Purposeful activity, however, may be accompanied by tension in muscles whose action does nothing to promote the outcome, such as grimacing while writing. This is referred to by Jacobson as 'secondary activity'. Differential relaxation calls for the recognition and elimination of all secondary activity and of any excessive tension in the muscles performing or helping to perform the primary activity.

The approach is underpinned by the same theoretical principles as progressive relaxation (see Ch. 5). A thorough knowledge of progressive relaxation provides the skills to carry out differential relaxation.

Description

Jacobson's method

Jacobson has described a method in which he isolates the task, reduces muscle tension to below the level at which the task can be performed then, gradually, reintroduces tension to the minimum level where the task can be carried out efficiently. He gives an example (Jacobson 1976).

Sit holding an open book on your lap. Reduce the tension in your posture so that the book nearly falls off your lap. Relax your eye and speech muscles so that you are unable to follow the words. Then little by little, increase the tension until the book is secure on your lap and you can see the words ... then, gradually increase the tension enough to take in their meaning.

A similar routine can be applied to writing.

Take up a pen with the intention of writing your name, but using too little energy to make a mark on the paper. Repeat the action, this time putting a little more force into it. Continue putting slightly more force into it until you reach a point where you are able to write in a way which you recognize as your style. Keep it relaxed. You are now combining effective outcome with economy of effort.

A good time to test for the presence of secondary tensions is when opening the morning mail. The anticipation and apprehension of what it might reveal can raise tension levels far beyond what is necessary for the simple task of opening envelopes.

Bernstein & Borkovec's method

In their manual on progressive relaxation training, Bernstein & Borkovec (1973) develop the idea of differential relaxation. They single out three aspects of complexity: position of the body, level of activity and the situation in which the activity takes place. Variations of each are worked into an eight-step schedule, starting with 'sitting, doing nothing in a quiet room' and ending with 'standing, performing some activity in a busy environment'. Four of the items occur in the sitting position while the level of activity and the situation are varied; the other four occur in the standing position. During the performance of these exercises the pupil is asked to monitor his tension levels, using 'recall' (Ch. 8, p72) to relax herself.

Öst's method

This approach is described in Chapter 9.

Examples of the use of differential relaxation

Seated at a desk typing

Using just enough power in the hands to control the keys, type a few sentences. Then break off to check your body for tension. If you find any, relax it away using 'recall' (p72) or cue-controlled breathing (p83). Resume typing, checking again for tension. Make a telephone call, maintaining a relaxed posture, using only enough tension to hold the receiver.

Driving to the supermarket

As you settle yourself into the driving seat, spend a minute checking all your muscle groups for tension. Identify the muscles you need for driving. If you notice excess tension in any of these muscles, relax it. Check that the muscles you don't need, such as the face muscles, are relaxed. Maintain relaxation while steering and changing gear until you arrive at the store. Park the car and walk towards the entrance, relaxing any tension in your face and shoulders. Pick a trolley and as you push it around, continue to check your body, relaxing those muscles you do not need and putting the minimum of tension into the ones you need for the task. Pause regularly to scan your body for unnecessary tension.

Digging the garden

As you pick up the spade, feel the weight of it in your hand, fleetingly judging the degree of muscle work required to use it. Remind yourself that you can put too much effort into tasks of this nature. Relax your face muscles while you carry out the digging.

Stressful situations

Differential relaxation is relatively easy to achieve in activities which do not pose any threat but is more difficult in situations of stress, e.g. delivering a speech. In such cases additional strategies may need to be employed, such as mental rehearsal of the event and positive self-talk, to help reduce excessive tension (see Ch. 19).

Standing and walking

The principles of differential relaxation can also be applied to the postures of standing and walking, where certain muscle groups, such as those of the back and the legs, hold the body vertical and propel it along while uninvolved groups, such as those of the face, can be relaxed. The following two examples illustrate these ideas.

Standing

Have your eyes open. Stand with shoes off, feet parallel and 5 or 6 cm apart. Release excess tension with cue-controlled breathing. Unlock your knees, slightly bending and stretching them a few times to feel the weight falling evenly down through them to your feet. Rock forwards and backwards over them until you find a comfortable position for your hips. Feel your spine rising above your hips ... feel it supporting your head, and let your head reach up as high as it wants to go. Nod it gently to find its best position. Relax your face muscles. Let your arms hang down by your sides with your shoulders dropped. Feel your body relaxed and resilient. Enjoy being inside it. There should be no effort involved. When the posture feels as comfortable as possible, notice what makes it feel like that.

Walking

One way of finding your own energy-economical way of walking is to experiment with different kinds of walking. Marching, sailor's roll and tiptoeing are, of course, artificial ways of walking but by exploring different styles, you may find it easier to distinguish between unnatural and natural forms, and be helped to find your own natural way of walking. This will be the one that gives you most comfort and ease. Practise it, enjoy it. Feel your whole body relaxing into the rhythm of your step. Feel that the muscles responsible for carrying you along are no more tense than they need to be ... and that your face and shoulder muscles are relaxed.

Prerequisites

Differential relaxation is thus concerned with minimum tension levels during activity and task performance. There are two prerequisites: knowing which muscle groups are needed for each activity and which are not; and possessing the skill of muscle relaxation.

Comparison with other methods

The Alexander technique, with its concept of 'balanced use' (Ch. 12, p110), is grounded in the principle of differential relaxation. Here, the crucial elements are the relationships of head, neck and spine which, when correct, allow the body to adopt balanced and relaxed postures while engaged in activity. Alexander's procedures for the actions of sitting down and rising are essentially techniques of differential relaxation.

Mitchell (1987) is advocating differential relaxation when she urges the partial use of her schedule during task performance; for example, practising 'joint changes' for the shoulders and the jaw while driving or typing. Her 'key changes' can also be seen as a differential technique, in that they are directed at switching off unnecessary global tension while allowing specific movements to take place (Ch. 11, p102).

Poppen's mini-relaxation (1998) is another differential form. Here, relaxed-looking postures are adopted in the muscle groups not engaged in the task; for example, the legs can be relaxed while writing a letter (Ch. 10, p90).

KEY MESSAGES

- Differential relaxation is a form of applied relaxation in which actions are performed with the minimum of energy.
- The muscles employed in carrying out the task are working with just enough effort to accomplish the task while the muscles not directly employed are as relaxed as possible.
- The approach can be illustrated in all activities. Examples given here are typing, driving and garden digging.
- Practice is essential in order for the action to become automatic.

Stretchings

CHAPTER CONTENTS

Introduction and rationale

Flexibility is one of the properties of muscle tissue which mild stretching helps to maintain. Gentle stretchings also help to promote the mobility of the joints and stimulate the flow of synovial fluid. This fluid lubricates the joint and creates a smooth action.

In the case of the spinal joints, stretchings help the discs to recover after activity which changes their shape. The intervertebral discs are soft structures whose shape is altered when the spine is moved. Bending in any direction transforms the discs into wedge-shaped bodies with their fluid content squeezed towards the thick end of the wedge. When a body position such as leaning over a desk, for example, is held for long periods and under load, even the load of the body's own weight, this effect becomes more pronounced (Twomey 1993). This is known as 'creep' and is defined as the progressive deformation of a structure under constant load by forces which are not large enough to cause permanent damage (Kazarian 1975). The condition rights itself as the body resumes its normal position, but it takes time. Stretchings in the opposite direction can aid the recovery and may help to reduce the risk of injury, since the spine is vulnerable during the interval.

For this reason, motorists who have driven long distances, creating conditions in which creep occurs, should avoid lifting heavy loads immediately afterwards and should perform stretchings, not only at the end of the journey but at regular intervals throughout its course (Twomey & Taylor 1987). Stretchings will not guarantee protection from injury but they may make it less likely to occur. (See the sections on Back arching and Crouching/squatting.)

Many jobs require work postures which put strain on body structures. Stretches help to relieve this strain. The stretch exercise is designed to carry the body or body part in the opposite direction from the posture determined by the work; for example, a seated worker could stand and stretch upwards, whereas a standing operator might arch himself backwards or crouch down on his haunches. Activities which involve precision movements with flexed arms and fingers would call for wide arm stretches.

Stretching is something we do unconsciously after being in one position for a long time. The body seems to ask for it. We stretch after sleeping, after working at a desk, after bending down to weed a flower bed. All three trigger the need or the desire to stretch the body. Subjectively, stretches result in a feeling of comfort, pleasure and relief.

Stretching is essentially a physical action. The process of stretching links in with physiological principles in that the stretched group is responding in a reciprocal way to the action of the prime mover. Charles Carlson, a psychologist at the University of Kentucky, has looked at the effects of stretching and suggests mechanisms by which it might help to promote relaxation (Carlson et al 1990).

1. It has been found that a stronger contrast can be obtained between stretching and releasing than between tensing and releasing, because more length-sensitive receptors in the muscle are activated during stretching than during tensing (Anderson 1983). This more pronounced contrast effect might make it easier for individuals to release body tensions.

2. Stretch-based exercises have been found to lower the excitability of the motor neuron pool (Scholz & Campbell 1980), a finding which suggests a resulting decrease in levels of muscle tension, pain and ischaemia.

Description

Carlson and colleagues have devised a procedure consisting of muscle stretchings on the lines of progressive relaxation training; that is to say, the tensing routines in the abbreviated version of Bernstein & Borkovec's protocol are replaced by stretch-based actions. Each stretch lasts 10 seconds and is followed by a relaxation period of 60 seconds (Carlson et al 1990). The purpose is to induce an overall sense of relaxation.

Stretchings presented here consist of a range of large body movements and are similar to those in Carlson's schedule. Each stretch is carried out slowly, held for 5–10 seconds, then released quickly. An interval of approximately 30 seconds can be allowed between each stretch (Heptinstall 1995) . Participants are asked to notice the feelings in the relevant body part and to compare the sensations during and after the action.

Introductory talk to participants

The method you are about to learn consists of a series of stretches. It is believed that stretching a muscle helps to relax it and there is evidence to support this idea. The exercises are arranged so that each stretch lasts about 5 seconds after which there is a rest period of 30 seconds. Please don't overdo the actions – they should be comfortable, even pleasant. Let the stretch build up slowly and take note of the sensations that accompany it. Then, when you release it, register the feelings of relaxation and notice how they contrast with the feelings of the stretch. I'd like you to settle into a comfortable position before we start.

Procedure

The exercises are arranged according to their starting positions.

Lying

The floor or ground provides the best surface, softened by a mat or a carpet. Grass or firm sand also give the degree of hardness required. A bed is too soft.

Body rotations (Fig. 14.1)

Lie flat on your back. Bend both knees and place the feet flat on the ground. Now roll your bent knees to one side; roll them as far as they will easily go. At the same time, carry both your arms and your head to the other side. You are now twisting your body and stretching one set of oblique trunk muscles. Make it a comfortable stretch. Hold the position for a few seconds. Then bring your knees back to midline, resting your feet on the ground and your arms by your sides. Repeat the exercise in the other direction.

Curling into a ball (Fig. 14.2)

Lie flat on your back. Draw your knees up. Gather them in your hands and gently pull them towards your face. Still holding your knees, release the pull. Repeat the pull a few times.

Here the soft structures on the posterior aspect of the spine are being stretched. Some lower back conditions respond favourably to this exercise and the previous one, Body rotations.

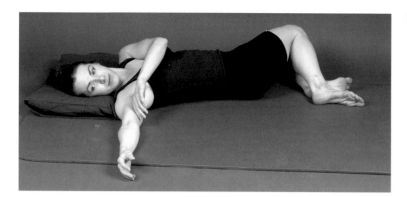

Figure 14.1 • Body rotations.

Hip joint stretches (Fig. 14.3)

Sit on the ground (cushion optional) and draw your legs into a bent position with your knees pointing sideways. Have the soles of your feet facing each other and in contact. Place your hands around your ankles and rest your elbows on your thighs. Apply pressure to your thighs, gently and slowly. You should feel a comfortable stretching in the hip area. However, the range of movement in hip joints varies greatly, so do not compare yourself with other people. Perform the exercise just to the point where you feel it is giving you a comfortable stretching sensation and no further. Then take a rest. Reapply the pressure.

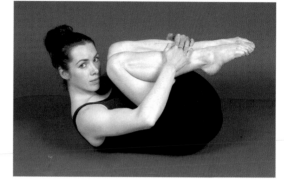

Figure 14.2 • Curling into a ball.

Sitting

An upright chair or stool is used for this group of stretchings. For the first item, a long stick such as a broom handle is needed, in an exercise which stretches the trunk and shoulder muscles. Other exercises in this group stretch the shoulder area in different ways.

Body turning (Fig. 14.4)

Sit with your feet flat on the ground. Grasp the broom handle with your hands 90 cm (3 ft) apart and raise your arms so that the stick just clears your head (your elbows are bent). Turn the upper part of your body to the right. This moves the stick through about 90°. Just go as far as you need to in order to get a comfortable stretch. Do not overstretch or bounce. Then return to the starting position. Repeat in the other direction.

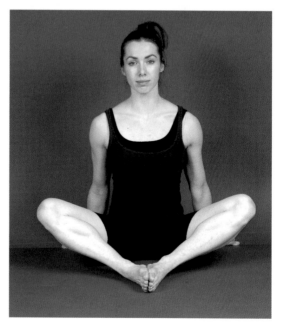

Figure 14.3 • Hip joint stretches.

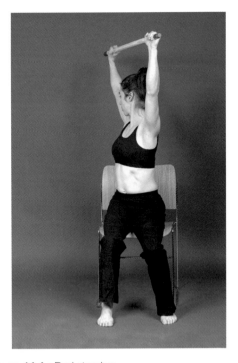

Figure 14.4 • Body turning.

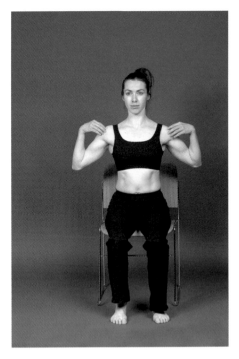

Figure 14.5 • Shoulder circling: 1.

Shoulder circling (Figs. 14.5 and 14.6)

Bend your elbows and place your fingertips on your shoulders. With your elbows, slowly draw circles in the air. After two or three circles, break off and repeat in the opposite diection.

Arms stretching above head (Fig. 14.7)

Bend your elbows and lift your arms above your head. Feel yourself pushing the air above you with your open hands. When your elbows are straight, spread your arms sideways and lower them to your sides. Let them rest limply. Repeat once or twice.

Head pressing backwards (Fig. 14.8)

Clasp your hands behind your head and, resting your head in them, arch backwards. Take care not to lean back too far if you are in a lightweight chair. Return your body to a vertical position.

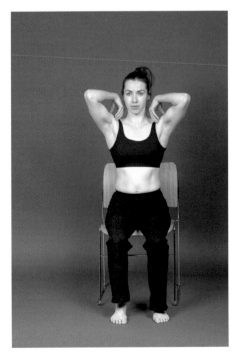

Figure 14.6 • Shoulder circling: 2.

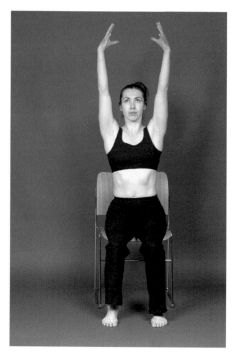

Figure 14.7 • Arms stretching above head.

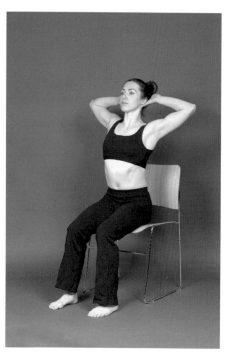

Figure 14.8 • Head pressing backwards.

Standing

Trunk bending sideways (Fig. 14.9)

Stand with your feet apart and your hands by your sides. Bend your body sideways, giving it a good stretch. Return to the upright position and repeat on the other side.

Arm and trunk bending sideways (Fig. 14.10)

This exercise resembles the previous one except that the sideways bend is performed with one hand over your head. Maintain an easy stretch in each direction.

Arms stretching back (Fig. 14.11)

Clasp both hands behind your back and straighten your elbows, drawing your shoulders back at the same time. Feel a stretch in the shoulder area, but do not overdo it. Then relax your arms and repeat the exercise.

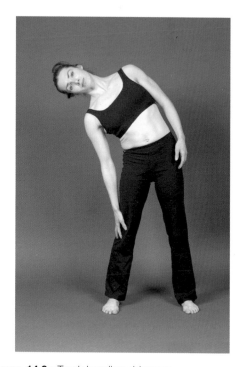

Figure 14.9 • Trunk bending sideways.

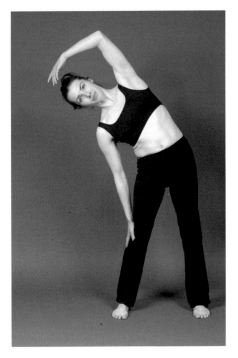

Figure 14.10 • Arm and trunk bending sideways.

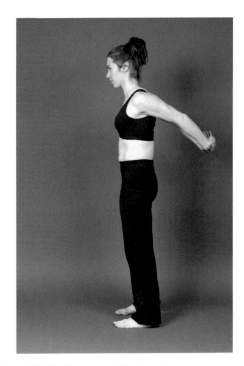

Figure 14.11 • Arms stretching back.

Arms reaching upwards (Fig. 14.12)

Stand with your feet slightly apart. Clasp your hands, then raise your arms above your head, turning the palms towards the ceiling as you straighten your elbows. Hold them there a few seconds, then lower them.

Arms stretching sideways (Figs. 14.13, 14.14)

Stand with your feet apart, and your arms bent at the elbow and raised to shoulder level. Gently swing one arm sideways and as you do so, allow your elbow to straighten. Return your arm to the bent position. Repeat with the other arm.

The previous five exercises are particularly useful for people who are leaning over a desk or a workbench. The last two can also be performed in a sitting position.

Trunk twisting (Fig. 14.15)

Stand with your hands on your hips. Slightly bend your knees and twist the upper part of your body to the left. Feel a comfortable stretch, then return to the starting position. Repeat on the other side.

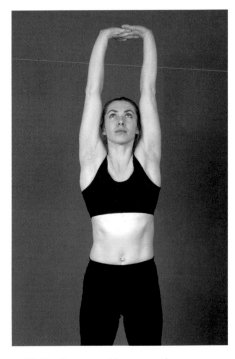

Figure 14.12 • Arms reaching upwards.

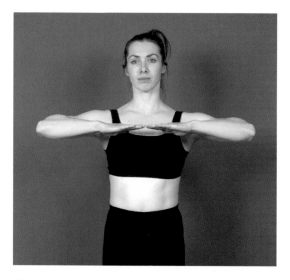

Figure 14.13 • Arms stretching sideways: 1.

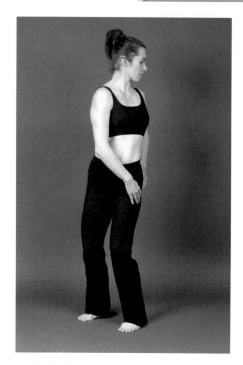

Figure 14.15 • Trunk twisting.

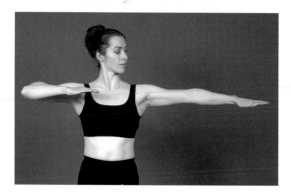

Figure 14.14 • Arms stretching sideways: 2.

Back arching (Fig. 14.16)

Place the palms of your hands over the bones that run sideways from your lumbar spine. Using that point as a fulcrum, bend over backwards. Go as far as is comfortable. No further! Then return to an upright position. Repeat. If the exercise makes you feel dizzy, keep your head and eyes looking forwards as you perform it.

Benefit can be gained from this exercise when driving long distances, brushing paths, vacuuming carpets or leaning over a table to sort papers.

Crouching/squatting (Fig. 14.17)

Get into a crouching or squatting position. Hold the position for 10–20 seconds. If you can, lay your feet flat on the ground; otherwise, perch on your toes. That is all that most people can do.

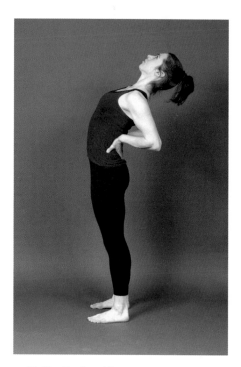

Figure 14.16 • Back arching.

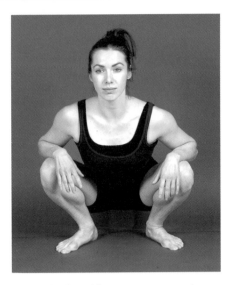

Figure 14.17 • Crouching.

This is another exercise which may be found to ease the lumbar spine during long-distance drives. Its somewhat bizarre appearance will escape attention if the driver pretends to be examining the tyres of his vehicle. The squat position seems to be beneficial for back health in general since it has been found that in populations where it is habitually adopted, lumbar disc degeneration is rare (Fahrni & Trueman 1965). For people with painful knees, however, it may not be advisable.

Calf stretching (Fig. 14.18)

Take your shoes off and stand facing a wall with your toes about 30 cm (12 in) away from it. Have your feet parallel and 10 cm (4 in) apart. Raise your arms and lean your forearms vertically on the wall. Rest your body weight on your forearms. With your heels on the ground and your knees straight, let your hips sink forwards.

You will feel a stretching in the calf muscles. Let it be a comfortable stretch, not a punishment. If you do not feel any stretching, take your feet further back until you do. As you stretch the calf muscles, hold the position for 5 seconds, then release it. Repeat a few times.

Inner thigh stretching (adductor stretching) (Fig. 14.19)

Stand with your feet about 50 cm (20 in) apart, hands on your hips. Swing your weight over the left knee, bending it as you do so. This

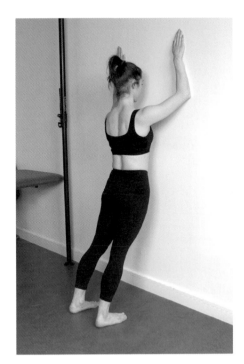

Figure 14.18 • Calf stretching.

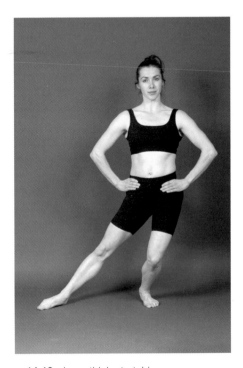

Figure 14.19 • Inner thigh stretching.

puts a stretch on the inside of the right thigh. Hold the position for about 5 seconds, then release the stretch. Repeat. Then swing your weight over the other leg.

Evidence of effectiveness

Relaxation training can take the form of stretch-release. This approach was adopted in a study to explore stress and relaxation in Hong Kong hospitals. Sixty-five nurse managers were randomly assigned to three groups: stretch-release, cognitive and test control. Mental health status was assessed using the Chinese versions of the State-Trait Anxiety Inventory and the General Hospital Questionnaire at three time points: pretreatment, after four sessions and at 1-month follow-up. In the results, both intervention groups were shown to derive benefit but no statistical analysis was reported (Yung et al 2004).

POTENTIAL PITFALLS

1. A participant may be undergoing medical treatment which contraindicates a particular stretching exercise. Priority should always be given to any medical instructions he has received.

2. The stretching must be done slowly to avoid causing microscopic tearing of the connective tissue (Anderson 1983). It should also be done without straining. At no time should any exercise feel uncomfortable. If it does, it should be stopped. Reasons for possible discomfort are that:
   a. the trainee is overdoing it
   b. the has an innate restriction of joint movement
   c. he has an incipient disorder

3. The number of repetitions carried out is a matter for the individual to decide. Only he knows if he is still benefiting from the exercise.

4. When working in a group of people there is often a temptation to do better than, or at least as well as, the others. Minor injuries can occur when participants feel challenged by neighbours (perhaps older than they) who outshine them. People often feel they have a duty to prove themselves. This of course is mistaken thinking. The only 'duty' imposed on the individual in this context is to make his body feel as comfortable as possible.

It has long been held that stretching a muscle before use confers benefit; conventional wisdom has suggested it provided protection against muscle soreness, but this claim has often been challenged. In their systematic review, Herbert & Gabriel (2002) found no evidence to support the claim. These same researchers drew similar conclusions in a subsequent systematic review (Herbert & de Noronha 2007), adding, however, that stretching may have other advantages such as reducing injury and enhancing performance. The latter benefits suggest that stretching should be an established part of a warm-up session.

KEY MESSAGES

- Gentle stretchings can make the body feel more comfortable. The increased comfort can promote relaxation.
- A full programme of body stretches should include all the major groups of voluntary muscles.
- Reductions in muscle tension have been noted in some studies following a course of stretchings.
- It is suggested that stretch-based procedures be viewed as effective alternatives to tense-release.

Physical activity

CHAPTER CONTENTS

Physical activity is an effective way of relieving stress, whether the activity is practised on its own or as part of a stress management programme (Tsatsoulis & Fountoulakis 2006). The effect of exercise on body systems resembles the effect of a stressful event or situation in that the same autonomic, musculoskeletal and endocrine systems are involved. The smooth integrated functioning of these systems, which takes place during exercise, can help to resolve the stress-related effects of adverse events or situations. Thus, exercise enhances the body's ability to deal with stress.

Any movement of the body which involves the expenditure of energy constitutes physical activity. It includes routines of daily living, domestic chores, gardening and walking. Exercise is a subset of physical activity and may be practised for health reasons or for leisure where it covers such activities as swimming, jogging, brisk walking, physical workouts and sport. The topic has been included to provide

the reader with the evidence in favour of physical activity as a means of promoting mental and physical health. Throughout this chapter, the words 'physical activity' will be used synonymously with 'exercise'.

A lifestyle which incorporates exercise has the potential to promote physical and psychological well-being, limiting the risk of life-threatening disease and common mental health disorders (see also Ch. 26). Such a programme is not only intuitively appealing, it is now supported by strong evidence. Physically active lifestyles are beneficial to health and well-being (WHO 2004).

Initially, research focused on vigorous exercise, such as running (Blair 1995); however, in the last 10 years, the emphasis has shifted to moderate-intensity physical activity (such as brisk walking) since this has been linked to a reduction in the incidence of coronary heart disease, colon cancer, obesity and diabetes (Department of Health 2004, United States Department of Health and Human Services 1999, Warburton et al 2006).

Physical inactivity is a major public health concern because it is now known that people who lead sedentary lives are at much higher risk of developing life-threatening conditions such as heart disease and cancer. In acknowledging these public health risks, the Chief Medical Officer (CMO) in the UK published a position paper about physical activity entitled *At least five a week* which emphasizes the strength of the evidence for the relationship between physical activity and health (Department of Health 2004). The guidelines for adults are summarized in Box 15.1.

Alongside the prevention of life-threatening diseases, regular physical activity provides some protection

Box 15.1

Recommended physical activity guidelines for adults (Department of Health 2004)

- At least 30 minutes a day of moderate intensity physical activity on five or more days of the week will provide general health benefits
- This can be achieved by undertaking one daily session of physical activity or splitting it into several shorter bouts of ten minutes' duration across the day. Activity can be part of lifestyle, for example, walking; alternatively it can take the form of structured exercise such as gym class, sport or a combination of these.
- All movement involves energy expenditure; consequently it plays an important part in weight management. For many people 45-60 minutes a day of physical activity at a moderate level of exertion may be necessary to prevent obesity. For bone health, physical activity which involves putting physical stress on the bones is necessary, e.g. using weights and/ or taking part in a low- to- moderate impact aerobic class
- These recommendations are also appropriate for older adults. It is important for older adults to maintain mobility through daily physical activity. Activities to increase strength, coordination and balance can be especially beneficial to older adults.

from depression. The evidence for this has been made available over the last 20 years from longitudinal studies undertaken with men and women in different countries: in the USA, examples include Paffenbarger et al (1994) and Motl et al (2004); in The Netherlands, van Gool et al (2003) and Bernaards et al (2006); in Germany, Weyerer (1992); and in Finland, Lampinen et al (2006).

The evidence for the psychological benefits of exercise suggests that it is an effective treatment for common mental health problems such as anxiety and depression either as a treatment in its own right or as an adjunct to cognitive–behavioural therapy or medication (Biddle & Mutrie 2008, Donaghy 2007).

Psychological well-being

Rationale

Why is physical activity important for mental well-being? On reviewing the existing research evidence in both healthy and clinical populations, a panel of experts, which included one of the authors of this book, found that regular physical activity decreased depression and stress; it also improved cognitive function in fit older adults and had positive effects on mood, physical self-perceptions and body image (Biddle et al 2000).

Regular participation in physical activity is linked to mental well-being. There is evidence of the link in healthy populations, but in clinical populations the link is even stronger (Donaghy 2007). Psychological outcome measures suggest that a sense of well-being is derived from regular physical activity, with participants reporting less tension, fatigue, aggression, depression and insomnia (Biddle & Mutrie 2008). The psychological benefits of exercise include distraction from worries, release of frustrations, sense of achievement, a feeling of improved physical appearance, self-confidence, and enjoyment in the company of other individuals in the pleasant surroundings of the exercise activity. In addition to the above benefits, exercise is inexpensive, non-invasive and has few side-effects.

As a therapy, physical activity is not underpinned by any particular theory. However, rather than being conceptualized as an atheoretical approach, Mutrie & Faulkner (2003) suggest it should be viewed as a process through which therapeutic goals can be reached.

How does exercise help in preventing and alleviating mental health problems?

Many explanations, both physiological and psychological, are put forward in an attempt to explain the mechanism underlying the association between physical activity and mental well-being. For example, the increased blood flow to the brain stimulates the release of naturally occurring mood-enhancing chemicals which are similar to morphine and have been linked to the 'runner's high'. Their presence in blood samples of people following a bout of exercise has been demonstrated (Mutrie & Faulkner 2003). Studies on animals have also shown that chemicals associated with mood elevation are released into the bloodstream during exercise (Chaouloff 1997). Antidepressant medication such as Prozac works by boosting these chemicals. The finding may also partly explain why exercise offers protection against depression and is effective as a treatment intervention. A further benefit is an increase in levels of the brain-derived neurotrophic factor (BDNF). This is a substance associated with the enhancement of mood and the longer survival of brain cells and may be linked to improved cognitive function (Donaghy 2007). It has also been suggested that increased levels of phenylethylamine, a known stimulant in the brain occurring during exercise, is linked to the release of dopamine and endorphins, which act as natural antidepressants (Donaghy 2007).

Explanations from psychology suggest links between exercise and physical self-perceptions such as body image, physical self-worth and self-esteem (Mutrie & Faulkner 2003). The findings from a survey undertaken by the charity MIND support this explanation, with 50% of the participants stating that exercise boosted their self-esteem (MIND 2002). Central to the exercise and its planning is the setting and achieving of goals, the development of skills and the resulting increase in self-confidence; exercise may also provide a mechanism for social support if the exercise includes other people. In addition, the anxiety-reducing effects of exercise have been linked to improved cardiovascular fitness since they reduce the reactivity to psychosocial stressors and help to promote recovery from them (Biddle et al 2000).

This creates a persuasive picture but leaves many questions unanswered. For example, does the sense of physical well-being transfer to the psychological sphere, making the thoughts more positive? Does the active coping strategy engender a feeling of mastery? Mutrie & Faulkner (2003) refer to the association of regular exercise with raised self-esteem, but it is not known whether this is brought about by virtue of weight reduction, improved physical health or sense of achievement.

Then again, is there some connection with people's expectations? Do people feel positive mood changes following a bout of exercise because they expect to? Does distraction play a part?

La Forge (1995) has reviewed all the possible mechanisms. He sees them as integrated rather than separate. His model shows the mechanisms as overlapping, sharing the same neural pathways. In this light, an approach which addresses them as linked processes would seem more appropriate than one which studies them in isolation.

Anxiety

Anxiety can refer either to an emotional state or to a personality disposition. The first is called 'state' anxiety, the second is 'trait' anxiety. *State* anxiety occurs as a temporary reaction to an event perceived as adverse or threatening; it refers to the experience of apprehension in a precise moment. Such feelings are normal reactions to life circumstances and are often accompanied by worry and physical symptoms such as dry mouth, raised heart rate, sweating and butterflies in the stomach. *Trait* anxiety, by contrast, is characterized by the individual's tendency to view all neutral events as potentially stressful and to experience state anxiety as a response to them (Spielberger 1980). State anxiety tends to accompany most disorders and is a natural concomitant of adverse conditions.

In a recent review of four meta-analyses on exercise and anxiety, Biddle and Mutrie (2008) conclude that exercise has a small to moderate positive effect on non-clinical levels of anxiety. There is also some evidence to suggest that people with high levels of aerobic fitness have reduced levels of physiological arousal in reaction to psychological stressors (Biddle & Mutrie 2008), indicating the possibility of a protective factor for those who regularly participate in aerobic exercise.

It is perhaps easier to accept that exercise (a high arousal activity) could relieve depression (a low arousal state) than that it could relieve anxiety, itself a high arousal state. Nevertheless, exercise has been fairly consistently associated with decreased levels of state anxiety. Experimental studies support an anxiety-reducing effect for exercise, with benefits resulting from moderate exercise during activity, and from moderate- and high-intensity exercise, after activity (Biddle & Mutrie 2008, Scully et al 1998).

The most persuasive results have been found in the field of generalized anxiety, where a marked treatment response often occurs. Martinsen (1990) found that little benefit was gained in the field of panic disorder or agoraphobia. However, this conclusion has subsequently been challenged by the findings of Broocks et al (1998) in their study of 46 outpatients with moderate to severe degrees of panic disorder, where symptoms were reduced by a programme of exercise. Although exercise (aerobic) was found to be less effective than medication (clomipramine), its effect after 10 weeks was significant.

Persistent and untreated anxiety can lead to generalized anxiety disorder which can itself be associated with panic and phobia. These and other forms of anxiety are discussed in Chapter 2 (p22). With regard to the effects of exercise in specific anxiety disorders, such as panic, reviewers find the evidence inconclusive (Biddle & Mutrie 2008,

Donaghy & Durward 2000). However, the research base is small compared with that of depression. Future work will cast more light on this area where, in many instances, anxiety and depression occur in the same individual.

Depression

The evidence associating exercise with relief from symptoms of depression has been gathering strength over the last two decades. This association has been demonstrated in randomized controlled studies looking at the efficacy of exercise in the treatment of adults with mild-to-moderate levels of clinical depression (Blumenthal et al 2007, Mead et al 2008). The consistency of the evidence makes a persuasive argument in the case of mild-to-moderate depression, (Biddle & Mutrie 2008, Donaghy 2007).

Exercise as a treatment for depression has not only been found effective but its results compare well with those of psychotherapy and cognitive-behavioural therapy (Fremont & Craighead 1987, Greist et al 1979, Klein et al 1985). Furthermore, when drug intervention is added to exercise and compared to exercise alone, no difference is shown (Blumenthal et al 1999, Babyak et al 2000).

Patients themselves have reported favourably on exercise, many of them adding that they would choose it as an intervention for clinical depression. The survey by the charity MIND found that 83% of people with mental health problems looked to exercise to lift their mood or reduce their stress, while two-thirds of them indicated that it helped to relieve their depressive symptoms (MIND 2002). A recently commissioned report in the UK also came out strongly in favour of exercise as a first-line treatment for depression. This led to a raising of awareness through the publication of leaflets and posters distributed to GP surgeries in England (Mental Health Foundation 2005).

Non-clinical populations have also been studied, showing that symptoms of depression in this population group can also be reduced by physical activity. The evidence comes from randomized controlled trials as well as cross-sectional and large-scale epidemiological studies (Biddle & Mutrie 2008).

Evidence for the benefit of exercise in general has, in recent years, accumulated to the point where guidelines endorse its use as a treatment in its own right or as an adjunctive treatment for mild-to-moderate depression (NICE 2003, SIGN 2009).

Exercise as a preventive measure

Since exercise has been shown to confer substantial benefit as a treatment for depression, it has been hypothesized that it might also have some protective value in psychologically healthy members of the community. In a recent review of 11 prospective longitudinal studies, Donaghy (2007) found a positive association between physical activity and the reduced risk of depression. (These studies included measures of exercise and depression at two or more time points.) Research carried out in the USA, Netherlands and Finland (which includes populations of community dwellers, workers, adults, adolescents and older people) has produced similar results. These show that people who are physically active and exercise regularly are less likely to be diagnosed with depression in the period between baseline and follow-up.

One of the earliest prospective studies (Farmer et al 1988) produced findings which suggest that women who had engaged in little or no recreational activity were twice as likely to develop depression as women who had engaged in moderate or high levels of activity. The Harvard Alumni (Paffenbarger et al 1994), one of the largest longitudinal studies of its kind, confirms the protective effects of physical activity and the lowered risk of developing depression for men. Thus, exercise has been found to be a protective factor for both men and women.

Evidence for the protective action of exercise has also been demonstrated in studies of older people. Adults over the age of 65 who took part in a daily walking programme were followed up for 3 years, providing evidence that exercise in this form reduced their risk of depression (Mobily et al 1996). Another study in the USA with middle-aged and older adults confirmed these findings (Strawbridge et al 2002). Protective factors have also been found in studies undertaken in Europe: van Gool and colleagues, in The Netherlands (2003), found that study participants who became depressed between baseline and follow-up had changed from an active to a sedentary lifestyle, and research undertaken in Finland (Lampinen et al 2006) found that mental well-being in later life is associated with mobility and physical activity.

This research raises the question of whether these benefits are only available to people with a long-standing active lifestyle. Motl et al (2005) looked at vulnerability to depression when physical activity was introduced to formerly sedentary, older adults. Study participants were randomly assigned to 6-month conditions of either walking or low-intensity resistance and/or flexibility training. Findings showed that depressive symptom scores decreased after the 6-month intervention; this was followed by a sustained reduction over 1–5 years. The effect for both types of physical activity was found to be similar (Motl et al 2005). The authors concluded that there may be gains for previously sedentary populations. A study in The Netherlands, looking at how much exercise was needed to offer protection, found that those with sedentary jobs only needed to engage in strenuous physical activity once or twice a week to reduce their risk of depression and emotional exhaustion (Bernaards et al 2006). Interestingly, higher levels of activity, three or more times a week, did not offer this protection.

Adolescents also benefit from the protective effects of physical activity (Motl et al 2004). Findings indicate that a decrease in the frequency of leisure-time physical activity is related to an increase in depressive symptoms. Studies have been undertaken in a variety of community settings and workplaces, and provide support for the transferability of findings across different populations. Some studies have followed up formerly clinically depressed populations to see if maintaining physical activity offers protection from recurring incidents. Harris et al (2006) investigated a clinical sample of 424 previously depressed patients (with a 1, 4 and 10-year follow-up). They found that more physical activity was associated with less concurrent depression; physical activity appeared to be countering the effects of negative life events.

Not all studies concur with these results, however. Cooper-Patrick et al (1997) carried out a prospective study on 973 middle-aged physicians to explore the preventive capacity of exercise, but results did not indicate that exercise reduced the risk of developing depression.

Prescribing exercise

Before prescribing exercise or participating in increased levels of physical activity, it is important to undertake an assessment on readiness to exercise. This should consider the individual's current and past patterns of physical activity and her preferred forms of activity. It should also identify goals and assess the risks. There should be a discussion with the patient/participant about her beliefs regarding the benefits and risks of exercise, and an acknowledgement of any concurrent disease. Motivation and barriers should be considered together with the availability of social support throughout the programme. Finally, time and scheduling matters need to be agreed.

It is important to develop a realistic programme of physical activity and to monitor compliance and progress at regular intervals. The Par Q is an easy-to-complete questionnaire which can offer some guidance to potential health risks and is used widely in leisure centres for new and visiting members (see Appendix 4).

Type of exercise

Exercise may have a variety of effects: it may strengthen a muscle, increase its flexibility, improve its endurance, refine its co-ordination ability, to mention a few. It may also fall into one of two categories or types: aerobic and anaerobic. Aerobic exercise consists of sustained rhythmic activity such as walking, swimming, cycling, jogging, distance running and dancing. It involves large muscle groups contracting in a repetitive manner at low-to-moderate levels of energy expenditure for long periods of time. This kind of exercise strengthens the cardiovascular system and increases overall strength and stamina. Anaerobic exercise, on the other hand, improves muscle strength and flexibility.

There are three kinds of anaerobic exercise: isotonic, isometric and calisthenic. The first two single out particular muscle groups for the purpose of building up their strength. Isotonics are exercises where the muscles contract against a resistant object with movement, as in weight-lifting; this type of resistance exercise increases muscle bulk. Isometrics are exercises where the muscles contract against resistance but without movement as in squeezing a tennis ball; this increases strength without building bulk. Calisthenics are stretching exercises which increase flexibility and joint mobility. Examples include raising the arms above the head and other exercises to be found in Chapter 14.

Many forms of exercise achieve aerobic and strengthening effects, and both kinds have been found useful in the context of mental health. Stretching exercises are frequently used to warm up the muscles before starting the exercise.

Dosage of exercise

A general principle of exercise prescription is that it should be introduced gradually and progress by small stages covering a period of several weeks. This is to ensure that the activity designed to benefit the body is matched by the body's capacity to tolerate the exercise. The chosen activity and setting should be attractive to the individual and one that she believes will be enjoyable. Personal preference should influence whether it is performed in a group or as an individual activity. Important aspects at the outset are fitness for participation in the chosen activity and willingness to continue exercising in the future.

Dimensions of exercise

It is conventional to describe exercise in terms of its three dimensions:

- intensity
- duration
- frequency.

Intensity

Intensity, which can be high, medium or low, has received particular attention from researchers. Although results have not been consistent, there seems to be a consensus that moderate-intensity activity produces the greatest benefit. 'Moderate', in this context, means that the exercise should be vigorous enough to create a physical effect but not so strenuous that the person feels unduly challenged. Extremely high intensities can have negative effects by inducing a degree of stress (Gauvin & Spence 1996).

Duration

The exercise may be taken either in one 30-minute period or broken up into short multiple periods. One advantage of the short, frequent exercise period is that it can be fitted into break times, which makes it ideally suited for people experiencing work stress. In setting the duration, much depends, first, on the nature of the exercise, in that lighter activities are easier to sustain for longer periods, and second, on the physical health and age of the individual, both of which will affect his exercise tolerance.

Frequency

On the matter of frequency, programmes vary in their specifications from three to seven times a week. Certainly a high frequency of practice is

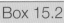

Box 15.2

Grades of exercise intensity
Vigorous

Activity in which the individual exerts himself to the point of getting out of breath and sweating. It includes squash, football, tennis, strong sustained swimming, long distance running, cycling over difficult terrain and energetic aerobics (Allied Dunbar National Fitness Survey 1992).

Moderate

Activity which makes the individual feel comfortably challenged (Young & Dinan 2005). Less demanding activities such as golf, social dancing, table tennis, garden digging, long brisk walks, climbing stairs or gentle uphill gradients are included, performed at an intensity which causes breathing to be somewhat harder than normal and sweating to occur for some of the time.

Light

Activity of an unchallenging nature which has little effect on the breathing. A few of the above activities such as golf, social dancing and table tennis are performed in a light manner; also included are fishing, darts, snooker, bowls, weeding, planting, light DIY and long walks at an average pace.

advocated, but whether seven times a week confers more benefit than five times a week has not been established. Most researchers suggest that daily exercising has merit.

The amount of energy expended during exercise relates to the balance between these three variables. Andrea Dunn and colleagues (2005) have been investigating the amount of energy expenditure required to gain health benefits in the relief of symptoms of depression. Their findings suggest that energy expenditure of 17 kcal/kg/week should be attempted. This can be achieved by exercising for at least 30–60 minutes a day (depending on intensity) for a minimum of 3 days a week. Alternatively, 30 minutes of moderate-intensity exercise, 5 days a week, will have the same effect. Guidance on these matters can be found in Box 15.2.

Using a consultation approach for increasing physical activity

Many people find difficulty in starting an exercise programme. They may be vague about the choice of activity or lack the confidence to begin. Motivation to get started in an exercise programme, maintaining exercise over time and overcoming barriers to exercise has been extensively studied (Biddle & Mutrie 2008). This has led to the development of different theoretical models that provide plausible explanations for the choices people make. To provide the reader with some knowledge of the factors that influence decision-making with regard to exercise participation, we have selected the transtheoretical model which also provides a framework for intervention strategies.

The transtheoretical model (DiClemente et al 1985) contains three key ideas. First, behaviour change in the individual is seen as a dynamic process that occurs in the following *stages*: 'precontemplation' (the person is not considering exercising), 'contemplation' (he is considering exercise and is seeking information from the doctor, physiotherapist or others), 'preparation' (he makes efforts to start exercising by joining a class or planning a personal routine of physical activity), 'action' (he attends the exercise class/starts the programme of physical activity) and 'maintenance' (he maintains attendance at the class or keeps up the programme of physical activity). These stages represent different levels of behaviour change.

The second key idea is that progress through these stages is driven by a series of 10 *processes* specific to particular stages, including 'consciousness raising' (receiving information on how exercise may help or how exercise classes can be accessed), 'counter-conditioning' (using the positive aspects of exercise to counter fears and anxieties about future health) and 'stimulus control' (controlling situations that may trigger dropping out from the exercise class).

A third key idea refers to the individual's experience of accompanying problems such as his symptoms, the situational constraints, maladaptive cognitions, interpersonal conflicts and family problems. These may occur during any of the stages specified above. The advantage of this model is that it indicates the individual's readiness for change.

The above knowledge can be applied by healthcare professionals and exercise instructors to enhance the likelihood of participants' continued attendance in an exercise programme. It is an approach which has been well received by healthcare professionals. However, while it is one of the most researched models, some misclassification of

---

Box 15.3

Steps in a typical physical activity consultation session

Step 1: Determine physical activity history: what the person previously enjoyed doing, why she wants to increase physical activity and the kind of activities she may now wish to engage in.

Step 2: Discuss what she sees as being the 'pros' and 'cons' of increasing her physical activity. Discuss how the 'cons' may be managed.

Step 3: Ask him what kind of support she will need and who can provide it, both for getting started and for continuing with the exercise.

Step 4: Help her identify appropriate goals for gradually increasing physical activity. Write out action-related goals, e.g. in 4 weeks' time I would like to be walking for 30 minutes at moderate level of intensity (slightly out of breath) on at least 5 days of the week.

Step 5: It is helpful also to discuss relapse strategies, i.e. what to do if she misses sessions or if her motivation to continue wanes.

Step 6: Provide local information about leisure centres, sporting activities, walking paths, swimming pools. This makes a useful supplement to the discussion.

---

stages may occur as a result of the way those stages are operationally defined (Bulley et al 2007).

The typical content of a physical activity consultation session has been outlined in step form by Biddle & Mutrie (2008) and appears in Box 15.3.

Conclusion

There is strong evidence that regular physical activity at the recommended level offers protection from life-threatening physical diseases and prolongs life expectancy (Department of Health 2004). It is therefore in everyone's interest to promote these key targets and messages. The evidence for protection against depression is less strong but there exist a number of randomized controlled trials that suggest that exercise is a useful intervention to reduce symptoms of depression. Exercise may also offer some protection against anxiety. Getting started and maintaining programmes of physical activity depend on motivational factors and social support; it is therefore recommended that people seek advice from a relevant healthcare professional or exercise consultant.

POTENTIAL PITFALLS AND RECOMMENDATIONS

In recommending exercise to participants, the health care professional/exercise instructor needs to be aware of its hazards. Exercise can be excessive and beyond the capacity of the individual. There have been instances of muscles and tendons being injured and even death occurring in the course of exercise. It is important, therefore, to keep the activity within safe limits. The following points should be borne in mind.

1. Exercise should not be seen as a substitute for medical help in the presence of disease or suspected disease. People with cardiovascular problems should first consult their doctor before taking up exercise.

2. Any programme of exercise should be introduced gradually and progress in small stages in order to allow the organs to adapt to the new demands. Walking or swimming are useful ways to start. Unaccustomed strenuous activity is potentially hazardous.

3. All exercise should be preceded by some kind of 'warming up' activity to prepare the muscles for action (Safran et al 1989). Warming up takes the form of mild activity such as running on the spot, gentle contractions against resistance and balance exercises performed for 5–10 minutes. The effect of this procedure is to open up the blood vessels in the working part, thus protecting against ischaemia (inadequacy of local blood supply), which can occur in unprepared muscles.

4. Cooling down is also important. During vigorous or moderate exercise a higher than normal proportion of the total blood volume circulates through the voluntary muscles. This state continues for some while after the exercise has come to an end and causes a lowering of the blood pressure. It is potentially hazardous in the elderly, but should be guarded against even in the very fit. As a remedy, the exercise can be slowly reduced in intensity or, alternatively, some lighter activity such as slow walking can be performed to bring about a gradual return of normal blood distribution (Hough 2001).

5. Exercise should not be too strenuous. To be safe, exercise should be well within the capacity of the individual and performed regularly. The individual should never feel he is exercising to the limit of his strength. He should also know how to recognize signs of fatigue. Warnings of overwork in the form of chest pain or faintness, for example, should never be ignored.

6. While team sports and marathons can be fun, they involve a spirit of competition which may be stressful. Non-competitive activities, on the other hand, impose less pressure on the individual, who can pace himself in a way that takes account of his reactions.

7. The capacity of the individual to carry out exercise may be compromised by medical problems or by the drugs she is taking. It is advisable to check that these do not conflict with the effects of exercise. If an individual is in doubt about her health, she should seek advice before taking up exercise.

8. The cardiovascular benefit of jogging has to be balanced against the physical stress it imposes on the weight-bearing joints (US Preventive Services Task Force 1989), although hard evidence of any association between running and the risk of osteoarthritis in weight-bearing joints is slight (Blair et al 1992). However, if there is a family history of joint problems, it may be advisable to consider an alternative form of aerobic exercise such as cycling or swimming.

9. Exercise is contraindicated during any kind of fever and should be avoided during viral infections such as influenza.

KEY MESSAGES

- Regular physical activity offers protection from life-threatening diseases such as heart attack, stroke and some cancers and may offer protection from depression.

- Exercise can be offered as a treatment in its own right for mild-to-moderate depression or as an adjunct to medication and/or cognitive–behavioural therapy.

- Exercise may be helpful in managing state anxiety as it reduces the stress response.

- The minimum requirement for general health benefits is 30 minutes of moderate activity on at least 5 days of the week.

- Getting started in exercise where there are health problems should involve an appropriate assessment by a GP, health professional or exercise instructor. Previous medical and exercise history is important to ensure fitness to start exercising and to provide appropriate guidance on type, frequency, intensity and duration.

- Support is needed in maintaining motivation. Goals should identify where support is being provided and indicate how feedback will be monitored.

Section **Three**

Cognitive approaches

Chapter Sixteen

16

Cognitive–behavioural approaches

Introduction

Cognitive–behavioural therapy (CBT) is an approach designed to alleviate symptoms and to help people learn more effective ways of overcoming the problems and difficulties that contribute to their distress (Davidson 2008). It seeks to address the individual's difficulties from her point of view and to equip her with the information and confidence to become an active participant in the management of her condition (Marshall & Turnbull 1996). It thus lends itself to conditions such as anxiety, depression, psychotic disorders, eating disorders, chronic fatigue syndrome and chronic pain and is relevant in many other illnesses and dysfunctions. The theory behind it also has a major role to play in the field of prevention.

Description and rationale

The origins of the approach lie in cognitive and behaviour theories (see Ch. 1). Cognitive theory is based on the premise that individuals constantly process information gathered from their surroundings and that problems arise as a result of the way the individual interprets a situation or event (Beck 1976). Knowledge, previous experience and memories of situations or events all play a part, influencing these interpretations. An inaccurate or biased interpretation of an event or experience can lead to faulty patterns of thinking and unrealistic beliefs. This can cause symptoms of stress, anxiety and depression and can be linked to other physical and mental health problems (Donaghy et al 2008). The individual needs to recognize the negative content and bias in her thinking before she can learn ways of challenging it. This involves a re-evaluation of her perception of vulnerability or danger, whether she is dealing with full-blown anxiety or day-by-day stress (Beck 1976, Greenberger & Padesky 1995).

Cognitive theory views the individual as a self-determining agent in life, which means that, when receiving treatment, she needs to feel a degree of control over the management of her condition. This aspect makes the approach particularly applicable in the field of chronic disorder.

Behaviour theory, on the other hand, views human behaviour as a result of environmental conditioning, and when this behaviour is maladaptive, employs methods such as reinforcement, distraction and exposure to modify it. Positive and negative reinforcement are methods for increasing the likelihood of desired behaviours. Distraction, i.e. holding the attention elsewhere, can be a useful strategy particularly for people in chronic pain. Exposure, i.e. facing the anxiety-provoking situation itself, can be a useful tool for people who experience panic attacks or various forms of social anxiety.

The cognitive–behavioural approach combines both theories. Developed by Aaron Beck, it emphasizes the importance of thought processes while acknowledging that they can be influenced by reinforcement. This highlights the inter-relationship of thoughts, feelings and behaviour, creating a unifying philosophy with a strong psychosocial emphasis (Marshall & Turnbull 1996).

Procedure

Client assessment

Central to the method is the collaborative relationship that is developed between client and therapist (Ralston 2008). This begins with a first assessment to determine whether the client has the motivation and commitment to be an active participant, and also to determine whether CBT is the most appropriate path to follow. The approach can be illustrated in the handling of anxiety, for example, where a first step would be to discover the situation or event which triggers the anxiety and to review it alongside the various symptoms it provokes, i.e. physiological, cognitive, behavioural and emotional. The client is encouraged to articulate her beliefs and interpretations of that situation or event. Through dialogue with the therapist, she explores the factors which make the symptoms of anxiety better or worse, and examines the ways in which she copes with them. This person-centred approach helps the client to gain a sense of personal empowerment. Initially, the client may need to be guided into active participation as she may not be aware that she has that power; she may not realize that any change in her symptoms will be the result of her own actions. With continued collaboration, however, information will emerge and be used in planning the treatment.

Cognitive restructuring

Clients are introduced to the format for each session, including agenda setting, shared goal setting and home-based tasks. In early sessions, general examples of links between thoughts, feelings, physical symptoms and behaviour are presented alongside examples specific to the client. It is important that the links between fear, anxiety and worry become evident since constant worrying intensifies anxiety and extends the associations which trigger it.

The next step is to help the client to recognize the negative content and bias in her thinking so that she can learn ways of challenging it. This process is termed cognitive restructuring. Both clinical dialogue and diary keeping are important in guiding the client to recognize negative thinking. Between sessions, the client will keep a note of any anxiety-provoking events, describing the situation, the emotion elicited and what was going through her mind at the time, whether it was a distressing image or a negative thought about herself, her situation or the future.

With the information gathered from the interviews, negative thoughts, beliefs and assumptions are set out alongside the evidence that challenges them. For example, abdominal pain experienced with anxiety may be associated with the belief that she has cancer; people with cancer suffer pain. This negative thought can be challenged by different kinds of evidence, such as pain being confined to anxiety attacks, an absence of other symptoms or non-existent family history of cancer. Moreover, pain linked to anxiety can itself have a physiological explanation.

Learning about automatic negative thinking errors also helps her to understand that it is her thinking, not the event itself, which is causing her distress. In common with others who display negative thinking habits, she tends to overestimate danger and underestimate her own coping abilities.

Useful cognitive techniques to employ include the following: considering how other people would view the situation (an indication that other perspectives exist); reviewing past experiences where she has coped successfully; and considering what might happen if her worst fears came true. This helps the client to see that her fears are unlikely to be realized. However, if the fear is plausible an action plan can be drawn up for use, should the event occur.

Yet another cognitive–behavioural technique is getting the client to confine worrying to pre-agreed times. Specific worries are identified and a time and location set aside for addressing them. When worry occurs outside these times, the client is asked to note the item in the diary but not to dwell on it at that point. She is encouraged to wait until the pre-arranged 'worry time' when she picks up the item and works on it with the use of the cognitive restructuring techniques outlined above.

A relaxation technique to deal with the physical symptoms can also be offered to the client. It is helpful for her to learn brief techniques which can be used at times when panic or fear is experienced (see Ch. 24). The client is also encouraged to face situations previously avoided, having first discussed them with the therapist. Such exposure is likely to be time-limited, progressing in a phased manner. If managed appropriately, her beliefs and assumptions will change, her anxiety will be extinguished, she will experience the absence of any catastrophic

outcome and begin to recognize her ability to cope with challenging situations.

Cognitive–behavioural interventions were first used clinically with mental disorders such as anxiety and depression, acknowledging that mood is regulated through cognition and behaviour and the interaction between these systems. More recently, the application of CBT has been extended to areas where anxiety and depression are associated with other clinical conditions such as pain, fibromyalgia and chronic fatigue. For a detailed account of the application of cognitive–behavioural interventions in these and other conditions, see Donaghy et al (2008).

In the case study below homework includes a range of cognitive techniques which challenge Barbara's beliefs about cancer. One of these is thought stopping (see Ch. 24, p201), a technique which intercepts the intrusive thoughts and replaces cancer fears with a vision of her two children, healthy and laughing. Six weeks from starting treatment, Barbara's symptoms of severe anxiety are extinguished and she is pain free.

Case study Heightened anxiety after the birth of a child

Barbara is a 28-year-old mother of two children under the age of 5. She describes having experienced feelings of heightened anxiety after the birth of her first child (a girl) 4 years ago. At that time she also developed pain in her neck and right shoulder and she associated the pain with a belief that she may have cancer (her friend had been diagnosed with a brain tumour 9 months previously). Barbara gradually recovered from her anxiety and from the pain with its associated beliefs but states that her self-confidence never returned to its level prior to the birth of her daughter. However, she managed to hold a job as manager in a large sports outlet, where she worked until the birth, 18 months ago, of her second child (a boy).

She had no anxious feelings after the birth of her second child and she has enjoyed her time as a mother, meeting other mothers and their children. However, in the last 10 weeks, Barbara has felt that her anxiety has returned and it seems to have been triggered by her daughter being hospitalised for 4 days with pneumonia.

Although the little girl has now fully recovered, Barbara's anxiety is not subsiding. Alongside this anxiety, she has again developed pain in her neck and shoulders. She referred herself to a physiotherapist, describing her symptoms as pain which intensifies as the day goes on.

Following an initial assessment, Barbara explores with the physiotherapist her thoughts and beliefs about her

pain and anxiety. They discuss how anxiety creates changes in the muscles, making them tense, and how this can cause pain. They discover that the pain is aggravated by lifting and carrying her son. Added to this, she is suffering from sleep disturbance and intense worry. Barbara also shares her thoughts about the possibility of having cancer, basing her thoughts on the experience of her friend with the brain tumour who had similar physical symptoms and died from the tumour 12 months ago. Barbara agrees to keep a diary and to note when anxiety afflicts her, what happened immediately before feeling anxious, what she is thinking, how it affects her pain, what helps to reduce the anxiety/pain and what makes it worse. She learns to recognize a negative bias in her thinking and challenges it by reminding herself that she has never had a serious illness, that the chances of her getting cancer are very slim and that she has no other symptoms which might justify such a fear. She now appreciates that anxiety can trigger pain.

Together, Barbara and the physiotherapist develop a plan to help her relax by learning a relaxation technique which she agrees to practise every day. Using the information gathered from the interviews and diaries, the process of 'restructuring' her thoughts continues over a period of 4 weeks. Barbara also learns a brief relaxation technique for use during periods of anxiety when the worry about having cancer intrudes into her thoughts.

Evidence of effectiveness

The effectiveness of CBT has been clearly demonstrated (Butler et al 2006, Roth & Fonagy 1996). It is now the most widely endorsed form of psychological therapy (Rachman 2003) and has broad application in both physical and mental health. Despite the huge scientific impact that CBT has made, it is still a relatively new approach. It is only in the last 30 years, with the theoretical and practical integration of cognitive and behavioural strategies, that CBT has become influential in terms of health service delivery. As a clinical intervention, CBT not only works but we know *how* it works (Salkovskis 2002).

However, while many of the cognitive–behavioural interventions currently in use contain elements which are transferable across conditions, research indicates that specific clinical problems require different approaches. For example, CBT in the treatment of depression is quite different from the treatment for obsessive compulsive disorder or the management of chronic pain.

Cognitive–behavioural therapy has been found to be effective in the treatment and management of major mental health problems. Recent meta-analyses undertaken by Butler et al (2006) found large effect sizes for CBT in a range of mental health disorders including unipolar depression, anxiety, panic disorder (with or without agoraphobia), social phobia, post-traumatic stress disorder, and childhood depressive and anxiety disorders. Moderate effect sizes for CBT were found in the treatment of marital stress, anger, childhood somatic disorders and chronic pain. CBT was also found to be as effective as behaviour therapy in the treatment of adult depression and obsessive compulsive disorder, and as effective as antidepressants for the initial treatment of moderate-to-severe depression (Hollon et al 2005).

A recent Cochrane review found that CBT was effective in the treatment of anxiety and more effective than psychodynamic therapy (Hunot et al 2007). Öst & Breitholtz (2000), comparing CBT with applied relaxation in a small study of 36 outpatients with generalized anxiety disorder, found no significant differences between the two methods, although both demonstrated improvements. There was, however, a lack of evidence for the longer term effectiveness of CBT in treating generalised anxiety disorder (Hunot et al 2007).

Evidence for the effectiveness of CBT in patients with alcohol disorders consists of findings from meta-analyses and randomized controlled studies (Longabaugh et al 2005) The strongest evidence is linked to social skills training, community reinforcement approaches and relapse prevention (Miller & Hester 1995). In a large study comparing CBT with the Twelve Steps Alcoholics Anonymous programme and motivational enhancement therapy (Project MATCH 1998), all treatments were equally effective.

Many other clinical conditions have benefited from CBT. The literature is extensive, as the following studies indicate. A Cochrane review of CBT found it more effective than orthodox medical management or other interventions for adults with chronic fatigue syndrome; here, benefits were equal to those of graded exercise (Price & Couper 1999). CBT has also been found effective in reducing symptoms of pain, anxiety and fatigue in children with fibromyalgia (Degotardi et al 2006). Meta-analysis of studies of breast cancer found CBT effective in managing the distress and pain associated with this condition (Tatrow & Montgomery 2006).

Opinion suggests that cognitive–behavioural interventions are valuable in the treatment and management of chronic pain (Keefe et al 2004, Morley 2004, Vlaeyen & Morley 2005), an opinion which is based on published research trials and systematic reviews (Guzman et al 2001, Morley et al 1999, van Tulder et al 2000). The systematic review undertaken by Morley et al (1999) found CBT to be beneficial in exploring the components of the pain experience such as thoughts and feelings; it also improved social functioning.

Who should use cognitive–behavioural therapy?

Who should be using these techniques? Although CBT is a psychological specialty, many of its techniques are highly accessible to the healthcare professional, and since healthcare professionals have been asked to broaden their approach by taking account of psychosocial aspects of assessment and treatment, they will find in cognitive–behavioural techniques a means of achieving this (Everett 2003, Johnstone et al 2002). CBT approaches now feature in occupational and physiotherapy treatment programmes, although relatively few studies of effectiveness in these professions have so far been carried out (Duncan 2003). Health care professionals can acquire CBT expertise from a variety of postgraduate courses, many of which are condition focused, such as CBT for chronic pain. These programmes allow people to get a basic training but for further competence, supervision with an experienced cognitive–behavioural therapist is required.

Conclusion

In summary, CBT helps people to challenge their beliefs and thoughts and to develop positive coping strategies. Relaxation is taught to reduce the physiological symptoms and is a component of the cognitive-behavioural strategies used in many of the conditions mentioned in this chapter. The overall effect of CBT, however, goes far beyond the strict bounds of relaxation.

KEY MESSAGES

- Cognitive–behavioural treatments combine a wide range of strategies drawn from both cognitive and behavioural approaches.
- Treatment programmes are designed and carried out with the client in the role of active participant.
- Self-management by the client is a characterizing feature, particularly in chronic disease.
- Although CBT is a psychological specialty, many of its techniques are highly accessible to the healthcare professional.
- Strong evidence exists for the effectiveness of CBT.

Further reading

Donaghy, M., Davidson, K., Nicol, M. (Eds.), 2008. Cognitive Behavioural Interventions in Physiotherapy and Occupational Therapy. Butterworth-Heinemann Elsevier, Oxford.

17

Self-awareness

CHAPTER CONTENTS

Introduction and rationale

'Being aware' or 'being conscious' convey similar ideas. Their use when applied to the self, however, is very different. Being aware of the self is defined as 'the tendency to focus attention on the private aspects of the self' (West 1987). This signifies a process of self-exploration, a getting to know oneself, recognizing one's strengths and weaknesses. Being conscious of the self as we use the phrase in everyday language, on the other hand, implies the sense of being 'painfully aware of being observed by others' (Burnard 1991). A person who is self-conscious sees herself as being critically scrutinized by other people. The result of self-consciousness is embarrassment; the result of self-awareness is self-knowledge.

  Increased self-knowledge comes from listening to ourselves: to who we are, what we are and how we are (Tschudin 1991). It relates to questions such as

'Am I the person I want to be?' and if not, 'What is stopping me becoming that person?' or 'Why don't I allow myself to develop to my fullest?'. The answers help us to understand ourselves. The better we know ourselves, the easier it is to make decisions which further our life plans. Without this knowledge, we may find decisions being made for us.

  Self-awareness also puts us in touch with our outward behaviour and the way others may be responding to it. In this way, self-awareness can enhance our personal relationships.

  The notion of self-awareness is fundamentally linked to the notion of living in the present, responding in the here-and-now and being aware of the present moment, since that is where we express ourselves and make our impact on life. Of course, we need to take into account lessons learned from the past and goals set for the future, but it is all too easy to dwell on these and let the present take care of itself. This can lead to our losing whatever control we had of it. Being aware of the self helps us perform in the present.

  Greater control of our lives, enhanced relationships and improved self-knowledge all contribute to our peace of mind. Self-awareness exercises can thus be seen as relaxation techniques.

  Authors have structured self-awareness in different ways. Stevens (1971) divided it into three parts: an outer world of sensory information, one inner world of feelings (visceral and emotional) and a second inner world of mental activity (thoughts and images). Burnard (1992) sees the internal part as corresponding with Jung's four functions of the mind (thinking, feeling, sensing and intuiting), to which he adds a visceral component which includes muscle tension and bodily relaxation. The external part refers to what other people see: our verbal and non-verbal behaviour together with other aspects of the way we present ourselves.

To Tschudin (1991), the inner world consists of thoughts and emotions and the outer world of people and environments, with a 'go-between' world relating to the senses. A further version of this categorization appears in the current development of Wellness Centres in Thailand (Pothongsunun 2006). These focus on an awareness of what has to be managed to maintain physical and mental health. Their key feature is self-image consisting, in this case, of sensation, feeling, thought and movement. Sensation includes the five senses plus a proprioceptive component which registers the body's orientation in space. It also includes perception of pain and the passage of time. Feeling covers the field of emotions such as joy, anger, grief, self-respect. Thinking embraces all cognitive functions: intellectual, intuitive, moral as well as imagination and memory. Finally, movement includes all actions of the body, from breathing to athletics.

A composite view is presented in Figure 17.1. The inner aspect covers thinking, intuition, emotions and bodily sensations which include those of muscle tension; the outer aspect refers to the way we relate to other people and to society in general. The social level refers to the context of our lives as well as the events which take place on a daily basis. On an individual level, it refers to the way we relate to our work, family and important others, including the way we spend our leisure time. Allowing us to experience the world are the five senses which can be seen to play an intermediate role.

Self-awareness exercises are essentially of the mind, being concerned with the thoughts in the head. The approach is thus underpinned by cognitive theory; it also has a behavioural component. Exercises presented here are adapted from a variety of sources.

Exercises in self-awareness

Awareness of thinking style

We have different ways of thinking; sometimes we think in a vertical or focused way, as when doing arithmetic. At other times our thinking may be more inclined to a lateral style, as, for instance, when we are engaged in creative work. We also have our own personal styles of thinking: some people tend towards a cause–effect style, others to a broader canvas style.

Other modes of thinking relate to self-esteem. For example, thinking strategies which direct the individual into areas likely to lead to successful outcomes are associated with high self-esteem, while those which direct her into areas with a low probability of success tend to be associated with low self-esteem (Fox 1997). Self-esteem can also be promoted by attributing successful outcomes to one's own efforts and poor outcomes to external factors over which one had no control (Blaine & Crocker 1993).

Or again, thinking can be influenced by the individual's locus of control (see Ch. 2 , p21): an internal locus, with its accompanying sense of self-reliance, seems to be related to high self-esteem, whereas an external locus seems to be related to lower levels of self-esteem (Fox 1997). Although our self-esteem owes much to value systems set up by the culture and society we belong to, it is also governed by our use of self-serving strategies such as the way we present ourselves (Carless & Fox 2003). To Carless & Fox, low self-esteem is more a defect in the use of self-enhancement strategies than a reflection of any deep sense of disregard.

The individual can review her own style in the following manner.

Take a few moments off to make a list of the thoughts that are going through your head and the dialogue that accompanies them. Write them down. Repeat this twice later in the day. Compare the items on your three lists and notice if a pattern emerges. Is some particular thought claiming your attention? If so, how do you approach it? Do you see it as a problem to be solved or do you let it dominate you? If you are trying to solve it, are you using a focused method or are you keeping your mind open and receptive to fresh ideas? Both approaches are useful. Do you have a tendency to favour one more than the other?

Do you tend to think in ways which enhance your self-esteem such as steering the self in directions likely to lead to success? Or do you tend to cling to areas where success is less likely to occur? Do you make a point of interpreting outcomes in ways which show yourself in the best possible light or do you let negative interpretations assert themselves?

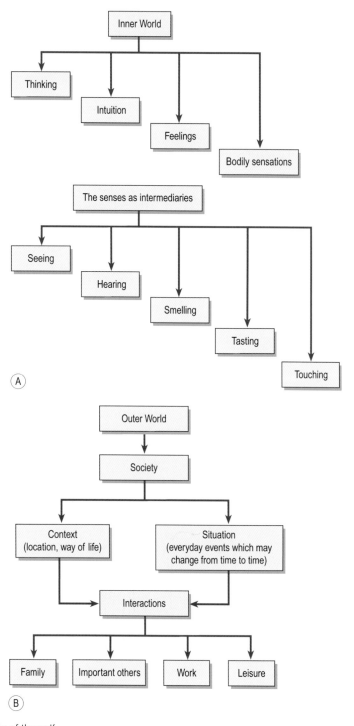

Figure 17.1•Aspects of the self.

Again, do you see most problems as being surmountable and, to some extent, within your control? Or do you, generally speaking, feel yourself to be a pawn in the hands of fate and a victim of events? This is an opportunity to examine your attitude towards yourself and to ask if it is serving you well.

Awareness of intuitive powers

Our glorification of the rational has all but eclipsed the imagination in everyday affairs. We distrust intuition or, at best, give it short shrift. Our belief in the undeniable value of logical thinking does not, however, mean we must stifle the imagination, and those who underestimate its power may do so at their peril for it communicates with the inner self.

Sit quietly and allow yourself to become relaxed. Follow your breathing, and next time you breathe out, release all your tension in a long sigh. Scan your body, checking that all your muscles are relaxed. Imagine yourself in a place of beauty and peace. Allow your thoughts to drift in and out. Focus on a matter that has been claiming your attention recently … keep it light … there's no compulsion to resolve it at this moment … just listen to yourself … tune into yourself … be receptive to any ideas that float into your head … listen to your gut feeling; you can judge its merits later … just be open to yourself … When you are ready, bring your visualization to an end.

Awareness of feelings (emotions)

The capacity to use our mental abilities is strongly influenced by the emotional state of the individual, whose thinking brain can be overwhelmed, even paralysed by the emotional brain (Goleman 1996). Goleman emphasizes the importance of self-awareness in this area.

To focus on emotions need not be seen as self-indulgence. Rather, it is a form of self-examination which can provide us with insights and perhaps indicate useful paths of change. While our emotions may be said to enrich our lives on the one hand, they give us trouble on the other; some feelings can be so strong that they cloud our judgement and

others may be so uncomfortable that we repress the thought that gives rise to them. Anger and grief are two examples.

The handling of emotions requires skills which we have in varying degrees. In this connection Heron (1977) has picked out some salient points, which include the following:

- the degree to which we are aware of our emotional patterns
- whether we are inclined to express ourselves in controlled or in spontaneous ways
- our tendency either to share our feelings with other people or to withhold them.

1. Awareness of emotional patterns

We need to recognize our feeling patterns and tendencies to react in certain ways. Only when we are aware of them can we see how they may be influencing our behaviour.

2. Control or spontaneity

Many situations require us to hide our feelings, but there are other occasions when a more spontaneous response is called for. Whether we express our emotion or hold it back is governed not only by the circumstances but also by our general inclination. Some individuals have a tendency to respond in one way rather than another. If so, are they aware of it?

3. Sharing our feelings

Self-disclosure is part of the process of deepening a relationship and this applies whether the individual is making the disclosure or listening to another making hers. Although the sharing of feelings involves taking a risk, the relationship is unlikely to develop without it. Most relationships are enriched by some degree of self-disclosure; the extent to which it occurs depends partly on the nature of the relationship and partly on the inclination of the individual. Is she *inclined* to share her feelings?

Awareness of the body

From time to time, the body needs attention. In between, we spend periods of varying length without giving it a thought. Breathing, digestion, skin sensations can all be ignored; muscle tension also passes unnoticed. If we are interested in reducing muscle tension, it can be useful to make a point of listening to the body occasionally.

Allow your thoughts to focus on your body. Notice any sensations, such as stomach rumblings, joint discomfort, itches or the tendency to sigh … things you normally disregard as you concentrate on your work. Perhaps you are also ignoring feelings of tension in your muscles, in your back, your shoulders, your face or your writing arm … try focusing on those areas and releasing the tension … realize that you could just as easily increase it … try for a moment deliberately exaggerating the tension in the muscles. . . notice that you have the power to switch it on or off … simply by making a conscious effort you can increase or decrease those feelings of tension. Explore that idea for a few moments.

Awareness of the environment

This aspect of the self is concerned with information from the five senses: sight, sound, smell, taste and touch. Much of this activity never gets through to our consciousness, which may be to our advantage if we are concentrating on a piece of work. However, it is through our senses that we experience our environment and are able to relate to the world.

Sit on your own. Allow the breath out to carry all your tensions with it. Bring your mind to focus on what is happening around you: the sounds inside the building and outside … the smells of the kitchen/office/shop/classroom/ factory … the taste of the coffee you just drank … the arrangement of the furniture in the room … the colour of the decoration … the temperature of the room … the feel of the chair underneath you, the pen or the peeler in your hand … focus on each one separately for a few moments. If you are driving, notice the countryside. If you are waiting in a bus queue, pick out the different sounds in the street … if you are walking to the letterbox, notice the front gardens along the way …

Notice how the exercise has the effect of taking you away from your preoccupations and giving you an acute experience of the present moment.

Awareness of the way we relate to others

People can only know about us from what we show of ourselves: our appearance, general demeanour and what we say. These are outer aspects of the individual and disclose much or little of the inner self, depending on the level of intimacy. All that can be known about a person is what she consciously or unconsciously reveals, so that what we reveal is important since it establishes our identity in the world. Our behaviour, whether verbal or non-verbal, creates us as individuals in other people's eyes.

Verbal behaviour refers to the actual words spoken. Non-verbal behaviour includes aspects of speech such as tone of voice, timing, emphasis, accent (para-linguistic features), as well as facial expression, eye contact, gesture, posture, physical proximity, clothes and appearance (Argyle 1978). The way we respond within the interaction provides a further level of behaviour: how we prompt, cut in and listen.

Assertiveness

We also define ourselves by our readiness to be assertive or not (see Ch. 1). Assertiveness involves knowing how to advance our life goals while respecting the interests of other people. Put another way, it means insisting on having our *own* interests respected while other people advance *their* goals. For example, are we able to refuse a request which we feel is unreasonable?

Do you find it easy to say 'No' to a request in a situation where saying 'Yes' makes you feel you are being taken advantage of? Can you think of an occasion when this occurred? How did you react? Were you happy with the outcome? If not, how did you feel? In your imagination, go back to the occasion. Recreate the scene and rescript your part with you saying 'No'. What effect does this have on the other person? What effect does it have on you? Now ask yourself why you said 'Yes' in the first place. How would you deal with a similar request in the future?

Promoting a relationship while retaining a feeling of self is one of the social skills. This feeling of self is tied up with our self-esteem, i.e. the degree to which we feel we have worth. Low self-esteem is linked with non-assertive behaviour, high self-esteem with assertive behaviour. To increase her assertiveness, the individual needs to recognize her personal strengths and qualities; she has to question the appropriateness of the role she is playing and explore new possibilities. This will give her more rewarding personal experiences.

A script for an individual assessing her own assertiveness (or non-assertiveness) might run as follows.

Allow yourself to feel relaxed before you begin. Run through a relaxing procedure until you feel very calm and tuned in to yourself. Let your thoughts focus on a person you know … someone you are not close to … someone with whom you have had difficulties but are obliged to see from time to time …

Let your mind gently focus on this person … let her take shape … notice how she looks: her expression … what she is wearing … spend a little time creating her presence … then see yourself also, including your expression, posture and clothes, as you, in your mind's eye, greet this person.

Observe your actions … do they strike the right note? … is the conversation balanced in the sense that neither person is acting aggressively to the other's submissive behaviour? … if it is unbalanced what, if anything, do you think you should do about it? … it may be that you feel your behaviour is appropriate … on the other hand, you may wish to modify your style, to make it more assertive … you will know best what is needed in the situation . . .

If you decide to modify your style, consider ways in which you might begin … test these out in your imagination … notice how your new behaviour feels … spend a few minutes mentally experiencing the scene …

Evidence relevant to rehabilitation

Brain injury can result in self-awareness deficits. Bach & David (2006) reviewed the literature on self-awareness deficits following acquired brain injury and found that lack of social self-awareness was a predictor of behavioural disturbance. These findings were independent of cognitive and executive function. Such deficits can persist for months, even years after severe injury and greatly impede the rehabilitation process (Prigatano 2005). Self-awareness re-education may help to restore normality.

BENEFITS AND POTENTIAL PITFALLS

1. Exercises such as those described above can heighten our awareness of ourselves and the way we relate to other people. We also, in the process, deepen our self-knowledge. Through self-awareness exercises we learn to 'listen' to the self in all its aspects, and to tune in to its nuances. Self-awareness exercises, by their emphasis on 'exploring, experimenting, experiencing', thus lead us to a better understanding of ourselves (Stevens 1971).

2. Getting to know oneself can be a painful process, while changing oneself is difficult. Our efforts are, however, rewarded by the discovery that we have more power than we realized to control our lives, a thought which itself engenders a sense of calm.

3. As a relaxation technique, self-awareness might be said to be at the other end of the scale from distraction (the diversion of attention away from the self). Each is effective on its own but together they complement one another, self-awareness protecting the individual from the hazards of denial while distraction protects her from too much introspection.

KEY MESSAGES

- Awareness of the self leads to an increase in self-knowledge.
- Self-awareness helps us to see ourselves as we really are. This insight helps to enhance personal relationships.
- Being aware of the self involves living in the present, responding in the here-and-now. This helps the individual to achieve successful outcomes.
- Exercises to raise self-awareness are broadly classified into inner world and outer world domains – the inner concerned with thinking and feelings, the outer with how we relate to other people.
- Through these exercises we learn to 'listen' to the self and to others.
- Self-awareness helps us discover sources of inner strength which enhance self-confidence and peace of mind.

Chapter Eighteen

18

Imagery

This chapter is addressed to healthcare professionals who wish to use imagery to enhance the relaxation experience. It is different from the use of imagery in psychotherapy and other forms of counselling where it may be used to get in touch with repressed thoughts and feelings. The aim of imagery, as represented in this chapter, is to encourage people to have positive emotions.

Introduction and rationale

Imagery has already been mentioned during discussion of breathing, passive relaxation, the Alexander technique and self-awareness. Here imagery is considered in its own right.

Achterberg (1985) defines imagery as 'the thought process that invokes and uses the senses'. Sight, sound, smell, taste and touch modalities can all be involved in this activity, which may take place in the absence of any external stimulus. It could be said that imagery is thinking in pictures as opposed to thinking with words.

The importance of the image was underlined by Aristotle who said that without it, thought is impossible. Einstein also found imagery an essential component of thought. It is particularly associated with the creative aspect of thinking. However, we are forming images all the time, whether making plans for the future, remembering items from the past or creating fantasy in realms beyond our experience.

How can imagery relieve stress? A cognitive explanation was advanced by Dossey (1988) who suggested that imagery brought about a change in the individual's perceptions. Many researchers, on the other hand, consider that the mechanism lies in the distraction created by the pleasant imagery which can divert the mind from intrusive thoughts. There are also physiological explanations; for example, McCance & Heuther (1998) proposed that pleasant images could trigger the release of endorphins and create an analgesic effect, and Melzack & Wall (1983) put forward their theory whereby pain messages are blocked from consciousness by a 'gate' mechanism which shuts them off when the neural pathways are loaded with other information (which may include imagery).

Although the precise mechanism of imagery is unknown, it is believed to involve the right cerebral hemisphere. Consequently, this chapter contains a short discussion on the concept of laterality which is followed by a section on the unconscious mind. Examples of different kinds of imagery will be found in a later part of the chapter.

Laterality

The cerebral cortex is divided into two hemispheres, each of which has four lobes: frontal, parietal, temporal and occipital. Research indicates that the hemispheres have specialized roles (Fig. 18.1). One side, usually the left, is believed to process logical thought and language. It is involved in linear, analytic and rational thinking, reading, writing and mathematical activity and is normally the dominant hemisphere. The right hemisphere is seen as dealing with information of a non-rational nature,

being concerned with creative thinking, fantasy, metaphor, imagery, dreams, analogies, intuition and emotion, including feelings of stress, and is normally the non-dominant hemisphere. However, it is believed to acquire dominance during altered states of consciousness, i.e. states of mental functioning which seem different to the individual from the ordinary pattern experienced by her (Atkinson et al 1999). Deep relaxation is one such state. Others include dreaming, drug-induced states, hypnosis, meditation, day-dreaming and guided imagery. During these states, the influence of the left brain is reduced which allows material from the right hemisphere, normally hidden, to become accessible. Thus, the altered state is seen as providing a path to the interior of the self.

Lyman et al (1980) claim to have found a connection between images and emotions, having shown experimentally that emotionally charged situations are more likely than neutral ones to be accompanied by imagery. They posit a direct relationship between the right hemisphere (which is associated with imagery) and the autonomic system (which governs the physiological responses associated with emotion).

The link between imagery and physiological processes can be demonstrated by imagining a lemon (Barber et al 1964).

Visualize its exterior shape, colour, scent and texture; then slice it across the middle, look at the pale, glistening flesh, squeeze it gently and watch the juice dripping from it; take the cut end to your mouth and lick it. Notice your mouth watering.

Electromyographic recordings also demonstrate associations between visualization and physiological activity: positive imagery has been shown to lower muscle tension levels and negative imagery to raise them (Jacobson 1938, McGuigan 1971).

In applying these findings, it is suggested that a useful approach to stress relief and relaxation is through methods which involve the right hemisphere (Davis et al 2000).

The unconscious

Freud (1973) viewed the unconscious as a repository of repressed fears and unresolved emotions.

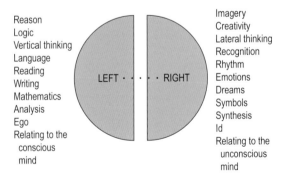

Reason
Logic
Vertical thinking
Language
Reading
Writing
Mathematics
Analysis
Ego
Relating to the conscious mind

LEFT · · · · RIGHT

Imagery
Creativity
Lateral thinking
Recognition
Rhythm
Emotions
Dreams
Symbols
Synthesis
Id
Relating to the unconscious mind

Figure 18.1 • Left and right hemisphere activities. (Adapted from Shone 1982.)

It thus represented aspects of ourselves which we wished to forget. Its contents were only available in certain states such as dreaming, when the conscious mind was less dominant. A Jungian view of the unconscious, however, saw it as also containing the seed of infinite new possibilities deriving from insight, intuition and inspiration (Fordham 1966, Jung 1963). Thus, while Freud viewed it in negative terms, Jung's view was primarily positive.

Whatever their theoretical position, writers in general agree that the unconscious operates not with the language of logic but through pictures, emotions, senses, symbols and imagery, i.e. the concerns of the right hemisphere. Hidden and elusive, the unconscious does not lend itself to direct investigation, either from the scientist or from the self-analysing individual. It is this quality of elusiveness that moves Jung to speak of the difficulty of penetrating one's own being. His archetypal figures (earth mother, wise man, persona, shadow, anima and animus) are the expression of attempts to find new ways of gaining access to the unconscious.

The inner guide

Arising out of these ideas is the concept of the 'inner guide', a mental construct that links the individual with her inner self. In its role as channeller of information from the unconscious, the inner guide may be seen as the personification of the intuitive self. It can take forms other than those of archetypal figures and may appear as any person or animal whose attributes have appealed to the individual's imagination.

Typically the inner guide evolves in the mind during a session of deep relaxation, using an imagined setting of rich sensory quality. Oyle (1976) suggests a place of peace and beauty such as a mountain lake or a natural grotto, while Ferrucci (1982) prefers an Alpine peak reached after an arduous climb. A figure is conjured up; it advances slowly. The visualizer welcomes the approaching figure, noticing everything about it: what it looks like, how it is dressed, who, if anyone, it resembles. A dialogue ensues. Ferrucci warns against the possibility of the guide being no more than a self-deceiving fantasy and suggests criteria for testing its authenticity.

- Does it bring answers which come from the self?
- Does it bring understanding?
- Does it carry a sense of rightness?
- Does its message make sense in the light of reason and morality?

- Will its advice stand up in real-life situations?

Even after acceptance of the guide as authentic, its advice should always be scrutinized and not blindly accepted. Although the guide is an aspect of the inner self, it may not be working in the individual's best interests. On the other hand, too sceptical an attitude will tend to generate fewer ideas than a trusting one.

The individual need not feel restricted to one guide and may find it useful to have one male and one female, each supplying complementary wisdom. A hazard of working with a number of inner guides, however, is that the personality may come to be seen as a collection of separate entities when the aim of the exercise is to achieve integration.

Any meeting with an inner guide should be rounded off with words of gratitude, respect and appreciation as this helps to strengthen the individual's respect for her inner self. Continuity also is important and may be established by a contract to meet on another occasion.

Therapeutic effects of imagery

Imagery can be used in a therapeutic sense to promote the following:

- Self-development and psychological change. These effects are expanded in Chapter 19.
- Relaxation. Zahourek (1988), working in a nursing context, sees imagery as a therapeutic tool which can reinforce the message to relax.
- Healing. This is an area not covered in the present work.

Procedure of a therapeutic imagery session

Relaxation

For the imagery to be effective, the individual should first be in a state of relaxation. Fanning (1988) regards relaxation as 'an absolute prerequisite' of effective imagery. The individual may use any method she finds helpful, but passive approaches are seen as being the most appropriate (Achterberg 1985). Thus relaxation is a precondition as well as a result of therapeutic imagery.

Introductory remarks to participants

As with other approaches, a short passage of explanation is necessary.

Imagery is about building pictures in the mind. The pictures can be pleasant or unpleasant. The first kind induce a feeling of calm, the second, of unease.

The relaxing effect of pleasant imagery is partly due to the distraction it creates from stressful thoughts. Day-dreaming is an example of this kind of imagery. However, the imagination can also bring us nearer to our inner selves, and this aspect of it is used to help people discover new possibilities within themselves, thereby enriching their lives. This kind of imagery is more structured than day-dreaming.

You'll find it helpful to make yourself relaxed before you begin.

Exercises in imagery

Exercises which use different kinds of imagery are then presented. They may include any of the following:

- Single sense
- Imagery as symbol
- Imagery as metaphor
- Colour imagery
- Guided imagery

Termination

A session of imagery should be gradually brought to an end. First, the image is deliberately allowed to fade. Then the visualizer slowly brings her attention back to the room in which she is lying, and in her own time opens her eyes. In the next few minutes she gives her limbs a gentle stretch and then resumes normal activity.

Exploring single senses

Some people find it easier than others to conjure up images. Not only do people differ in the vividness and clarity of the images they create, but they also differ in their ability to control the image once formed (Finke 1989). Image making is thus a skill with more than one facet.

There is some evidence to suggest that image forming can be improved with practice, although the extent of any such improvement has not been determined (Kosslyn 1983, Lichstein 1988). Nevertheless, exercises are often used in the belief that they help to develop innate potential. A difficulty in imaging should not, however, be seen as a deficit but rather as a manifestation of the many ways in which human beings differ from one another. People who report difficulty in forming images may also describe a sensation which fulfils the same function in their thought processes.

For those who wish to explore their capacity to create images, however, the following exercises are presented. They use the modalities of sight, sound, smell, taste, touch, temperature and kinaesthetic sense. A total of 15–20 seconds can be spent on each item.

Sight

Visualize:
- a shape: circle/triangle/square
- an oak tree
- a snail
- a sailing boat
- a button
- a strand of hair.

Sound

Since auditory images tend to be less dominant than visual ones, it can be useful, when evoking the former, to surround oneself with an imaginary mist or darkness which swallows up any visual images and releases sounds in isolation. Imagine:
- the wind blowing through the trees/through river sedges/through sheets on a clothes line
- the ring of your telephone
- different people calling your name
- horses' hooves on different surfaces: cobblestone/tarmac/hard sand/deep mud
- scales played on the piano
- traffic starting off
- water flowing along a rocky stream bed/lapping on a lake shore/cascading from a height.

Smell

Slowly conjure up, one by one, the following smells:
- thyme trodden underfoot
- petrol fumes
- newly baked bread
- hyacinth scent
- chlorine
- new mown grass
- vanilla.

Taste

Imagine the taste of:
- sprouts
- figs
- banana
- mayonnaise
- grapefruit
- toothpaste.

Touch

Let other sensory images fade as you turn your attention to those of touch. Evoke the following tactile images:
- shaking hands
- standing barefoot on loose/dry sand
- running your fingers over satin/velvet/sacking
- brushing past fur
- holding a smooth pebble
- threading a needle.

Temperature

Imagine sensations of heat and cold:
- drinking a hot liquid
- sunlight falling on your arm
- moving from a warm room to a cool one
- holding an ice-cube
- stepping into a warm bath.

Kinaesthetic sense

This sense is the perception of body movement. Feel yourself engaged in a form of activity:
- swimming
- running on grass

- sawing wood
- throwing a ball
- climbing a sand dune
- hanging a coat on a peg
- stirring syrup.

Imagery drawn from all sense modalities

Fanning (1988) suggests an exercise which draws on a variety of sense modalities.

> Take a fruit that you like, say an orange. Feel its texture … weight … size … notice its shape … colour and surface markings … is it firm or soft? … smell it … then dig your nail into the peel and begin to tear it off. Listen to the faint sound of the tearing. As you peel the orange, notice how the flesh gets exposed here and there, releasing a new smell. Separate the segments and put one in your mouth … bite through its juicy flesh … feel the sensation of the juice running over your tongue … recognize the taste of orange …

From the above exercise it can be seen that variety of sensory detail helps to build a vivid mental image. When we visualize a scene we usually draw on more than one sense modality, and we can make the scene still more vivid by adding further sensory information. Images of sight, sound, smell, texture, temperature and the sensation of body movement can all be used to enrich the mental picture. Guided imagery (p157) develops these ideas.

Symbolic imagery

Jung (1963) writes that symbols serve to connect us with the unconscious; they are keys which can unlock the deeper parts of the psyche. Symbols also feature in the writings of Assagioli where he notes the tendency for people to project meaningful ideas onto them. One of Assagioli's best known examples is his visualization of a rose (1965), paraphrased below.

> Picture in your mind a rose bush … see its root … its stem … its leaves. Crowning the stem is a rose in tight bud. See it folded inside its protective sepals. As you watch, the sepals

begin to roll back, revealing the closed flower, firmly and intricately packed … gradually, the petals begin to unfold and as they do, you may feel a blossoming also taking place within you … the rose continues to open and as you gaze at it, and smell its perfume, perhaps you can feel its rhythm resonating with your own rhythm … stay with the rose and as it opens further, revealing its centre, allow an image to take shape – one that represents whatever is creative and meaningful within you … focus on the image … and let it speak to you …

The symbol is seen here as a phenomenon to be experienced rather than decoded. It is suggested that by identifying with the symbol, the individual can discover new aspects of herself. This idea has been developed by Ferrucci, a student of Assagioli's. Two examples of Ferrucci's visualizations (1982) are presented below (in slightly altered form).

The fount

Imagine a rocky cleft in which a natural spring rises. It is a warm summer day. See the bubbling jet of water sparkling in the sunlight … listen to its gurgling and splashing … the water is clear and pure … cup your hands and drink from it … imagine the liquid travelling down your throat and into your body … in your mind's eye step into the spring and feel the water flowing over you … your feet, legs and the whole of your body … imagine it also flowing through your thoughts … and through your emotions … feel the water cleansing you … let its purity unite with your purity … let its energy become your energy … and as the fount continues to renew itself, feel life within you also renewing itself …

The bell

Picture a meadow on a warm day. Perhaps you are lying in the soft grass, surrounded by scented wild flowers. In a nearby village church, a bell begins to peal. The sound it makes is pure and clear and as it reaches you, it seems to arouse within you a deep, hidden joy … the sound fades for a moment as the wind changes … then … it returns … carried back to you, this time with renewed force … filling the air and echoing through the valley … and

as you listen, the sound seems to vibrate inside you … resonating with your own melody … and awakening new possibilities within you …

The use of metaphor

Imagery lies at the heart of metaphor. Metaphor itself, by describing one thing in terms of another, offers a fresh approach – a new and more telling interpretation.

Three items which illustrate the use of metaphor in relaxation imagery follow. In each one, the individual identifies with the image.

The rag doll

Sit in an armchair. Close your eyes. Take one deep breath low down in your chest. Then let your breathing set its own rhythm … listen to it … and as you listen to it, imagine a rag doll … see its soft floppy arms and legs … its lolling head … its slumped body … inert … immobile.

Now, try seeing yourself as that rag doll. Conjure up a feeling of being slumped … the weight of your arms dragging your shoulders down … your head rolling into the chairback … your face expressionless … your jaw relaxed … feel the passive quality of the rag doll … and as you continue to sit there … enjoy the feeling of being passive …

The fragment of seaweed

Lie down in a quiet place. Close your eyes. Breathe in deeply once … then relax into the rhythm of your natural breathing …

Picture a length of seaweed, rich, dark green, leafy seaweed, floating in the shallows. Air pockets keep it buoyant and allow it to bob up and down. As it floats, it changes shape, drawn this way and that as the currents swirl beneath it … pulling it … twisting it … stretching it … bunching it …

Now, picture yourself as that piece of seaweed … notice how limp your body feels … your outstretched arms and legs gently swept to and fro … imagine the wave passing underneath you … lifting you up as it rises, and lowering you as it dips, but always buoying you up … feel your body giving to the movement of the water …

The jelly

Settle yourself in a peaceful place. Close your eyes and listen to your breathing ... listen to it getting calmer with every moment that passes ...

Imagine a jelly not quite set. It has been turned out of its mould and stands, holding itself together but not yet firm. Every time the plate is moved, it wobbles.

Now, think of yourself as that jelly. You are standing on a dish, and every time someone knocks the table, a ripple runs through you. You yourself are not able to initiate the movement; only others can do that by bumping into your table or moving your dish ... and, every time this happens, you wobble. One bump, and you wobble several times ... imagine you are about to be bumped into ... feel your body limp ... let all the tension go out of it ... let yourself become a wobbly jelly ...

Transformations

Images can also undergo transformations: harsh images can give way to smooth ones. Fanning (1988) shows how negative emotions, represented by harsh images, can be influenced to move in a more positive direction, when the harsh images are transformed into smooth ones.

Imagine the sound of discordant music ... listen to its harsh tones ... and as you do, let your painful thought express itself in terms of the dissonant notes ... feel the mood of your difficulty resonating with the sound. Then gradually allow the image to undergo a transformation ... follow the music as it slowly resolves into harmonies ... and, as the harmonies fill the air, experience the beginnings of a change in your feelings ...

Other examples of negative imagery resolving into more pleasant forms are:
- sour lemon juice into sweet lemon sorbet
- sandpaper into silky fabric.

Both come from Fanning (1988). The next two are drawn from Davis et al (1988):
- a screaming siren into a woodwind melody
- the glare of a searchlight into the soft glow of a lamp.

Four of the sense modalities (taste, touch, sound and sight) are represented in these examples. The fifth, smell, is illustrated in the transformation from burning rubber into smouldering pine logs.

The above are simply examples. The most effective imagery is that which the individual creates for herself, choosing the context to which she can best relate.

Distancing

The distress caused by unpleasant events can be overwhelming. Moreover, the intensity of the emotion aroused by them may cloud the individual's judgement. In order to gain a more objective view, she may find it useful to draw back from the scene mentally: in effect, to distance herself. Certain images promote the feeling of being able to put a distance between herself and the situation:
- a leaf floating downstream
- clouds moving across the sky
- helium-filled balloons rising
- bubbles being blown away
- a train receding along a straight track.

Colour

People say they have favourite colours. Is this because certain colours make them feel good? And is this governed by the association that those colours have with pleasant events in their lives? It is generally believed that red is a stimulating colour and blue a soothing one but to what extent is the preference for one over the other tied up with the mood of the moment? Such notions might help to explain why a person does not always choose the same colour. Or does she simply become sated with one colour and feel the need to replace it with another (as in decorations, clothes, etc.)? These are psychological considerations, although the aesthetic aspects of colour give the topic a further dimension.

However, in the present context we are concerned with psychological aspects. Certainly colours can create strong effects. Some of these can be explored through exercises in colour imagery. The following example is adapted from the work of an autogenic therapist, Kai Kermani (1990).

With your eyes closed let the word 'colour' float into your mind. The word may first evoke one particular colour although others will quickly follow. Take the one that first appears. Stay with it. Let it develop in any way it wants to: flooding your field of vision, appearing in patches, little flecks or any other arrangement. Concentrate on the colour in a passive way, letting it speak to you. Does it remind you of anything? Does it trigger any special feelings or memories? If it has no effect on you, try 'stepping into' it and allowing it to surround you … notice any effect it now has on you …

After a few minutes, or when you are ready, allow the colour to draw itself away from you. In your mind's eye, watch it resuming the form it had in the beginning.

If colour can indeed influence our mood, then colour visualization could have particular value. We could mentally surround ourselves with single colours to gain specific effects, soothing our feelings when we are anxious and raising our mood when we are depressed. Single colours are again explored in the following two exercises.

Imagine finding yourself in a room decorated exclusively in a colour of your choice. See the entire room in this one colour, the walls, ceiling, paintwork, carpet, upholstery. If you have difficulty, try going through the motions of painting the walls and hanging the curtains. Totally immerse yourself in this colour and notice the effect it has on you … does it relax you or give you a lift? … why did you pick it? … what associations does it have for you? … stay with it long enough to absorb its full effect … then let it fade.

Now picture yourself in a room decorated in a colour you don't like … Surround yourself with this colour, let it permeate your consciousness (so long as it doesn't disturb you, in which case stop the exercise) … Ask yourself why you dislike this colour and what effect it is having on you … When you are ready, let the colour fade and be replaced by the colour of your choice before ending the visualization.

It is preferable to end colour imagery sessions with a colour that the visualizer feels comfortable with, in order to carry away a rewarding sensation.

Ernst & Goodison (1981) present a sequence in which colour flows to and from the visualizer. It is reproduced here in modified form.

First relax yourself using any method you find works for you. Close your eyes if they are not already closed. Let your mind be as still as possible. Pick a colour that feels right for you. Pick it spontaneously and see it before your eyes. You can picture it as brushstrokes of paint, coloured cloth, tinted smoke or coloured atmosphere. Let it extend all round you. Notice its quality, its tone and be aware of any associations it has for you. Feel yourself relating to this colour, harmonizing with it, becoming infused with it. Imagine yourself absorbing the colour through every pore of your skin until your body is filled with it …

Now … let the colour begin to radiate from you … feel yourself releasing it … making it expand all round you until it gradually comes to fill the room you are in. As you continue to generate more colour, see if you can fill the building you are in … pause for a moment … then slowly begin to draw the colour back, first from the building … then from the room … watching it get more condensed … until it gathers in a cloud around you … feel yourself bathed in this colour … now … absorb it back into your being … into the very organs of your body … pause again … then watch it drawing itself away from all parts of you … feel yourself being emptied of the colour. Convert it back to the paint, cloth or smoke in which it started. Be aware of how you feel after doing the exercise. Notice any effect it had on you.

Chakras

In hatha yoga vital energy is seen as being focused in specified areas of the body known as 'chakras'. These are situated at:

- the base of the spine
- the lower abdomen
- the navel
- the heart
- the throat
- the brow
- the crown of the head.

Each chakra is associated with one of the colours of the spectrum: the base of the spine with red, the lower abdomen with orange, the navel with yellow, the heart with green, the throat with blue, the brow with indigo and the crown of the head with violet.

Kermani (1990) presents a passage of healing imagery based on the chakras, which is reproduced here in slightly altered form.

See yourself lying in a natural setting of your choice. The sun is shining and it is warm and pleasant. Look around you ... build the scene. What plants are growing? Do they have a scent? What sounds can you hear? Feel the sun on your body. Imagine its rays bringing warmth to all parts of you. Imagine, also, the light broken up into its component parts so that it lies in a coloured spectrum across your body: warm red rays falling on your legs and hips, relaxing and warming them; orange rays casting a gentle light over your lower trunk; a soft yellow light glowing across your stomach; green rays casting a soothing light over your heart; blue light bathing your throat and lower face, a cool indigo light falling on your brow and violet light around your head.

Picture a ray of blue light travelling from each eye ... allow these twin rays to carry away any tension ... carrying it into the vastness of space ... as it recedes, feel yourself relaxing ... finally, a silver light appears ... let it gather up all the colours and ... as it does, let it draw away any remaining tension from your body, dissolving it and leaving you in a state of deep calmness ... imagine the silver light spreading around you to form a circle ... allow the circle to include others who also wish to share this peace. They stay for a few moments and as they leave, you notice they have left a gift for you ... it is a gift which you will recognize ...

When you are ready, gently allow the scene to fade ... slowly, bring your attention back to the room in which you are lying. Feel the floor beneath you as you open your eyes.

White light

The Rosicrucians, a brotherhood formed during the Renaissance, regarded white light as a symbol of guidance, inspiration and healing. The idea has been developed by Samuels & Samuels (1975).

Take yourself in your mind's eye to a place that is special for you. Imagine it filled with brilliant white light ... let that light flow through you ... filling your body and your mind ... healing you ... strengthening you ... renewing you.

Guided imagery

Definition and description

Guided imagery is a therapeutic technique which uses the imagination to achieve desirable outcomes such as decreased pain perception and reduced anxiety (Ackerman & Turkoski 2000). It has been described as an inner communication involving all the senses and is believed to form an emotional connection between the mind and the body (Tusek & Cwynar 2000). Typically, the participant is led through a scene enriched by sensual descriptions in the belief that the state induced creates access to a deeper concsiousness which will release latent healing abilities. The method can be used in most situations of pain and distress and is a useful adjunct to conventional medical and psychiatric treatments (Tusek & Cwynar 2000).

The visualizer conjures up a naturalistic scene, often of her own choosing, and moves around within it, noticing particularly its sensory content. A meadow, forest, beach or garden makes a suitable setting. Within this context, it is helpful to introduce a path and for three reasons: it can suggest a goal, provide a passage for the inner guide or simply carry the visualizer through the scene.

Where imagery is being presented to a group, it is convenient for the instructor to decide on a particular scene and to suggest its basic structure. For example, if a meadow is decided on, the instructor can suggest other features such as a stream and a backdrop of distant hills. The time of year and the weather can make the scene more vivid. The visualizer is asked to notice the scents and sounds as well as the appearance of the scene. It is left to the instructor as to how much information is offered. The participant fills in the detail.

The following paragraphs (adapted from Lichstein 1988) give the flavour of guided imagery.

Please get comfortable and close your eyes. As your mind becomes more peaceful, your body will also lose some of its tension. I am going to ask you to imagine a scene which you find pleasant and relaxing. Take a moment to choose the setting ...

Let your scene take shape ... do not force it in any way... just allow it to form by building its sensory detail ... create it visually ... making it as vivid as you can ... imagine the sounds that accompany it ... the scents that float in the air ... the textures that surround you ... feel the warmth of the sun on your skin ... find a path and experience the sensation of moving through the scene ... feel the tension leaving your body ... feel it being carried away each time you breathe out ... and enjoy the peace and calm of the scene you've created ...

For those who are looking for more specific scenes, try a sunny beach, a country meadow or a scented garden. (If the trainee suffers from hay fever, the first item is the best choice.)

A sunny beach

Imagine a stretch of shoreline ... make it rocky or smooth as you like ... notice the ground underfoot, is the sand wet and hard or is it dry and soft? ... if the sun is shining perhaps you can feel its warmth on your skin ... and see the light dancing on the water ... perhaps you can smell the sea air as it fills your nostrils ... what sounds can you hear? ... the gulls calling? ... the waves breaking? ... a motor chugging? ... you may decide to take a walk along the beach and, as you travel, notice how the scenery changes ... perhaps rocks begin to break up the surface of the beach, with pools beneath them ... you might feel you want to dip your hand into one of them ... and are surprised to find how warm this shallow water is ...

A country meadow

Picture yourself in the country ... perhaps you are in a field in early summer ... notice how long the grass is ... notice also how green it is ... are there wild flowers growing in it? ... which ones? ... can you smell their scent rising up? ... and is there a gentle breeze? ... enough to rustle the leaves on the trees? ... you may decide to wander along a narrow sheeptrack ... and as you cross the ground, perhaps you can hear the sound of water ... if it's a stream, notice how it runs ... whether smoothly or bubbling over rocks ... and how soon does it swing out of sight? ...

A scented garden

Let your mind conjure up the scene of a beautiful garden ... notice the way it is laid out ... the

trees, shrubs and flower beds ... perhaps it has just rained ... a gentle summer rain ... can you smell the air, warm and moist? ... in your imagination notice the scents around you ... is it honeysuckle? ... or is it thyme? ... or perhaps it's newly mown grass ... you may decide to walk through the garden, along a path which perhaps carries you under some trees ... notice how cool it is in their shade ... and how warm when you step out into the sunlight again ... notice also the trees which line the path ... and the texture of their bark ... in your mind's eye reach out to touch one of them ... was it smooth or deeply incised? ...

Evidence from research

Imagery is a safe, non-invasive and inexpensive procedure which requires no elaborate equipment. It is often employed together with other mind–body techniques as an adjunct to medical and psychological treatment and sometimes as sole therapy in the self-management of some mild conditions.

Pain is an area which has attracted much research. Here imagery has been used successfully in a wide range of conditions, including postoperative pain, (Laurion & Fetzer 2003), fibromyalgia (Fors et al 2002) and osteoarthritis (Baird & Sands 2004). Imagery has also been found useful in studies with children. A randomized controlled trial compared a combination of imagery and progressive relaxation with breathing routines in children with abdominal pain. It resulted in significantly fewer days with pain in the imagery group than in the breathing group (Weydert 2006). In these and other conditions it has been shown to be an effective self-management strategy for reducing the intensity of pain.

Guided imagery is a form of mind–body technique which is often used in the care of patients with cancer. Roffe et al (2005) conducted a systematic review to determine the effectiveness of guided imagery in the treatment of symptoms resulting from chemotherapy, such as nausea and vomiting. The researchers in this case found no strong evidence to indicate effectiveness of the intervention although they found some evidence to suggest that the imagery increased comfort and provided psychological support. Imagery training as an adjuvant therapy has also been found to reduce depression in community-dwelling cancer patients living in Sydney (Sloman 2002).

Halpin et al (2002) investigated the effects of guided imagery on cardiac surgery patients in a study in the USA and found that patients who practised the method had a shorter length of hospital stay and took fewer pain-killers than patients who did not practise it. This supports the earlier work of Tusek and Cwynar (2000) who found that imagery enhanced the experience of hospital patients.

However, imagery alone has rarely been studied as a treatment (Luskin et al 2000). It is usually combined with muscle relaxation techniques in the treatment of clinical conditions. For example, Cupal & Brewer (2001) found significantly less pain and re-injury anxiety following a course of relaxation and imagery among individuals undergoing rehabilitation after anterior cruciate reconstruction; and Johnson (2000) showed that the mood levels of competitive adults with long-term injuries could be significantly raised by relaxation and guided imagery. Sordoni and colleagues (2002) discuss different kinds of imagery in relation to athletic injury (p221).

Further evidence of the benefit of imagery may be found in Chapter 26 where reported trials involve the use of imagery and help to justify its widespread use in the clinical field.

 POTENTIAL PITFALLS

A cautious attitude is advised when using imagery. Potential pitfalls for imagery and goal-directed visualisation include the following.

1. Training in imagery and visualization should never be viewed as a substitute for medical treatment; wherever a disorder is present or suspected, medical help should be sought.
2. Imagery and visualization should only be used within the professional boundaries of the trainer.
3. People differ in their ability to form images. For those who find it difficult, a muscular approach might be more useful. On the other hand, since visualization is thought by some to be a learnable skill, practice may increase proficiency.
4. It is not the object of the exercise to create a hypnotic trance. Neither is it likely that one will occur. However, since some individuals are more susceptible than others, the possibility exists that the instructor may inadvertently create one. When a person is in a hypnotic trance, the power of suggestion becomes greater. That

being so, the instructor needs to be aware of the phenomenon of posthypnotic suggestion.

Posthypnotic suggestion results in the individual blindly carrying out injunctions outside the trance situation. For example, a statement such as 'When you go home you will assert yourself' would be indiscriminately applied. This would leave no room for reassessment of the situation which might, in changing circumstances, call for a modified approach.

Any suggestion which could be applied inappropriately outside the relaxation session should be avoided. Generally speaking, however, posthypnotic suggestion is not a problem since the individual tends to resist any exhortation that runs counter to her personal goals and moral principles (Lynn & Rhue 1977).

Larkin (1988) has useful advice for the health care professional who is offering imagery and is concerned to avoid hypnotizing the client: suggestion should be indirect, incorporating words like 'can', 'may', 'might' and 'perhaps'. Larkin emphasizes the importance of presenting the client with options, so that the suggestion finally adopted comes from the client herself.

However, if the instructor is in doubt as to the effect of her words, she can terminate the session with a cancelling statement (Shone 1982) along the lines of: 'Before you bring your visualization to an end, cancel any suggestion you do not wish to take effect in your waking life'.

As mentioned earlier, it is unlikely that unintentional hypnosis will occur.

5. Occasionally, a participant has difficulty returning from his visualization. Repeating the termination procedure usually resolves the problem. Another device is to include in the termination procedure some reference to feeling alert and refreshed.

KEY MESSAGES

- Imagery can enhance the relaxation experience.
- Symbolic imagery, metaphor, transformation and distancing are different ways in which imagery can be employed.
- Imagery should only be taught within the professional boundaries of the trainer.
- Imagery is a safe, non-invasive and low-cost form of treatment.
- Research suggests that this approach is potentially effective as an adjunct in some conditions.

Chapter Nineteen

19

Goal-directed visualization

Definition

Goal-directed visualization is a form of imagery which requires purposeful thinking leading to the fulfilment of self- directed goals.

In their book *Seeing with the mind's eye*, Samuels & Samuels (1975) describe a technique using imagery which has two phases, receptive and programmed. In the receptive phase, the individual passively listens to her inner self, drawing on her own wisdom. In the programmed phase, she engages in an active and deliberate thought process for the purpose of improving a situation or resolving a problem in her life. This is based on the assumption that, by repeatedly experiencing an outcome in the imagination, we increase the likelihood of it taking place in real life.

The Samuels' work has been developed by Achterberg (1985), Simonton et al (1986) and others in areas of medicine and healing, and by Shone (1984) and Fanning (1988) among others in areas of self-development and relaxation. Since in this book we are concerned with the latter area, the definitions of Fanning and Shone are appropriate. Fanning describes this kind of imagery as 'the conscious, volitional creation of mental sense impressions for the purpose of changing oneself'; Shone refers to it as a mental experience which helps to bring about desired outcomes. Implicit in both definitions is the notion of a goal.

How does this form of imagery differ from other forms? One answer is that it is more explicit than techniques which rely on metaphor and symbolism; it is also more purposeful than reverie states such as day-dreaming. How is it different from talking to yourself, reflecting and giving yourself advice? It may not *be* very different, but it does seek to offer a structured, step-by-step approach.

Rationale

The mechanism of visualization as a method for enhancing well-being is incompletely understood.

However, its success is often explained by the belief that the body cannot distinguish between the event as experienced and the event as imagined, a notion which is supported by a finding that the same physiological responses occur in each case (Dalloway 1992). As a result, new cognitive responses can be learned and practised in a safe environment from which, it is proposed, they can later be transferred to the event in real life; and if not wholly transferred, at least their liklihood of occurring is strengthened (Dalloway 1992).

Thus, tasks perceived to be difficult can lose some of their threat after being visualized with a successful outcome. This is mental rehearsal, a procedure which allows the individual to familiarize herself with the feared event and, in her imagination, to achieve her goal. Impending stressful events such as athletic competitions and performances of various kinds can be approached in this way (Farmer 1995).

The method

The method, which incorporates other techniques such as progressive relaxation and guided imagery (see Chs. 5 and 18), lends itself to a variety of conditions and situations, of which smoking cessation is one, and this topic is considered in some detail. The chapter opens with a general description of the procedure under the following headings:

- position
- preparatory relaxation
- special place
- receptive visualization
- positive self-statements or affirmations
- programmed visualization
- termination
- an additional technique.

Position

The visualizer lies down in a comfortable position in a dimly lit, warm room, free from noise and interruption. She closes her eyes.

Preparatory relaxation

Imagery is preceded by a short session of relaxation, since relaxation is generally regarded as a precondition

as well as an effect of visualization. Its role here is to create a 'state of balance, quietude and peace, free of negativity' (Ryman 1994). It allows the mind to be receptive to new information and tends to enhance the formation of images (Tusek & Cwynar 2000). The technique employed can be chosen by the individual, although Achterberg (1985) suggests that passive forms of muscle relaxation are more appropriate than tense–release, which she claims is ineffective for imagery work. Slow, gentle abdominal breathing will also help to induce deep relaxation. The visualizer may recite appropriate phrases such as 'My mind is calm and clear', 'I am open to images that will help me'.

Although this preliminary relaxation is common practice, there is little evidence to support its value as a facilitator of imagery (Lichstein 1988). Indeed, there are those who claim the opposite, i.e. that a totally relaxed body is accompanied by a mind devoid of images (Jacobson 1938). If muscular relaxation clears the mind of images, how can it also promote them? Lichstein (1988) refers to this as a matter yet to be resolved. Perhaps the answer lies in finding a level of relaxation which is deep enough to release tension but not so deep that images cannot form.

Special place

Lying quietly, the visualizer builds an imaginary scene or 'special place' as a retreat for relaxation and guidance (Davis et al 2000). The scene is rich in sensory images of sight, sound, smell, taste, texture, temperature, and gives her a feeling of peace and tranquillity. A beach, meadow, lake or forest all offer possibilities. The visualizer is encouraged to imagine how the body would feel in the special place, emphasizing sensations like sinking into springy turf or soft sand. Some time is spent initially setting the scene so that it can easily be recreated in subsequent visualizations. Since imagery is a right hemisphere activity, the constraints of logic do not apply. Thus, the special place may contain any figment of the imagination which the visualizer finds useful, as, for example, a permanent sunset in the background, a viewing screen in a forest clearing or a crystal ball in a mountain spring. It is in such a scene that the inner guide could appear (see Ch. 18, p151) and so there should be a clearly defined way in.

Some people prefer an indoor special place such as an attic room or a garden shed; others like to have both, using them on different occasions. There is no right or wrong way: whatever works for the individual is right.

Receptive visualization

The visualizer imagines herself in her special place. This is where she can feel in tune with herself and where she will be likely to gain insights. She is in a state of mind that allows her to listen to the part of herself which is normally beyond conscious awareness. It is a passive state of mind which in some ways resembles day-dreaming, but differs from the latter in that the visualizer is asking specific questions of herself (Samuels & Samuels 1975). Whether she is making a choice, sorting out a conflict, uncovering motivations or exposing automatic thoughts, the receptive visualization is a way of allowing intuitive insights to be released and inner wisdom to be revealed.

The visualizer should be advised that if uncontrollable or unpleasant feelings arise which she is not ready to deal with, she can walk away or distance herself in some other manner. She can also end the visualization. Otherwise she quietly tunes in to her unconscious. If ideas do not flow, the inner guide can be called and asked for advice (see Ch. 18, p151).

An example of a receptive visualization script is given below. (Allow 10–15 minutes for it.)

Lie down. Get yourself comfortable and close your eyes. Run through a relaxing procedure until you feel very calm. Visualize yourself lying in your special place. Evoke its atmosphere by mentally experiencing its sights, sounds, smells and textures. Feel at home there. Let your attention gently focus on the item that preoccupies you … just keep an open mind … quietly listen to the thoughts that flow through it … if you are stuck, call on your inner guide … listen to the wisdom your inner guide brings … realize that it is your own wisdom, coming from your deeper self … spend a few minutes listening to yourself …

When you are ready, end your visualization and gently bring your attention back to the room.

Write down any ideas that came to you. Consider them. Have you gained any insights? Do you want to change your way of handling this situation? Are there more positive ways of dealing with it?

Receptive visualizations can be repeated as often as they continue to provide insights.

Positive self-statements or affirmations

The positive self-statement, often referred to as an affirmation, helps the visualizer to see herself as being capable of realizing her aspiration and achieving her goal. Inherent in the affirmation is the suspension of self-doubt. Examples include the following:

- I believe in myself
- I am in control of my life
- I can achieve my aim.

While the above statements are of a general nature, additional affirmations relevant to the matter in question can also be composed. Thus, for a person wishing to become more relaxed, the following statements may be included:

- I feel calm
- I am at peace
- I can cope in stressful situations.

Positive self-statements need to be short, in the first person and in the present tense; the best ones are those composed by the individual herself (Fanning 1988). When repeated, they act like self-hypnotic suggestions, influencing the individual's view of herself in a positive direction and adding force to the positive images of the programmed visualization (described below).

Programmed visualization

In this phase, the individual may work on images that emerged during the receptive phase, turning them over and trying them out in different forms in her imagination. When she finds the most effective solution to her problem, she visualizes herself as instrumental in achieving it. Actions are imagined which allow her to feel herself displaying the qualities she wants to possess. Goals are mentally reached with the individual operating as their successful agent. By daily repetition, the new images of herself start to blend with her self-image, tending to generate still more positive internal dialogue and, in the manner of a self-fulfilling prophecy, increasing the likelihood of the desired outcome in real life.

Sometimes, while in the programmed stage, the visualizer gets 'stuck'. In this case, returning to the receptive stage may help to clear the block.

On other occasions, the receptive and programmed phases may not be clearly separated. Not all visualization work falls neatly into receptive and programmed categories, and individuals should not feel under pressure to structure them separately if one continuous visualization seems more appropriate. There is no set pattern for the programmed visualization: the topic itself will determine the style.

Procedure for programmed visualization

The preliminaries are similar to those for receptive visualization; that is, the person relaxes herself using cue-controlled relaxation (see Ch. 9, p83) or passive muscular relaxation (see Ch. 8, p71).

She then evokes the scene of the situation she wants to resolve, whatever it might be. (This is not the special place but a real-life situation.) Again, rich sensory detail is essential to bring it to life. Time spent building the scene enables her to experience it more keenly. She then works on the item, experimenting with it until she finds a good solution which she then enacts in her imagination. She plays a role which succeeds.

The tone of the programmed visualization is demonstrated in the following passage.

Let your thoughts become quiet and bring your attention to focus on your goal. Believe in your capacity to reach it ... don't dwell on the difficulties; just think of the result. If there are problems, see them as a challenge ... feel an eagerness to achieve ... to be a person who has reached that goal ... feel yourself in the part ... imagine yourself as having arrived ... congratulate yourself for getting there ... enjoy it ...

Termination

When the visualization is over, the procedure is brought to an end with a termination on the following lines.

If you are ready, gradually bring your attention back to the room you are in ... slowly count one ... two ... three ... and, as you open your eyes, feel yourself alert and refreshed.

Goal-directed visualization thus consists of the individual opening herself to her own wisdom (receptive phase) and then using it in her imagination to bring about the desired outcome (programmed phase).

Additional technique

'Distancing', i.e. drawing back from the scene to examine her actions, is a technique which allows the visualizer to gain a more objective view. In an imaginary viewing screen or crystal ball she watches her behaviour patterns: how she copes with situations and relates to other people.

This approach may reveal maladaptive responses she might be making. She then modifies those responses and reruns the film in a way which leads to a successful outcome. The next move is for her to step into the scene in her imagination, in order to experience the skills she observed herself displaying on the screen.

Relaxation and goal-directed visualization

It can be seen that relaxation is related to goal-directed visualization in a variety of ways.

- It is used as a preparatory measure to induce a state of mind conducive to visualization. Before the individual begins her visualization, she should first become relaxed.
- It may be experienced as a secondary effect following mental rehearsal in which the individual sees herself successfully coping with an activity which has hitherto been associated with stress.
- A need for relaxation may be created while the goal is being achieved, such as during the struggle to withdraw from cigarettes or tranquillizers.

Goal-directed visualization is thus not a primary method of inducing relaxation, but it does have close links with it.

Applying the method of goal-directed visualization

Unlike most other methods described in this book, goal-directed visualization addresses the specific

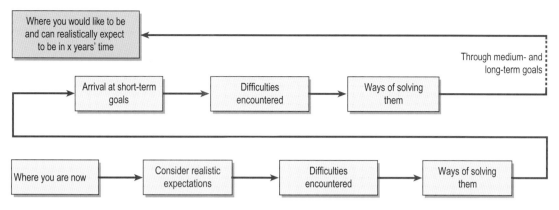

Figure 19.1 • Setting goals.

problems of a person. This feature is seen in both the receptive and the programmed components. Thus it is not possible to present a model script without a clear understanding of the background.

A key factor in the success of any plan is the motivation of the visualizer. While for some individuals this is not a problem, others may need encouragement. One way of fostering motivation is to make the goals specific. For example, having a timescale for a smoking abstinence plan defines it more clearly. Creating subgoals or intermediate stages is another useful strategy, since they act as stepping stones along the way. This has the effect of making the ultimate goal seem easier to reach, as well as providing rewards at intervals. Smoking one less cigarette a day can constitute a subgoal; so can taking one more step to a person recovering from leg injury. Difficulties can be considered in advance and ways of solving them worked out (Fig. 19.1).

Samuels & Samuels (1975) advise the individual not to confide her visualization to anyone who may not share her faith in the wisdom of the goal and in her capacity to reach it. Unshaken belief is vital for her success.

Of course, participants in some groups may be too demoralized to begin; they may feel they have little future, they may be angry or depressed. These are valid reactions which call for modification of the method and perhaps referral to a specialist agency. In general, however, the approach can be a useful one.

Although it is difficult to construct a model script without specific knowledge of the problem concerned, an attempt is made here to provide an example.

The reader is reminded of the principal items in the method:

- *Receptive visualization.* The individual tunes in to her own wisdom.
- *Self-statements.* She reaffirms herself through positive internal dialogue.
- *Programmed visualization.* She works on a plan for the future in which she sees herself surmounting obstacles, realizing possibilities and achieving goals. The keynote of this stage is seeing the self as succeeding.

When techniques are being learned and applied, one cannot count on instant success. As with any new skill, the most that can be expected is a trend in the desired direction. Frequent practice, however, strengthens this trend.

Visualizations for people who want to give up smoking

It could be argued that smoking has more to do with relaxation than smoking abstinence has, and many people become smokers because they perceive cigarettes as being a source of mental calm. However, many such people may then wish to quit smoking. Quitting is associated with stress, which means that the same people may be seeking an alternative means of obtaining relaxation. Health care professionals increasingly find themselves faced with groups of people who are struggling to give up cigarettes and for whom relaxation training has been prescribed. Although any of the methods in this book might help, a method which directly addresses the problem would seem to have particular advantages.

Within a single group of people who wish to reduce their smoking habits, there may be a wide variety of aspirations: one person may want to cut down from 40 cigarettes a day to 20, another may want to give up altogether. They may also have different ideas as to how to go about it: one may want to reduce by one cigarette a day, another may want to make a more abrupt change. Or again, the group may consist of people who are looking for ways of avoiding relapse after having successfully given up smoking. The following visualization and sequel (adapted from Fanning 1988) are designed for people who have decided to give up altogether.

Receptive visualization

Lie or sit in a position which you find comfortable. Close your eyes. Allow yourself to unwind. (The instructor presents either passive relaxation or slow breathing.) As your body and mind become calm, let your special place take shape in your imagination. Notice the sights, sounds and smell of the place. Put out your hand and feel the textures: the grass, the rug, the pine needles, etc. ... feel that you are there ... lying peacefully ... tuned in to yourself.

Gently bring your mind to focus on your smoking habit. Explore your feelings about it. Why do you smoke? Perhaps you hadn't thought about it before, just taken it for granted. In your mind's eye, take out a cigarette and light up ... what does it do for you?

Run through different situations during the day when you feel the need of a cigarette ... start with breakfast time ... what prompts you to reach for the first cigarette? ... then follow yourself to work ... smoking on the journey ... at work in your coffee break ... after the midday meal ... again in the afternoon ... on the way home ... to round off the evening meal ... last thing at night ... do you notice if you smoke for different reasons? ... do you get different rewards from smoking? ... when do you find you particularly want a cigarette? ...

Bring your visualization to an end when you are ready ...

The visualizer may feel she smokes for different reasons at different times. Some of the reasons why people smoke are:
- to feel reassured
- to relieve boredom
- to feel soothed
- to feel relaxed
- to give her hands something to do
- to give herself a lift
- to reward herself
- to keep her weight down.

She decides which of these applies to her and is then urged to think of alternative ways of meeting these needs.
- For reassurance, she tells herself she does not need a crutch.
- To relieve boredom, she gets out a crossword puzzle.
- To feel soothed, she reminds herself of the love of her partner.
- To feel relaxed, she runs through a relaxation sequence.
- To give her hands something to do, she carries a small, rounded pebble which she rolls in her hand.
- To give herself a lift, she remembers the prize she won for cookery/essay writing/athletics last year.
- To reward herself, she buys the salmon roll instead of the cheese roll.
- To keep her weight down, she eats an orange instead of a second helping of potatoes, or goes for a walk/workout, etc.

Positive self-statements or affirmations

The individual cultivates a view of herself as a healthy non-smoker by composing a few positive self-statements which she recites regularly to herself.
- I am healthy.
- I am a non-smoker.
- I have the strength to control my habits.
- I value the time when I am not smoking.

Additionally, she is gentle with herself for occasionally breaking her resolve.
- I can forgive myself for occasionally breaking my resolution.

Some people find it helpful to have one strong reason for changing their behaviour and to focus on this one idea whenever they feel in danger of weakening.

Programmed visualization

This takes the form of a mental rehearsal of coping activities which may focus on the goal itself (the end result) or on the means of achieving it (the process) (Ryman 1995). The example below is mainly concerned with the process.

At the start of the session the instructor can offer passive relaxation or relaxation through abdominal breathing.

Lie down and spend a few minutes relaxing quietly. Imagine yourself at the beginning of a normal day. Run through every moment when you think you might want to light up. Have an alternative way of dealing with every urge to smoke. Start with the moment when you would have the first cigarette of the day ... evoke the scene using sensory detail to bring it to life ... really live the moment in your imagination ... feel yourself craving a cigarette, then promptly use your alternative strategy ... and as you do so, encourage yourself with your positive self-statements ...

Move on to the next moment when you would want to light up ... and the next and so on ... making each moment come alive by recreating the scene as vividly as you can ... employing alternative strategies and encouraging yourself with positive self-statements ... remind yourself of the benefits of giving up smoking: clear lungs, no cough, extra change in your pocket ... and if you feel your resolution weakening, remind yourself why you made it in the first place.

Continue through the day, appreciating the experiences that not smoking opens up to you: the taste of your food ... the garden scents ... the fresh smell of your clothes ... and the easy way you climb the hill. See yourself as someone who doesn't smoke ...

At some point, feel your stress levels rising as something goes wrong at work ... you weaken and take out a cigarette ... but after a couple of puffs you stub it out ... allow yourself to feel pleased that you could have a slight relapse but not let it interfere with your determination to conquer your habit ... see yourself continuing to carry out your resolution and succeeding ... see yourself as someone who can cope without resorting to cigarettes ...

When you are ready, bring your visualization to an end with a count of one ... two ... three ... open your eyes ... look around you ... stretch your arms and legs ... and in your own time prepare to resume normal activity.

Some visualization therapists include an aversion component as a further incentive to give up smoking. This could take the form of images of dirty ash trays, blackened lungs, stained fingers or smoky atmospheres. Aversive measures work for some people; other people simply switch off if the image becomes too unpleasant.

The benefits of programmed visualization come from daily practice: the constant repetition of a routine in which the individual sees herself as successful in the task she has set herself. The above example is offered as a guideline or starting point from which the healthcare professional may wish to develop her own script. Alternatively, participants can be encouraged to compose their own visualizations since the most effective ones are those designed by individuals for their own use (Fanning 1988).

Where motivation needs strengthening, the following additional visualization may be found useful.

Find a quiet moment. Relax yourself and close your eyes. Imagine the house in which you expect to be living 10/5/2 years from now. Go inside ... explore it ... what does it tell you about the occupant: yourself? ... who else lives there? ... try identifying with your older self ... notice how it might feel to be that older self ... at work ... at her hobby ... with her family ... then, try looking back at yourself as you are now ... do you have anything to say to yourself? ...

When you are ready, allow your visualization to fade ... slowly, bring yourself back to the present ... counting one ... two ... three ... as you open your eyes ...

Evidence of effectiveness of imagery in changing smoking behaviour

Formal smoking cessation programmes have been shown to have varying degrees of success. Some of these have included guided imagery and visualizations. Tindle et al (2006) conducted a randomized pilot trial to test the efficacy of guided imagery for smoking cessation in adults. Results showed that 36% of intervention participants compared with 18% of controls had abstained at 6 weeks. At 1-year follow-up 24% of the intervention participants continued to be abstinent. Of those who attended the training classes in guided imagery, 94% reported that the technique was helpful. The authors concluded that a programme of guided imagery for smoking cessation was associated with a trend towards quitting.

Research tells us that those who do not smoke before they are 20 are less likely to take it up in adulthood. This suggests that targetting adolescents would be a fruitful enterprise. Grimshaw & Stanton (2006) have reviewed the evidence concerning tobacco consumption in young people. They found that some approaches show promise but the existing evidence base is too small for conclusions to be drawn in this area. However, as one in four British and American teenagers smoke, it would be useful to devise and conduct programmes which help to prevent them starting.

Quitting smoking is one thing. Maintaining abstinence is another. Relapse rates are high, either because people lose their motivation or because they lack the coping skills to continue. The resolve can be strengthened by cognitive strategies such as images of improved health or behavioural strategies such as removing oneself from a scene where others are smoking.

Other applications of goal-directed visualization

Goal-directed visualization can be used in a wide range of situations and conditions associated with stress. From insights gained during the receptive phase, a realistic solution can be worked out. This solution can then be mentally rehearsed during the programmed visualization, where a successful outcome is experienced in the imagination. A few examples follow:

1. alcohol and substance misuse
2. anger
3. cancer
4. childbirth
5. injury
6. losing weight
7. pain
8. performance fear
9. phobia and panic disorder
10. problem solving and decision making
11. sport and athletics.

Alcohol and substance misuse

In programmed visualization the individual mentally rehearses the successful achievement of her goal using positive self-talk and alternative strategies (p169). She also finds ways of relaxing herself during the period of dose tapering and beyond.

Anger

For an individual who wishes to reduce her tendency to become angry, alternative and preferred courses of action can be mapped out (see Ch. 2, p23). The programmed visualization is employed to familiarize the individual with her capacity to respond in these preferred ways. Relaxation and positive self-talk play a prominent part (Fanning 1988).

Cancer

Imagery in this context can be used in a number of ways. In one, attention is focused on reversing the physiological changes produced by the tumour. Mental pictures of the cancer cells being attacked by white blood cells are created by the visualizer. The scene is made as vivid as possible by casting the cancer cells as villains. They can play any role which the visualizer chooses, such as, for example, enemy infiltrators. In this scenario, the white blood cells could be represented as a vast army which slowly and inexorably overpowers the intruders and destroys them. The scene is imagined in every detail and the exercise repeated at frequent intervals.

It has been shown that heightened immune responses can occur in patients with cancer who have practised relaxation and healing imagery compared with those who have not practised these techniques (Gregerson et al 1996).

Childbirth

Visualization is often taught to expectant mothers in preparation for childbirth. Polden & Mantle (1990) offer several examples of imagery for use during the first stage of labour. Ocean waves and mountain peaks are used as metaphors to help women withstand the intensity of the contractions. The following is adapted from one of their suggested pieces.

Imagine a beautiful day out at sea ... with blue sky, still air and calm water. As the day wears on, the surface of the water begins to show the odd ripple. These ripples may be small so that at first you hardly notice them. Gradually, the tiny ripples turn into small waves, waves which you feel you can ride quite easily. After a while the waves get higher, and as they get higher, they also get closer together. You are beginning to find them difficult to ride. Still higher and closer together ... the waves seem almost to overwhelm you, but as they dip, you notice that they are carrying you nearer to the shore ... nearer to the shore where your baby will be born.

Injury

Provided a patient is receiving all necessary medical attention, she may find it helpful additionally to introduce a healing visualization.

Close your eyes. Let your injured part occupy your attention. See it as a part of your body which is being looked after by organs which control its recovery: your heart whch is pumping out nutrients, the blood vessels which are carrying them, the injury site which is receiving them. These nutrients are helping to rebuild the injured tissues. Let your mind focus on this healing process. Feel your mind willing it to take place. Flow with it. Nurse it with your thoughts.

Losing weight

In the case of people wishing to lose weight, alternative strategies may be found to take the place of eating. These are incorporated into daily programmed visualizations in which the individual sees herself successfully carrying out her plan (Fanning 1988). In the course of it she builds an image of herself as someone who looks nice whatever size she is, but has chosen to lose some weight. Any diet she is following should be medically approved.

Anorexia calls for more specialized treatment.

Pain

Imagery is used as a therapeutic aid in some types of pain, where it may have an adjunctive role alongside conventional medical treatment. It should not be viewed as a substitute for medical treatment. It can, however, be a useful coping device for chronic pain and minor ailments, such as aches and pains where it can sometimes help the individual get through difficult patches. In addressing pain, imagery is used in different ways. It can be a distraction, on the one hand, and on the other, it can provide a focus which undergoes transformation in a positive direction; for example, the pain can be identified as a mass of red which gradually has its intensity drained away to become light pink (see Ch. 18, p157). Its use in some forms of intractable pain is a specialized area not covered in the present work.

Performance fear

The programmed visualization can be used to take the individual through every moment of the event whether it is a stage performance, a speech or similar activity. The scene becomes familiar to her. She mentally experiences all possible occurrences and develops coping strategies for dealing with them. Above all, she experiences the successful achievement of her goal. This has the effect of building and maintaining her confidence.

Phobia and panic disorder

Programmed visualizations allow the individual to see herself overcoming fear and mastering the situation. They are often performed in a hierarchical fashion, i.e. a list of situations from low to high threat is drawn up. The individual starts with the lowest and, taking each one in turn, mentally goes through the experience of overcoming her fear, using slowed breathing, relaxation techniques and positive self-talk. This method is known as desensitization and was first introduced by Wolpe in 1958; it is only used under the expert guidance of psychologists and psychotherapists.

Problem solving and decision making

A receptive visualization can be used to collect ideas for solutions. After weighing them up, the unrealistic ideas are discarded and the realistic ones retained. Possible results are then predicted both

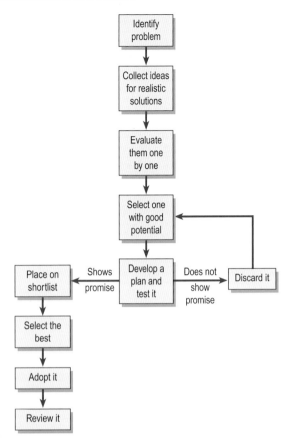

Figure 19.2 • Problem solving.

in the short term and in the longer term. These are then considered for their merits and disadvantages which together form the basis of the individual's final choice. Having picked what she considers to be the best solution, the individual mentally puts it into effect, experiencing its successful outcome in a programmed visualization. Figure 19.2 illustrates the process from identification of the problem to adoption of the best solution.

Vissing & Burke (1984) found that when faced with problems, individuals who regularly practised visualization had more success at solving them than those who did not.

Sport and athletics

Physical skills have a psychological dimension which is served by imagery in two ways, one cognitive, the other motivational (Paivio 1985). In the cognitive area, the player imagines successful routines in the game and rehearses appropriate strategies in her imagination. This leads to a strengthened integration between the physical and psychological elements of skill and helps to refine performance. In the motivational area, attention is given to the feelings of arousal and affect which accompany performance. The player trains herself to channel her emotional energy in positive directions such as imagining the experience of winning. In this way, the sensations of stress, pain and anxiety associated with the activity can be reduced.

A third type, healing imagery, is also practised by athletes following injury (Sordoni et al 2002) (see Ch. 26, p221).

Visualization has been employed to great effect in the field of sport and athletics, with numerous research findings supporting its use. The classic study was performed by Richardson (1969) who showed that basketball players who spent 3 weeks simply visualizing their throws achieved almost the same level of improvement (23%) as players who spent the time practising throws with a ball and whose level of improvement was 24%. A control group whose members did neither showed no improvement.

POTENTIAL PITFALLS

Goals, which should be set by the individual herself, need to be attainable. To set goals which are out of the individual's reach will only create additional stress. Goals may also be set too low to be constructive. These potential pitfalls should be considered alongside those found at the end of Chapter 18.

KEY MESSAGES

- Goal-directed visualization is a form of imagery which is structured to target particular behaviours.
- The client plays an active role in the achievement of a desired outcome.
- Affirmations are used to strengthen the resolutions.
- In imagining the event or situation, the same biochemical changes may be stimulated as occur in reality.
- As the visualization is repeated again and again, its message becomes stronger and more deeply embedded in the mind of the individual.

Chapter Twenty

Autogenic training

20

Autogenic training has been described as a method which uses easy mental exercises to bring about a meditative state of mind and deep relaxation (Bird & Pinch 2002). It has been used as a method of self-healing and is said to promote health and well-being.

Altered states of consciousness

An altered state of consciousness is often referred to as a 'trance'. It has been described as a condition in which critical faculties are suspended and the 'limits of … a person's … usual frame of reference and beliefs temporarily altered … making her … receptive to other patterns of association and modes of mental functioning' (Erickson & Rossi 1979).

The classic trance is the hypnotic trance, induced by procedures which create intense focal awareness, such as concentrating on a swinging pendulum. The participant becomes highly responsive to suggestion: 'the process whereby the individual accepts a proposition put to her by another, without having the slightest logical reason for doing so' (Hartland 1971). This is often described as 'uncritical acceptance'. Outwardly, the trance resembles drowsiness and dozing and is accompanied by a general reduction of muscle tone and a dilation of the capillaries; the person is, however, awake and highly focused although she may lose awareness of her surroundings.

Hypnosis may also be self-induced, in which case the individual herself governs the trance and plants the suggestions. The attention is again turned inwards, although this trance is described as a light one in which the individual retains awareness of her surroundings, being conscious of herself in all her senses (Rosa 1976). She does not, however, reflect on herself (Rosa 1976), which is to say that she does not distinguish between the self as subject (the 'I') and the self as object (the 'me') (Mead 1934).

Incomplete understanding of the mechanism of trance makes it difficult to draw further distinctions between trance states of differing depth. Some writers see altered states of consciousness as separate entities, different in kind from each other, while others view them as lying on a continuum between sleep at one end and wakefulness at the other. The latter view suggests that the altered states represent varying grades of trance, different only in degree and all part of the same entity (Barber 1969, 1970).

History and introduction of autogenic training

Autogenic training (AT) is an approach derived from self-hypnosis. It dates from the 1930s, when Johannes Schultz, a psychiatrist working at the Berlin Neurobiological Institute, discovered that some patients had learned to put themselves into a light trance by concentrating on images of heaviness and warmth. Even more interesting was the fact that they had seemed to benefit in terms of their mental health. Schultz called this self-generated trance state 'autogenic' and proceeded to develop a therapy based on it.

The goal of the procedure was attainment of this autogenic state, achieved by means of given phrases recited by the pupil. These phrases, by their imagery and autosuggestion, created what was called the 'autogenic shift' – a shift of the participant away from a stressed state towards the state known as autogenic. Exactly what, however, was the autogenic state?

A prominent exponent of the method, Luthe (1965), has described the autogenic state as being linked to drowsiness. In this work Luthe considers the nature of this 'drowsiness' and its relation to hypnosis, but without reaching any conclusion. These matters have still to be resolved. Today autogenic training (AT) is an established approach, but since the trainee is active in her own treatment, it is generally regarded as a relaxation technique rather than a form of hypnosis.

What is the difference between hypnosis and relaxation? Zahourek (1985) answers the question by pointing out that hypnosis purposefully aims at producing a trance; hypnosis also emphasizes therapeutic suggestion. In relaxation, by contrast, there is no striving for a state of trance and any suggestion made is under the control of the individual herself who, as a human being, is constantly making suggestions to herself anyway. Certainly, some of the devices used in relaxation, i.e. passive concentration, self-suggestion and imagery, are closely related to hypnosis but they are not confined to that practice and their effective use does not require the full knowledge of a formal hypnosis training (Zahourek 1985).

Imagery and autosuggestion form part of most relaxation approaches (Larkin 1988); indeed, many would say there are elements of suggestion in all stress reduction methods (Barber 1984). To ensure that they are used responsibly, however, it is necessary for the healthcare professional to have clear goals, to use techniques designed to promote those goals and to be aware of the hazards involved.

Davis et al (2000), addressing their book particularly to those who 'work with people who are in stress' (itemizing doctors, nurses, therapists, teachers and supervisors), present step-by-step directions for mastery of different approaches, one of which is self-hypnosis. They claim that no cases have been reported, even among the most inexperienced practitioners, of harm resulting from self-hypnosis (Davis et al 2000). This is an important point because, although self-hypnosis is not one of the methods contained in this book, there is no strict demarcation between self-hypnosis and relaxation. Pitfall number 4 in Chapter 18 (p159) is relevant to this discussion.

Rationale

Autogenic training is not underpinned by any theory; rather, it is based on principles of suggestion. It is claimed that the recited phrases, following many repetitions, create a light trance which increases the suggestibility of the participant and helps to promote a natural healing process. Possible explanations include the Freudian notion of lowered mental defences allowing communication with the interior. The method also has cognitive and physiological elements: cognitive ones in its attention-focusing phrases, and physiological, in the induced sensations of warmth which associate it with the parasympathetic branch of the autonomic nervous system, and a reduction in physiological arousal. The sensations of warmth are also associated with an improved blood flow which brings with it an augmented supply of oxygen. This can benefit a variety of conditions including rehabilitation following injury and recovery from surgery as well as providing relief from stress and anxiety.

In their search for an underlying mechanism, Henry et al (1993) suggest that AT may be re-establishing a balance between the sympathetic and parasympathetic systems.

Description

Autogenic training teaches the body and the mind to relax. It is based on four requirements.

1. Reduced external stimulation, i.e. a quiet environment with dim lighting.

2. An attitude of passive concentration, described by the British Autogenic Society as a state of mind which is relaxed, non-striving and unconcerned with the end product. This means not forcing any change, just letting the exercise work (Achterberg 1985): an 'allowing' rather than a 'doing' (Rosa 1976). If, while engaged in passive concentration, distracting thoughts enter the mind, they can be ignored or gently dismissed. Thoughts which carry insightful images, however, can be seen as a valuable product of the exercise. Passive concentration may be said to exist in other approaches such as meditation and some forms of progressive relaxation.

3. The repetition of relaxation-inducing phrases based on six main themes:

   a. heaviness in the arms and legs

   b. warmth in the arms and legs

   c. calm and regular heart beat

   d. calm breathing

   e. warm solar plexus/abdomen

   f. cool forehead.

These phrases are repeated to emphasize their effect and to draw the client's attention away from the external environment. The first two themes (heaviness and warmth in the limbs) are frequently presented on their own (by clinicians and researchers alike), although it is not known at what cost to the overall relaxation effect (Lichstein 1988).

4. Mental contact with the body part to which the phrase refers.

Central to AT is the principle of client control: the trainer describes the method, but it is the trainee who carries it out. To reinforce this notion, the phrases are styled in the first person. The instructor reads the relevant phrase using a slow and soothing tone and the trainee repeats it mentally or vocally three times. About 30 seconds are assigned to each phrase and a further 35–40 seconds for continued focusing of attention by the trainee. After working through the allotted phrase, a cancellation procedure is carried out as a safeguard against any deep trance state or physiological disturbance. The whole routine is then repeated, including the cancellation, three times. There may be several repetitions, at the end of which the trainees are seated for a debriefing or feedback session (see Ch. 3, p27).

In the feedback session clients are asked to describe their reaction. They are asked if they feel less anxious and if they feel this was a useful way of calming their thoughts. They are urged to keep a diary to record incidents which made them anxious and to describe how they coped with them. If they had difficulties evoking the sensations, images of lead could be used to deepen the sense of heaviness and images of sunshine or warm water to intensify the warmth.

Schultz & Luthe (1969) worked slowly through the schedule, taking 6 months to complete the instruction. The need to save time and money has, however, led to reductions in length and now the full programme is presented in a few weeks, depending on the aptitude of the trainee. The following version is adapted from the works of Bird & Pinch (2002), Brion (2003) and Welz (1991/2000).

As outlined here, the procedure is no substitute for a registered course on autogenic training. To acquire proficiency as a trainer, it is necessary to join such a course (Appendix 2). This chapter is included to inform the reader of the principles of autogenic courses and provide an introduction to their contents.

Procedure

Some schools start with a preparatory session to familiarize the client with the format prior to the course itself, but this is optional. On the second visit the concept of heaviness is put into practice.

Introductory talk to trainees

A short description introduces trainees to the method or reminds them of the procedure. For this talk they can be seated.

Autogenic training has been shown to help people overcome feelings of anxiety. It creates a state of extreme calmness which helps people to be in touch with deeper parts of their mind. As the mind becomes more receptive the individual can suggest changes to himself which he feels may enhance his life.

The method consists of short phrases describing sensations of heaviness and warmth. I'll be reading them out and as I do I'd like you to focus your attention on each one in turn, repeating the phrase under your breath. Concentrate on the phrase as completely as you can, imagining the words written down or relayed in the air, or in any way that holds your attention.

An important feature of this approach is that you should feel passive and casual about it; avoid forcing any response to occur. Let the sensations of heaviness and warmth arise on their own, rather than making an effort to bring them about. If other thoughts intrude, gently bring your attention back to the phrase; focusing on it will help to weaken their hold on you.

The images of heaviness and warmth will influence the circulation, so it is very important that you should return to your normal state after your session of autogenic training. This 'return' process or cancellation consists of a few exercises to normalize your body systems such as working your arms, taking a deep breath and only then, opening your eyes. This is a routine to be carried out after every group of exercises and every session of practice or instruction.

I'd like you now to settle into a relaxed position (lying or reclining) for the exercises … please close your eyes … imagine yourself in a place that makes you feel relaxed … perhaps a warm, sunny meadow …

The standard exercises

With the clients now in a supine or reclining position, the trainer leads with a short scanning procedure designed to relax the body. It is presented at the beginning of each lesson and should precede each practice session (see Ch. 8, p76). This is followed by the standard formulae of heaviness, beginning with the dominant arm.

Lesson 1

My right arm is heavy.
My left arm is heavy.

My right leg is heavy.
My left leg is heavy.
Both my arms and legs are heavy.

The trainer asks participants to continue to think about the heaviness in their limbs as they sink into the soft grass of the sunny meadow or other chosen place. After three repetitions the trainer carries out the cancellation procedure:

When you are ready, slowly allow yourself to become aware of the room. Make a few fists. Bend and stretch your limbs. Take one deep breath and then open your eyes. Let them scan the interior of the room. Tell yourself you are now feeling fresh and alert.

This is followed by the first of three repeats of the full routine. When these come to an end there is a discussion and feedback session with the participants in a seated position (see Ch. 3, p27).

Lesson 2

This starts with a recapitulation of the 'heaviness' phrases, then leads into the following 'warmth' formulae.

My right arm is warm.
My left arm is warm.
My right leg is warm.
My left leg is warm.
Both my arms and legs are warm.

At this point a calming phrase may be added on the lines of the following:

I am at peace.

Lesson 3

My right arm is heavy and warm.
All my limbs are heavy and warm.
My heart beat is calm and regula
I am at peace.

The programme continues in a similar vein to incorporate the remaining three standard exercises.

Exponents insist that the six basic phrases remain unchanged. The choice of imagery, however, is left to the participant; a sunny beach, a heated bath or a favourite chair in front of a log fire may be used as alternatives to the warm meadow scene. Having chosen her scene, however, the participant is advised to remain with it throughout the training period.

Running alongside the standard autogenic formulae are what are called 'intentional off-loading exercises' designed to provide opportunity for the release of emotions which have got locked up in the body. These exercises may take the form of limb shaking, shouting, sobbing or discharging pent-up emotions through verbal and written form and are practised when the trainee is alone.

Home practice

Written handouts enable trainees to continue with the standard autogenic exercises at home where it is suggested they practise three times a day. This home practice is essential and builds up the skill of being able to respond readily to the phrases. Eventually a single key phrase will have the capacity to switch on total relaxation.

After several weeks of practice the client is ready for the next stage in which she introduces phrases (personal statements) which help to lead her in a positive direction. Some of these personal statements take the form of affirmations which confirm her sense of self-worth such as 'I am an achieving person'. Others may strengthen her determination to make certain changes to her behaviour such as 'I can handle my anger'. Such personal statements are most effective when kept short and simple, expressed in the first person and in the present tense. Other examples, adapted from Davis et al (2000), are:

- I believe in myself (for those lacking in confidence)
- I have control over what I eat (for compulsive eaters)
- Smoking is an unhealthy habit (for people who wish to quit smoking)
- My mind is quiet and serene (for anxious individuals).

Certain physiological problems can be addressed through 'physical formulae' such as:

- My throat is cool (for a troublesome cough)
- My feet are warm (for a tendency to blush).

The trainee will incorporate particular phrases according to her personal requirements. AT should not, however, be viewed as a substitute for medical attention.

Other autogenic training exercises

Autogenic training also includes meditative exercises which involve colours, objects, concepts and personalities. Other exercises known as 'advanced' belong to an area described as therapy rather than training, and are beyond the scope of this book.

Evidence of effectiveness

The meta-analysis of Stetter & Kupper (2002) shows that AT is effective in the treatment of anxiety, mild to medium depression and functional sleep disorders. Positive effects have also been observed in psychosomatic disorders such as tension headache, migraine, essential hypertension, coronary heart disease, asthma, Raynaud's disease and certain kinds of pain.

Kanji and colleagues (2006) have conducted a series of systematic reviews to investigate the effectiveness of AT in different medical conditions. One of these reviews examined its effect on tension-type headache in adults. However, none of the seven controlled clinical trials reviewed found AT to be more effective than other relaxation interventions. The authors reported that the methodological quality of the studies was poor.

These same researchers had previously mounted a systematic review in the field of hypertension. Here they found conflicting evidence. Three randomized trials demonstrated significant reductions in systolic blood pressure in the AT group compared with no treatment. However, a placebo group was included in one of the studies and showed a similar significant fall in blood pressure to that of the AT group, suggesting that AT might be no more effective than placebo (Kanji et al 1999).

Results supporting the practice of AT emerged from a randomized clinical trial of the anxiety associated with coronary angioplasty, where the researchers compared AT with standard medical care. Findings showed a significant difference between the two groups, both at 2 months and again at 5 months, suggesting that AT is effective at reducing anxiety in this area (Kanji et al 2004).

Kanji & Ernst (2000) also studied the effectiveness of AT as a pain reliever in conditions such as childbirth, back pain, heart pain and cancer pain, and found the approach to be useful. As a result, they proposed that AT be introduced into the treatment of a wide range of pain-allied disorders where it could help to reduce the need for analgesic drugs.

In the field of anxiety disorders AT has been compared with progressive relaxation and found to be superior in terms of EMG decreases and effects on symptoms (Takaishi 2000). A further finding from this study indicated that the patients judged AT easier to carry out than progressive relaxation. This suggests that an approach which involves passive listening, i.e. AT, may be a more effective route to relaxation than one which demands active concentration, i.e. progressive relaxation, for people experiencing anxiety-related disorders.

Results should be viewed with caution since the evidence is equivocal and the methodological quality of the studies is variable (Stetter & Kupper 2002).

 POTENTIAL PITFALLS

1. Training in autogenic training should never be viewed as a substitute for medical treatment; wherever a disorder is present or suspected, medical help should be sought.
2. The phrase inducing abdominal warmth should be deleted for people suffering from abdominal problems.
3. AT is not suitable for children under 5 years of age.
4. Trainees should be advised to keep their personal formulae realistic. Creating unattainable goals will only lead to disappointment.

The pitfalls of visualization (Ch. 18, p159) are also relevant.

KEY MESSAGES

- A light trance state can be induced by images of heaviness and warmth
- This trance state is condusive to relaxation and also makes it easier for the individual to relate to his inner thoughts.
- The therapy entails the repetition of phrases based on six main themes, related to different areas of the body. They are accompanied by images of warmth and heaviness
- Individually designed affirmations can be woven into the schedule such as, 'My mind is quiet' for a person experiencing anxiety.
- Essential to the success of AT is an attitude of passive concentration
- Evidence of the effectiveness of AT has often shown it to be of benefit but results must be viewed with caution because of methodological problems in some of the research.

The British Autogenic Society runs training courses. Their contact information may be found in Appendix 2.

21

Meditation

CHAPTER CONTENTS

Introduction

The word 'meditation' is used to describe varied states of inner stillness. It is also used to describe different methods of attaining those states. Again, the many schools of meditation all have their own interpretation. Thus, with no universally agreed meaning, attempts to define the word fail. Common to all interpretations, however, is the concept of emptying the mind of thought; that is, letting go of the preoccupations that make up the mind's chatter.

If there is a general aim in meditation, it might be described as non-attachment, although some writers, such as Fontana (1991), feel that to have an aim at all tends to destroy the result since any kind of goal setting calls on rational powers and left-brain activity (see Ch. 18, p150).

Meditation could, therefore, be seen as an opening of the self to reveal its inner world, while at the same time conveying no hint of determination since that would be alien to the meditative state.

People come to meditation for many reasons:
* to find peace
* to achieve awareness
* to gain enlightenment
* to find themselves
* to empty the mind
* to experience true reality.

Since relaxation is one of the effects of all these pursuits, meditation is a relevant topic for inclusion in a book such as this.

Originating in the East, meditation is an integral part of the Hindu, Taoist and Buddhist religions. In the West, versions have been created which are simpler and these have, for the most part, evolved from Zen and yoga. The material presented here is of a non-religious form and comes from a variety of modern sources, notably the work of Fontana (1991, 1992).

It has been pointed out that meditation is both a state and a method. As a state, it is one in which the mind is stilled and listening to itself. The meditator is relaxed but at the same time alert. As a method, it consists of focusing attention on a chosen stimulus. This concentration is sustained but effortless and has the effect of detaching the meditator from external life events on the one hand and from her own mental activity on the other. Thoughts may enter her head but instead of examining their content, she allows them to drift away.

This attitude has been described as one of passive concentration and it implies that the meditator has a relaxed attitude while at the same time giving attention that is without criticism or judgement. Mental functions such as thinking and evaluating are inappropriate since they are processed by the left brain; rather, the meditator should cultivate what in Zen is called a 'don't know mind'; that is, a mind which is open and receptive to new, undreamed-of possibilities. Past and future associations are shed. The mind is emptied of all thought save awareness of the stimulus.

In common with hypnosis and day-dreaming, meditation is an altered state of consciousness. Fontana (1991) distinguishes it from other altered states, seeing it rather as a rediscovery of normal consciousness since it takes the individual to the core of the self.

The meditator does not fall into a trance, become drowsy or surrender control; on the contrary, she is in a state of heightened awareness, alert, aware of her surroundings and securely focused on the present moment.

Passive concentration, referred to above, is also a feature of autogenic training and receptive visualization, although not of programmed visualization which, as it is involved with the achievement of goals, is essentially a left-brain thinking activity and therefore remote from meditation. However, to say that meditation excludes the analytical thinking process does not imply that meditators consider left-brain activity to be of lesser value. Analytical thinking is an essential human function but its tendency generally to dominate mental activity has the effect of devaluing its counterpart, the imagination. Meditation enables the individual to redress the balance.

Rationale

It is claimed that meditation helps to quieten the mind and reduce the effect of stressful thoughts. It can thus contribute to a state of relaxation.

A number of theories have been put forward to account for the effect of meditation on the individual. Of these, Banquet's (1973) shift in hemispheric dominance is widely accepted. His research suggests that during meditation the left cerebral hemisphere loses its dominance, resulting in a more influential right hemisphere than occurs in everyday life. As a result, linear, verbal thinking plays a less prominent part, allowing intuitive, wordless thinking to express itself. By this means the individual may come to know and understand herself better and acquire a new peace of mind.

Benefits of meditation

Devotees of meditation claim that they benefit greatly from its practice. These are some of the advantages.

- A better understanding of the self is achieved through meditation. That is, through meditation the individual becomes more aware of herself and more receptive to the insights that arise from her deeper being.
- A new sense of relaxation and inner peace can be derived from meditation.
- The process itself promotes a clearer mind and improved powers of concentration. These extend outside the meditation session.
- The individual, by discovering her inner self, is able to live more in harmony with herself.
- By developing a sense of detachment, the individual comes to accept that many of her unpleasant emotional reactions are no more than short-lived bodily sensations created by her thoughts.
- The emphasis on self-awareness helps the individual to live in the present and to value the here-and-now. When the mind is concentrated in the moment, it becomes keenly alert.

A procedure for meditation

Introductory remarks to the novice meditator

A few words describing the procedure are required before starting the first session.

Meditation is an ancient method of quietening the mind. The method you are about to experience is a non-religious form. It is concerned with focusing the attention on different phenomena such as the breath, a visual object or a repeated phrase. The effect of the meditation will be to make you feel very peaceful. At no time will you lose consciousness or be controlled by any outside force. The state you reach will be entirely created by you. It is best to come to meditation without expectations; rather, to have an attitude which makes you content to be in tune with yourself.

A meditation session

A session may be seen to have four components:

1. attention to position

2. a winding-down procedure

3. concentration on a chosen stimulus

4. return to everyday activity.

Attention to position

In an environment that is quiet and warm, the meditator takes up a sitting or a lying position. Sitting is preferred since some people tend to fall asleep when lying down. The individual may sit in a straight-backed chair, sit cross-legged on a cushion on the floor or take up the lotus position (cross-legged with each foot resting on the opposite thigh). This position can be very uncomfortable for people who are not used to it; even in the East it has never been obligatory if the novice found it unbearable.

Whichever sitting position is chosen, the hands rest on the thighs, with the fingers gently curled or arranged in traditional symbolic postures. The head should be held in a relaxed position directly above the spinal column to release the neck muscles from strain while the eyes may be closed or slightly open.

Winding-down procedure

Participants are asked to direct their thoughts inwards.

The meditation session is preceded by a check for muscle tension, i.e. each participant checks all her muscle groups to make sure they are as relaxed as possible. It is often referred to as scanning and may be introduced in the following way.

I am going to ask you to check that your muscles are as relaxed as possible. Starting with your

feet, notice any tension ... then move up to your ankles, shifting them slightly if they are not relaxed ... now your legs ... and your hips ... settle them into the chair or the floor. Continue up through your body to your shoulders, letting them drop down. Allow your arms to fall comfortably, with your fingers free of tension. And now your head: relax your jaw and let your tongue rest in your mouth ... let all the muscles in your face feel smoothed out. Allow yourself to unwind, and as you unwind, feel in tune with yourself ... listening to yourself ... just being you ... experiencing what it is to be you ... being aware how it feels, without delving into reasons, explanations or even words ...

Irritating sounds or bodily discomfort may interrupt the meditation. Davis et al (2000) suggest 'softening' them by purposely giving them attention for a few moments instead of pretending that they do not exist.

Concentrating on a chosen stimulus

'All meditations are built upon concentration and tranquillity' (Fontana 1992). The individual quietly focuses attention on the chosen stimulus which may take the form of breath watching, gazing at a visual object or chanting a mantra. The purpose of the stimulus is to hold the attention of the participant.

This may be difficult at first since the mind is used to being engaged in a constant stream of images, memories and associations, all competing with one another. It will not help the individual to fight these distractions, but if she can accept their presence and continue her concentration on the stimulus, they will become weaker. Some people find it useful to regard intruding thoughts as clouds drifting by or leaves floating down a stream. The attention is then gently brought back to the item under focus.

The result of this meditation may be nothing more than a respite from stress for the individual. On the other hand, as the focused mind enters a state of clarity and tranquillity, a deeper part of the self may be reached whereby new insight is gained (Fontana 1991).

Grounding strategy

Any hint of depersonalization may be counteracted by a process known as 'grounding' or bringing the individual back to the here-and-now. It involves encouraging the meditator to return her attention to some form of body awareness. Fontana (1991) suggests concentrating on the breathing, while Titlebaum (1988) emphasizes the value of feeling the ground. The following passage is adapted from Titlebaum (1988).

> *Be aware of the ground beneath you. Feel it taking the weight of your body. Feel it supporting you. Notice the parts of your body which touch the ground or are in contact with the chair, if you are sitting. Concentrate on the sensations you are getting from these contact points and feel safely tethered to the ground.*

The duration of the session should depend on the experience of the meditator; 5 minutes is considered enough for the novice, 15–20 minutes for the experienced practitioner.

Return to everyday activity

The return to everyday activity, also known as arousal or termination, is a sequence which brings the meditation to a close.

> *When you are ready, let your meditation come to an end. If your eyes are open, remove your gaze from the point of focus. If your eyes are closed, allow the point of focus to fade until it disappears. Let it go with a feeling of gratitude towards it. Then turn your attention to your breathing, slowly counting three or four natural breaths.*
>
> *To help your muscles regain their tone, try slowly moving the body round in small circles before you get up. A few gentle stretches will also enliven the muscles.*

Home practice

Regular practice enhances the benefits gained from meditation. Lichstein (1988), reviewing the evidence, refers to numerous studies which indicate a direct association between the number of hours spent practising and the beneficial effects of meditation.

Focal points for meditation

Items on which the attention may be focused cover a wide range of objects, sounds and other phenomena. Included in this section are the following:

- the breath
- visual objects, i.e. circle, mandala, candle, china bowl
- parts of the body, i.e. space between the eyes, crown of the head, big toe
- mantras.

Concentration on the breath is mentioned first for a number of reasons (Fontana 1991):

- it is constantly available
- it has a rhythmical quality
- it is directly linked to the autonomic system
- it symbolizes the life force.

The breath

The practice of counting the breaths, with one count for every outbreath, is commonly used as a stimulus to hold the attention. On reaching the count of 10, the meditator reverts to 1 again, and continues the process for 5 minutes. The breaths should be natural and unhurried. Other forms of breathing meditation consist of focusing the attention on parts of the body involved in respiration such as the tip of the nose or the moving abdomen.

The tip of the nose

In the passage below, the meditator concentrates on the tip of her nose. It is assumed that she has already gone through a winding-down procedure (see above). Plenty of time should be allowed between the sentences.

> *Let your attention focus on your breathing and in particular, on the tip of your nose, that curved piece of cartilage that separates your nostrils. If you like, touch it with your fingertips to increase your awareness of it ... then concentrate on the feeling of air passing from the outside into your nostrils ... notice how cool it is ... notice also the warmth and moistness of the air that leaves your nostrils ... allow your breathing rhythm to be completely natural as you focus your attention on the tip of your nose ... feel the sensation of air being drawn in ... sweeping through your nostrils and, in its own time, passing out again ... if outside thoughts intrude, gently return to the sensation at the tip of the nose ... continue to focus your*

attention on that point ... feel your senses converging on that one spot.

On another occasion the meditator might wish to adopt a different focus, as in the next passage.

The moving abdomen

Here, a counting procedure is combined with focusing attention on the abdomen.

Gently turn your attention to your breathing. Begin by noticing it in a general kind of way, then slowly bring your mind to focus on the movement of your abdomen ... keep your attention fixed on the movement of your abdomen ... swelling as the air is breathed in and sinking as it is breathed out ... allow the air to pass in and out quite naturally while you are concentrating on the abdominal movement. Do not try to influence the breathing rhythm but let yourself flow with it ... if your mind wanders, gently bring it back to the swelling and sinking abdomen ... counting the breaths helps to hold the attention ... one count for every breath out ... and when you get to 10 or lose count, start again. Please continue on your own.

Visual object

Visual concentration on an object, sometimes referred to as gaze meditation, offers varied possibilities. Almost any object can become the focus of attention but typically the object is chosen for its symbolic value or its neutral associations: a geometric shape, a candle or a flower all have these characteristics.

The circle

A circle has the following symbolic qualities:
- it has substance in that it may be solid
- it has emptiness in that there may be nothing inside it
- it has motion in that it can roll and spin
- it has stillness in that it may come to rest
- it has wholeness by virtue of enclosing all its parts within it
- it has continuity in that any point along its circumference is both the end and the beginning.

If a circle is chosen as an object for meditation, the instructing meditator may produce one by drawing a thick-edged ring about 30 cm (1 foot) in diameter, emphasizing the centre with a dot, and hanging it on the wall. It should be level with the eyes of the seated participant, who positions herself at a comfortable distance from it (Fontana 1991).

The following script can then be used.

Let your gaze fall on the centre of the circle and then remain there ... consider the circle simply as a shape and let it speak to you in intuitive terms rather than in words ... try to keep your gaze focused on the centre while at the same time absorbing the whole image ... do not examine it but feel yourself experiencing it ... maintain the visual experience without reacting to it ... feel the image extending around your point of focus ... be aware of its extremities as your mind flows from the centre to the edges and from the edges to the centre ... if your attention should wander, gently bring it back to the centre point ... spend several minutes gazing at the image.

The mandala and the yantra

These serve a sacred purpose in the Buddhist religion. Their complexity, beauty and harmony enrich their symbolic quality and make them the supreme focal object for visual meditation. Although created for use by devotees, they can be meditated on at any philosophical level, and examples are shown in Figures 21.1 and 21.2. The mandala generally contains representations of living things while the yantra is predominantly geometric.

Both enclose symbolic motifs arranged in concentric rings around a clearly defined central point. This point symbolizes the inner self on the one hand and divine consciousness on the other, while the enclosing circles represent the cycle of life and the notion of Nature forever renewing herself. Thus the mandala/yantra stands for the personal as well as the transpersonal, for change within permanence, for life both in the present and in eternity, while affirming the fundamental unity of all things.

The candle

As mentioned above, the visual image can be used in different ways to clear the mind of thought.

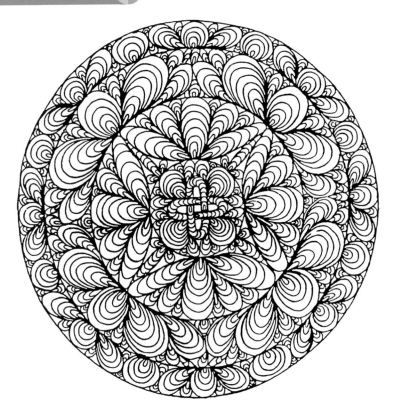

Figure 21.1 • A mandala.

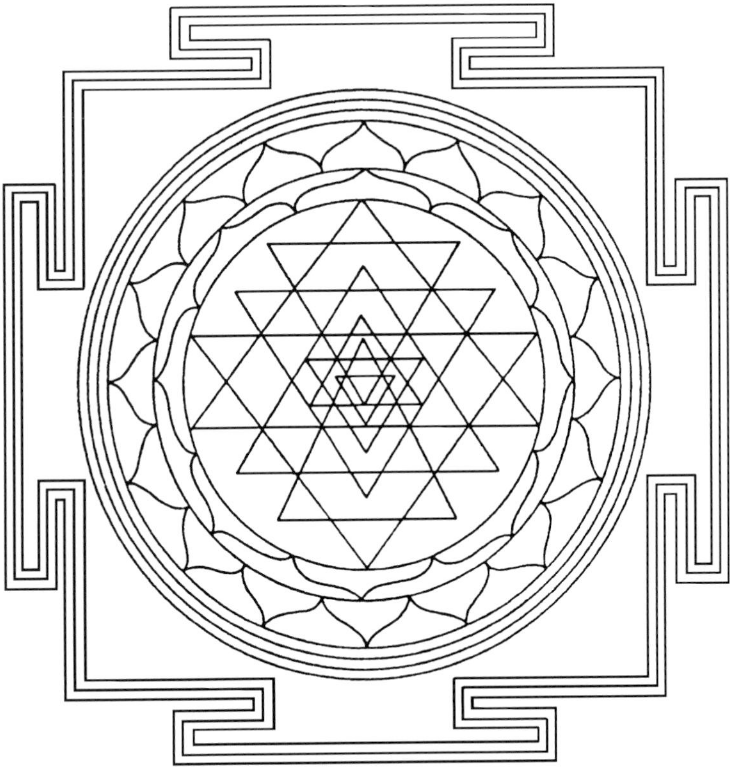

Figure 21.2 • A yantra.

into this category. For instance, Davis et al (2000)
suggest a china bowl.

Box 21.1

The after-image

When the gaze is fixed on a particular point for
about a minute and the eyes are subsequently
closed, the phenomenon of the after-image occurs.
This is the negative representation of the object
stared at. It immediately begins to fade and after
about 20 seconds or so has disappeared. It is
a physiological reaction which occurs when the
retinal cells get fatigued. Experiencing the after-
image is quite different from recreating forms in
the imagination, a practice which belongs more to
visualization than to meditation.

If the meditator is in doubt as to what she
is seeing behind her closed lids, there are two
questions she can ask herself.

1. Does the image fade or disappear within 20
   seconds? If so, it is likely to be an after-image.
2. Can she scan the image, i.e. trace its outlines?
   If every time she moves her eyes to trace the
   outline the image moves too, it is behaving like
   an after-image (Samuels & Samuels 1975).

For instance, while the individual is gazing at the
object, she can intermittently close her eyes and
allow the image to recreate itself in her mind, as in
the following meditation on a candle burning in a
darkened room.

*Let the lighted candle hold your attention …
settle your eyes on the upper part of the wax
column rather than the flame itself … sit
without moving while you gaze at it … focus
on it in a relaxed but constant way, letting the
image fill your mind … continue for at least
a minute … Now close your eyes. Notice that
the image of the candle prints itself in the
darkness … hold the shape in your mind's eye,
accepting any change of colour … if it slips
to one side, gently bring it back … continue
to focus on it until it fades … then open your
eyes and resume your gaze on the candle …
continue, repeating the sequence in silence for
several minutes.*

The image that appears behind the closed eyes is
known as the 'after-image' (see Box 21.1).

A china bowl

Certain objects lend themselves to a more exploratory approach. A flower or a piece of porcelain falls

*Settle your gaze on the object … take it all
in … after a few moments, allow your eyes to
travel over the object, tracing its lines …
noticing its colours … its decoration … and
the way it glistens … do not dwell on who made
it, how or for what purpose, but see it simply
as a shape … experience its visual qualities
as if you were seeing it for the first time … if
your mind wanders, gently bring it back to the
object …*

Parts of the body

Other body parts as well as the breathing organs
can be used to provide a focus of attention. This
kind of meditation is a feature of yoga, where
energy centres (chakras) are represented by the
base of the spine, the lower abdomen, the navel,
the heart, the throat, the space between the eyebrows and the crown of the head. After meditating
on the sites in this order, the physical energies are
said to be transformed into spiritual energies.

Yoga is a separate subject and no attempt is
made here to present it. However, the symbolic
nature of the chakras makes them suitable sites for
meditations outside yoga. Two examples are given
here: the space between the eyebrows and the
crown of the head.

The space between the eyebrows

*Behind closed lids, let your eyes turn upwards
and settle on the space between your eyebrows …
relate to it … recognize its closeness to your
brain … feel its central position … imagine
viewing it from the outside … then, imagine
viewing it from the inside … continue to focus on
that one spot … feel drawn to it … and consider
that, as the space between your eyebrows is part
of you, so you are part of that space.*

(Pause)

*If outside thoughts drift into your mind,
mentally blow them away and return to your
point of focus … to the space between your
eyebrows.*

The crown of the head

With your eyes closed, focus your attention on the crown of your head, concentrating on it in a passive way ... let your inner eye be drawn to it and held there ... see it from the outside, noticing how it appears ... then imagine it from the inside, from under the dome of your head ...

(Pause)

Symbolically as well as literally, it represents the highest part of you ... if thoughts intrude, let them be carried away ... let them drift away from you as you gently return your attention to the crown of your head ... feel yourself identifying with it ... experiencing it ... feel yourself uniting with all that is highest within you.

On a simpler level, any part of the body can serve as the stimulus, for example, the big toe.

The big toe

With your eyes closed, your legs uncrossed and your muscles relaxed, draw your attention to your right big toe. See it in your mind's eye ... move it gently to make its presence felt ... notice how it feels when you move it ... focus on the sensations you get from bending and stretching it ... be aware of the feel of the sock or stocking over it, or of the shoe restricting it ... think of it carrying the full weight of the body ... think of its strength as well as its mobility ... if unwanted thoughts intrude, gently bring your attention back to the toe ... focusing on the toe ...

Mantras

A mantra is a verbal stimulus which can be used to concentrate the attention. Traditionally it embodies an ancient, sacred truth whose meaning may reveal itself to the meditator during the process of concentration. A well-known example is the Sanskrit word 'om' which is said to represent the primal sound. Pronounced like 'home' without the 'h' (Smith & Wilks 1988), the sound can be intensified by stretching the syllable to form 'a ... oo ... mmmm' (Fontana 1991). It is the *sound* of the mantra that has particular value for the novice meditator, although its meaning may also be

contemplated at a later stage. The following piece is adapted from a passage in Fontana (1991).

Breathe in gently and as you let the air out, recite the word 'om': a ... oo ... mmmm. Feel the sounds vibrating within your body: feel the 'a' ringing in your belly, feel the 'oo' resonating in your chest and the 'mmmm' resounding in the bones of your skull ... let these sounds provide a focus for your attention ... link them into your natural breathing rhythm ... keep the breathing calm and slow and avoid any inclination to deepen it ... after 10 breaths, gradually reduce the volume of the sound until the word is spoken under your breath ... lower it further ... keep your attention focused on the mantra ... eventually, you will come to a point where your lips cease to move and the syllables lose their form so that you are left with just an idea ... feel it clinging to your mind ... united with it ... if thoughts intrude, turn them into puffs of smoke and let them blow away.

Many other sounds or words can act as mantras, e.g. 'peace', 'harmony', 'calmness' or phrases such as 'God is love' and 'here-and-now'. It does not matter if the word has a meaning, since constantly reciting it will tend to divest it of that meaning, although the word may still retain its aura. It is advisable, however, to choose a word that has no emotional associations for the user, and one that is unlikely to stir up her thoughts. While the main purpose of the mantra is to hold the meditator's attention, its rhythmic repetition also has a soothing effect.

On the other hand, a mantra may be picked expressly *for* its meaning. In this kind of meditation the mantra is not reflected on philosophically so much as experienced. It is identified with, rather than analysed.

Lichstein (1988) compares mantra chanting with dwelling on the muscles in progressive relaxation (see Ch. 5) and to the silent recitation of phrases in autogenic training (see Ch. 20) and points out that in addition to their inherent relaxation properties, they all share the capacity to divert the attention from stressful thoughts.

Transcendental meditation

An approach which sets great store by the mantra is transcendental meditation (TM). Its central feature is the contemplation and repetition of a Sanskrit mantra bestowed by Maharishi Mahesh Yogi who brought the movement to the West in 1959. As well as gathering many disciples, TM attracted a great deal of research: from several hundred studies it emerged that TM created significant physiological changes associated with relaxation. However, lack of controls and the use of self-selected (volunteer) participants weakened the validity of some of these findings.

Proponents of TM insist on the mantra being chosen with ceremony and in secrecy by a master teacher, although this practice has not been shown to be any more effective than one which uses simple words (Benson 1976).

Evidence of effectiveness

Electroencephalographic changes during meditation suggest a state of decreased arousal in the cerebral cortex. This supports the view that mental activity is reduced. Certainly, meditation has been found to be effective in reducing tension and can often lead to deep states of physiological and phenomenological relaxation. However, it is unclear how much more effective it is than any other relaxation practice. Research findings are inconsistent; some point to the superior benefit of meditation, while others are unable to show that meditation is any more effective at lowering physiological arousal than ordinary rest.

Meditation has been investigated in a variety of conditions. A systematic review of its efficacy in the field of medical illness concluded that the strongest evidence in its favour lay in the areas of epilepsy, premenstrual syndrome and menopausal symptoms. A somewhat lesser benefit was found for mood and anxiety disorders, autoimmune disease and emotional disturbance in neoplastic disease (Arias et al 2006).

Existing research revolves mainly around TM whose effects have been studied extensively. One of the areas of investigation is hypertension where trials have shown a favourable association with meditation (Canter 2003, King et al 2002). Barnes and colleagues (2001) demonstrated significant decreases in systolic blood pressure following a 2-month daily course of TM in a randomized controlled trial of 35 American adolescents.

However, methodological weaknesses characterize many trials exploring the effect of TM on blood pressure. This is the view of Canter & Ernst (2004) who, in their systematic review, were unable to draw conclusions about the effect of TM on blood pressure owing to a lack of good-quality evidence.

In the case of heart disease, there is some evidence to suggest that risk factors such as high blood pressure, high cholesterol and psychosocial stress could be reduced and pathophysiological changes slowed or even reversed following a course of TM (Walton et al 2002, 2004). Results were found to resemble those of orthodox interventions.

Cancer also is an area where the effects of TM have been studied. Tacon (2003) has proposed and designed a meditation programme for people experiencing different forms of this disease.

Meditation is frequently offered to people with anxiety disorders since it helps to still the mind. However, very few studies are available. From those that exist, it can be seen that the effect of TM on anxiety is comparable with that of other relaxation approaches, as concluded in the systematic review of Krisanaprakornkit et al (2006).

Perceived stress has been shown to benefit from meditation in a randomized controlled trial on a healthy population of hospital professionals. Following a non-sectarian 8-week course, the researchers found significant reductions in stress levels which remained at that level 19 weeks later (Oman et al 2006).

It has been proposed that TM could improve cognitive function. Canter & Ernst (2003) conducted a systematic review to test this claim. They found that some trials did support it but the authors attributed this result to an expectation effect and concluded that there was insufficient evidence to support the claim that meditation could improve cognitive function.

Although many of the trials investigating the therapeutic effectiveness of meditation have produced positive results, a high proportion of them are flawed. In the absence of more rigorous testing, Canter (2003) does not, therefore, find the evidence in favour of meditation to be strong.

POTENTIAL PITFALLS

1. Training in meditation should never be viewed as a substitute for medical treatment; wherever a disorder is present or suspected, medical help should be sought.

2. Meditation may not be suitable for people in acute psychotic states.

3. Although the central idea of meditation is to keep the mind focused and aware, it does occasionally happen that an individual loses the sense of who and where she is or develops the feeling of being 'outside her body'. These are trance-like states of disorientation and depersonalization. In this event, a grounding strategy similar to the one referred to on p185 may provide a remedy. The instructor can safeguard against disorientation and depersonalization by regularly reminding participants to keep their attention focused on the stimulus (Fontana 1991).

4. Meditation creates an altered state of consciousness. The novice will not know in advance how she will respond. It is therefore recommended that, to begin with, sessions be kept short, no more than 5 minutes in length. This can be increased to 15 or 20 minutes for those with experience but not exceeded, as it is possible to meditate too much and run the risk of getting out of touch with day-to-day life. Benson (1976) reports that none of the participants in his studies displayed ill effects after meditating for 20 minutes twice a day.

5. The breathing meditations in this chapter do not seek to interfere with the natural breathing rate or rhythm. However, the mere request to become aware of the breathing can result in a slight alteration of its rhythm. It is therefore suggested that, before attempting breathing meditations, the reader become familiar with the section on hyperventilation in Ch. 4, p40.

6. Benson (1976) believed that it was better to practise meditation before a meal than directly after it. He considered that the process of digestion, by drawing the blood to the viscera, interfered with the physiological changes associated with meditation, and advised waiting for at least 2 hours after eating. More recent research, investigating the distribution of blood during meditation, supports Benson's view: Bricklin (1990) found that the blood flow to the brain during meditation increased dramatically, rising on average by 65% of its normal volume.

It would not, therefore, be constructive to practise meditation at a time when other demands were being made on the vascular system.

7. The lotus position has been referred to as the posture traditionally adopted in the East. This posture, however, was never obligatory even in its country of origin. In the West it may be inadvisable for novices even to attempt it because of the excessive stretching of the joint structures which accompanies it. Sitting cross-legged on a cushion is no less conducive to meditation, and many people practise meditation sitting in a chair.

8. Those who expect meditation to be a ready remedy for life's problems may become disillusioned. Meditation should be seen as a way of life, not as a panacea.

Guidance should be sought from an experienced teacher by those wishing to pursue more advanced forms of meditation since they are beyond the scope of this book.

_____

KEY MESSAGES

- Meditation can help to reduce an arousal state.
- A meditation session begins with a winding-down procedure consisting of a scan of the voluntary muscle groups.
- The session itself consists of focusing on an object such as the breath.
- If distracting thoughts intervene, the meditator should try to ignore them and bring his attention gently back to the breath or other focal point.
- Mantras may be used to augment the concentration.
- The effectiveness of meditation is unclear on account of the quality of much of the research. It is, however, widely used in a variety of conditions. Benefit is reported but does not appear to exceed that of other techniques.

Chapter Twenty Two

22

Benson's method

The relaxation response

In the 1970s, the physiologist Herbert Benson, who was studying aspects of high blood pressure at Harvard's Thorndike Laboratory, was approached by a group of transcendental meditators who believed that their meditations could lower their blood pressure. Unconvinced, Benson at first dismissed the idea but he later changed his mind. He and his colleagues then began to carry out a series of investigations which revealed that transcendental meditation (TM) was accompanied by marked physiological changes: there were reductions in the heart rate, breathing rate, oxygen consumption, blood lactate levels and, of particular interest to Benson, blood pressure. These changes reflected diminished activity in the sympathetic nervous system.

One study demonstrated drops in systolic and diastolic pressures from group averages of 146 and 93.5 mmHg respectively (borderline high pressure) to 137 and 88.9 mmHg (within normal range), following several weeks of practising TM. Oxygen consumption was found to be reduced by 10–20% within the first 3 minutes of meditation. (It is interesting to compare this result with work on the sleeping state where the oxygen consumption was found to be reduced by only 8% and not before the person had been sleeping for 4 or 5 hours.) These were impressive findings, particularly in the case of the blood pressure recordings which were not made during actual periods of meditation. The participants, however, were volunteers who had already applied to join a transcendental meditation course to reduce their blood pressure. This would suggest that their motivation was high.

Extensive study of other meditation practices led Benson to the belief that the above effects were not confined to the practice of TM but were the result of certain key elements common to all meditation practices. He set out to identify these elements, seeing them as responsible for eliciting what he called 'the relaxation response' or a state of decreased psychophysiological arousal. To Benson (1976), this was 'a natural and innate protective mechanism' that opposed the effects of the stress response. Viewed in these terms, the relaxation response appeared synonymous with parasympathetic nervous activity.

The key elements that Benson (1976) identified were:

* a quiet environment
* a comfortable position
* a mental device such as a word to focus on
* a passive attitude.

The key elements

Quiet environment. In the ideal setting there is an absence of any background stimulus, pleasant or unpleasant.

Comfortable position. Benson does not insist on any particular position since he feels that discomfort might draw the attention away from the mental device. The meditator should be allowed to choose her own position. She can, however, be too comfortable and tend to fall asleep; the orthodox lotus position (see Ch. 21, p179) is thought to have been introduced partly to prevent that happening. For the same reason Benson does not recommend a lying position.

Mental device. Since his studies had shown that TM was not unique in its ability to lower physiological arousal, Benson concluded that any repetitive, monotonous stimulus, capable of holding the attention, could fulfil the function of the Sanskrit mantra, i.e. that any emotionally neutral object, sound or other phenomenon could be used as a focal point of attention. Benson chose the word 'one', which has similar qualities of resonance to the primal sound 'om', but he felt the choice of word or words was best made by the individual herself. He refuted the idea that the mantra's meaning added to its effect.

Passive attitude. Passive acceptance is an essential feature of the approach. A 'let it happen' attitude should be adopted. Benson regards the passive attitude as 'perhaps the most important element in eliciting the relaxation response'. Distracting thoughts may intervene but they should be ignored and the meditator's attention returned to the recited mantra.

Rationale

By focusing the attention on a particular object, word or concept in a sustained and effortless way, meditators are able to detach themselves from daily events and induce a mental stillness. This stillness is reflected in reduced physiological responses, that is, diminished activity in the sympathetic nervous system (Benson 1976). Both cognitive and physical elements are present: the first relating to the focusing of attention on the mantra (or other stimulus) and the second, to the role of the breath. The theory underpinning the method is a unitary one in that the meditation creates a general, integrated

calming effect. Although the participant is engaged in the cognitive activity of focusing on the mantra, the effect on the system is global. This led Benson to coin the phrase 'relaxation response'.

Procedure

Introductory remarks to participants

A few words explaining the method are addressed to novices, who should be seated.

The relaxation method you are about to learn is a non-religious version of meditation. It has a very simple form, requiring that you sit comfortably in a quiet place, that you focus your attention on the word 'one' and that you adopt an attitude which is accepting and unconcerned.

These conditions will help you to experience what is called the relaxation response; a state which research shows is associated with reduced physiological activity. That means the heart rate will become slower and the blood pressure will fall. You'll notice that you feel calmer than usual and the whole sensation will be a pleasant one.

At no time will you lose consciousness or be controlled by an outside force. The state you reach is one which you will have induced in yourself.

Induction

When participants are ready, the induction sequence itself is carried out. The following version is adapted from Benson (1976). The '10 minutes' indicated can be extended to 20 as the meditator becomes more experienced.

Settle comfortably in whatever position you have chosen, and close your eyes. Relax all your muscles, starting with your feet and ending with your face. Feel yourself deeply relaxed.

Notice the rhythm of your breathing. Let the air in through your nose, allowing the breaths to take place quite naturally. Each time you exhale, recite the word 'one' under your breath. Repeat the word slowly every time you breathe out. If thoughts intrude, try to ignore them, and continue repeating the word 'one'.

Avoid any inclination to judge how successful you are being. Keep your attitude passive, and allow relaxation to occur in its own time. Please continue for 10 minutes …

When you are ready to end your meditation, continue to sit quietly for a few minutes with your eyes closed, then for a few minutes longer with them open.

Features of Benson's method

As shown above, the induction is short and simple. Benson writes that his method carries little embellishment. Perhaps he made it too simple; in excluding all but the essentials, he may have overlooked the value of ceremony and ritual, which are important factors for some individuals (Carrington 1984, Lichstein 1988).

In identifying what he considered to be key factors, Benson's purpose was not to create a rival approach, but to devise a standardized technique which could be used in scientific investigation. Apart from that, his method is very similar to transcendental meditation except that the word 'one' replaces the Sanskrit mantra and the process is entirely secularized (Lichstein 1988).

The emphasis placed on 'passive attitude' recalls the 'passive concentration' of autogenic training (see Ch. 20). It is also not far removed from the quiet observation that characterizes progressive relaxation (see Ch. 5). It would seem that, underneath their varying procedures, the approaches are saying much the same thing (Lichstein 1988), and that in their psychophysiological effects, they are all evoking the relaxation response.

Research has questioned the importance of a quiet environment and a comfortable position. De Leon (1999) argued that the relaxation response could be elicited in a variety of locations even if they were noisy. It could also be elicited in a variety of positions even if they were uncomfortable. According to this researcher, it was the passive attitude and the mental device which were the essential ingredients of this approach, while Benson himself placed greatest value on the passive attitude.

In common with the authors of other methods, Benson stressed the importance of regular practice, to be carried out once or twice a day. When practising at home, people are urged not to use an alarm but to guess when it is time to end the meditation.

Evidence of effectiveness

Meditation appears to have a role to play in the field of coronary heart disease and hypertension, where the approach increasingly features in both prevention and treatment (King et al 2002).

Among other cardiac conditions where benefit has been demonstrated is congestive cardiac failure. Veterans with this condition were trained in the relaxation response method and the effects compared with those of cardiac education and usual care. In terms of physical and emotional improvements, participants in the relaxation group experienced more benefit than those in the cardiac education group. No benefit was recorded in the usual care group, physically or emotionally. The authors concluded that the relaxation response may offer benefit to people experiencing congestive cardiac failure (Chang et al 2004).

Other research has examined many conditions, including pain management. Schaffer & Yucha (2004), in their review, find that non-pharmacological methods of pain management, such as Benson's relaxation response meditation, are able to reduce the emotional components of pain. Such methods can also strengthen coping abilities, give patients a sense of control, reduce fatigue and improve sleep. This is particularly so in the case of chronic pain and, to a lesser extent, in acute pain. One such painful condition is rheumatoid arthritis. Bagheri-Nesami et al (2006) conducted a pilot trial to investigate the effect of the relaxation response in this condition and found evidence to suggest a reduction in depression and anxiety and indications of a decline in the disease process (see Ch. 26, p220).

A review of the evidence was undertaken by Wright (2006) to determine the effectiveness of the relaxation response in serious illness. Results showed a tentative positive effect. This is supported by the systematic review undertaken by Arias et al (2006) who found that meditation techniques improved the treatment of autoimmune illness. However, while both these reviews highlight the safety and potential benefits of meditation, the authors indicate that many of these studies are methodologically limited by non-randomization, lack of intention to treat analysis, single cohort design and inadequate follow-up data; further research is therefore required.

POTENTIAL PITFALLS

These can be found at the end of the previous chapter.

KEY MESSAGES

- The relaxation response is a form of meditation introduced by Herbert Benson.
- It is based on the belief that all forms of meditation elicit the same response, i.e. a reduction in sympathetic nervous activity.

- It is characterized by a simple formula consisting of four elements: a quiet environment, a comfortable position, a mental device to hold the attention and a passive attitude.
- The induction procedure consists of gentle breathing which incorporates a soothing mantra.
- It is a widely used technique. Robust evidence for its effectiveness, however, is lacking.

Mindfulness-based meditation

What is mindfulness?

Buddhist principles of awareness and meditation lie at the core of mindfulness. The practice has also been studied by psychologists working in the area of stress and cognitions and this has led to the formation of a new structured approach in that discipline. Notable contributions have been made by Kabat-Zinn and others working in the field of anxiety and stress management, while Segal and colleagues (2004), combining mindfulness with cognitive principles, have investigated its application in the area of severe depression.

The key notion is that every moment should be seen as a celebration of life whether one is going through a marriage ceremony or simply washing the dishes. Mindfulness is cultivated by gently reminding yourself to be aware of the moment, whatever you happen to be doing; of being present in each moment with a sense of wakefulness, accepting and acknowledging it without judgement or criticism.

Psychological definitions include a 'moment-by-moment non-judgemental awareness' (Kabat-Zinn 2003), while Bishop (2002) sees it as a state in which the individual is highly aware of the reality of the present moment. The Buddhist mystic Gunaratana describes it as 'impartial watchfulness' (2002) and the monk Thich Nhan Hanh as 'keeping one's consciousness alive to the present reality' (Hanh 1991).

Experiencing the moment has the effect of separating the individual from any emotional reactions generated by the situation. Those reactions can then be seen as mental events which may have little to do with reality (Bishop 2002). Thus mindfulness urges the individual to stand aside from uninvited thoughts and to see them as entities separate from the self; to be aware of negative thoughts without responding to them. This lessens their hold on the individual as it tends to disempower them. A non-evaluative environment such as this also helps to promote the client's powers of perception by freeing a path to his inner resources (Whitfield 2006).

Kabat-Zinn, referring to his mindfulness-based stress reduction (MBSR) programme, describes the liberating feeling of treating thoughts as being outside the individual and not part of him. In his words: 'to see that your thoughts are just thoughts and that they are not you or reality'. Recognizing them in this way can free a person 'from the distorted reality they often create'. Thus, although mindfulness cannot change a person's thoughts and feelings, it can change his relationship to them (Segal et al 2004). This has implications for people experiencing negative thoughts such as occur in anxiety and depression.

What it is not

Mindfulness is a kind of meditation. However, it differs from other forms of meditation such as concentration. Concentration implies a focused attention on a particular item to the exclusion of other stimuli, in contrast to mindfulness which steps back and observes with a broad focus. It also differs from creative thinking such as occurs in visualization and problem solving where a deliberate intellectual effort is required and active solution-seeking skills called for. Conversely, mindfulness calls for a more observational approach, one that fosters a sense of total acceptance. Although mindfulness may lead to problem solving, its primary concern is to develop new insights. Its purpose is not to deal with problems but to create the state of mind which makes solutions possible (Gunaratana 2002). In this way, mindfulness is 'being' rather than 'doing' (Kabat-Zinn 2003).

To deepen one's understanding of mindfulness, Langer (1989) finds it useful to consider the reverse condition: mindlessness. In this state a person's attention is on outcome rather than process, on the future instead of the present. The task in question is carried out in an automatic manner using goal-based thinking styles with no thought as to how it is performed. These automatic responses may in the past have provided a convenient quick path for the individual but if they become a habit he will find himself unwittingly trapped in a rigid world where new possibilities are unlikely to occur to him. He has been wishing away the present moment because it stood in the way of carrying out the next task; he has been considering the end result at the expense of how to get there. His mindless approach has perhaps had the advantage of quickness and even a measure of effectiveness but it may leave him in a stressful state. He

has been rushing through the day to get everything done when a quiet moment of awareness might have revealed another way of managing the tasks, one which led to a more satisfying and less stressful outcome.

Thus, a preoccupation with outcome is associated with a state which is relatively mindless of the moment (Langer 1989) and may lead to an unfavourable outcome while an approach which considers process is more likely to improve outcome. Langer illustrates this point by referring to the sportsman who knows how to improve his game. His progress in mastering the sport is more likely to occur when he considers how he played that winning shot than when he rejoices in its success. Any kind of sport requires a focus on process rather than goal. Once attention to process falters, the chance of winning drops.

Mindsets dictate our reality and govern our behaviour (Langer 1989). By stepping aside from the situation and gently observing it without prejudice or criticism, a better solution may occur to the individual. With the insight gained, he may then be presented with a choice which was denied him in his mindless mode.

In emphasizing the means rather than the end, mindfulness techniques bear a slight resemblance to aspects of the Alexander technique where too much focus on goal achievement is seen as being detrimental to outcome, although in Alexander's case the entities are physical (see Ch. 12, p105).

Rationale

Awareness of the passing moment enables us to become fully engaged in it and detached from the thoughts and feelings triggered by it. This gives us space to question the validity of our immediate responses and to see our behaviour in a more objective light. We see that we need not be enslaved by our reactions since they are separate from and subordinate to our identity.

For people experiencing raised levels of stress in their lives, this offers a path which can lead to greater control of their stress and help to prevent subsequent states of anxiety and depression, while the meditation central to it helps to tap their inner resources.

The approach is underpinned by Buddhist principles of awareness and meditation.

Mindfulness-based stress reduction

Mindfulness-based therapies seek to help the client to manage the stress and distress associated with chronic illness (Bishop 2002). Their treatment programmes have a strong psycho-educational content. This is built around the central technique of mindful meditation with a focus on the breath. Awareness of the breath is seen as a way of 'anchoring' the individual to the present moment.

Procedure for mindfulness-based stress reduction

Mindfulness breathing is not an exercise where the rate and depth are regulated, as might occur in an aerobics class. Mindfulness breathing requires the client to do nothing since any attempt to control the breathing will interfere with its natural rhythm. The client is urged simply to be aware of the breath. Any distractions such as negative thoughts and bodily sensations should be observed in a passive manner and seen as mental or physical events quite separate from the meditator himself. The following passage contains ideas from Gunaratana (2002).

> *Turn your attention to the breath ... be aware of it ... follow its path ... in and out ... in awareness of each moment as it passes ... be gentle with yourself ... accept everything that arises ... feel yourself flowing with whatever comes your way ... don't expect anything ... if the attention wanders, simply acknowledge and accept each thought and feeling which intervenes ... then let them go, as you return to your contemplation of the breath ... be gentle with yourself ...*
>
> *You may become drowsy. That's because you are very relaxed. But try to stay awake. Insights only arise when you are awake. If you feel overwhelmed by negative thoughts just mentally 'step out of the way' and wait for them to subside. Try to accept the pain (or unpleasant thought). Accept what you cannot change. If you feel worn down by pain try 'breathing into it' or sliding into it'.*

Kabat-Zinn (2003) has set up a treatment programme called mindfulness-based stress reduction (MBSR).

This includes mental exercises in self-awareness. Gently reminding herself to be constantly aware of the moment, the client learns routines involving her experience of the moment; for example, viewing objects as if for the first time, devoid of their social and cultural associations and other memorized material, having to rely exclusively on the senses of sight, sound, smell, touch and taste. One of these routines is the 'raisin exercise'. Devised by Kabat-Zinn as an example of a mindfulness meditation, it is reproduced here in an adapted form (Box 23.1).

Training includes an educational component consisting of the psychophysiology of stress and the application of mindfulness skills to specific situations, gradually turning towards the difficult. These are taught once a week over an 8-week period during which the client spends 45 minutes a day practising her newly learned routines.

Evidence of effectiveness of mindfulness-based stress reduction

Cancer is an area where MBSR has been found to provide benefit in the form of improvements in mood and sleep quality (Carlson & Garland 2005, Matchim & Armer 2007, Ott et al 2006, Smith et al 2005). In a randomized controlled trial, Speca et al (2000) took a mixed sample of cancer patients and entered them for a course of MBSR. Results showed a 65% reduction in total mood disturbance and a 35% reduction in stress symptoms. Allowing for a degree of social desirability effect whereby participants tend to tell the interviewer what they think she wants to hear, these are still impressive results.

A recent study of patients with breast and prostate cancer indicated that participation in an MBSR training group was associated with decreased stress symptoms and enhanced quality of life as well as the physiological changes consistent with reduced stress (Carlson et al 2007).

Instruments for measuring the psychological impact on health among patients with cancer vary. In most studies a one-group pre- and post-test model was used. In a systematic review of these instruments it was found that they were useful and that MBSR was potentially beneficial as a nursing intervention in this field (Matchim & Armer 2007).

An area which seems particularly to respond to the benefits of mindfulness is chronic pain or disability. Focusing on this area is a system called the

The raisin exercise (based on an exercise created by Kabat-Zinn)

(The word 'PAUSE' indicates a 10-second silence; the three dots, a 3-second silence.)
The trainer asks the client to hold out one hand in which he or she places a raisin.

I have placed an object in your hand and I'd like you to imagine you have never seen it before. So, it does not have a name. Look at it – seeing it as if for the first time. It is an object with certain features. Notice its size, its shape, its colour … it has a certain texture … notice its folds and how the light catches them … moment by moment … PAUSE

Now, slowly turn it over … explore its underside … notice the feel of your palm being brushed by the moving object … let your eyes travel along the newly revealed contours of the object … taking in the kind of information you normally take for granted … hold the object in your gaze … moment by moment … PAUSE

And now, close your eyes … this emphasizes the feel of the object in your palm … if you are interrupted by such thoughts as: ' I wonder why I am doing this' remind yourself that it is just a thought and gently bring your attention back to the object … exploring it with your senses … moment by moment … PAUSE

And now, taking it with the thumb and finger of the other hand, lift it up to your nostrils … as you breathe, notice the faint aroma entering your nose … it is pleasant and perhaps your mouth begins to water … slowly transfer the object to your mouth, noticing how your hand knows how to reach your mouth … note the different feelings in your raised arm as the various muscles come into play … and now, the feelings as you slowly lower your arm … moment by moment … PAUSE

And now, turn the object over in your mouth, noting the feel of it on your tongue … feel it getting bathed in saliva … now, as your teeth bite through it, notice how the object changes, releasing its flavour as it gets crushed … moment by moment … PAUSE

And now, note the sensation in your jaw muscles and inside your mouth as you slowly chew the object … feel its consistency changing … preparing to be swallowed … then, note the feeling of swallowing …

Breathworks Self-Management Mindfulness-Based Pain Management Programme. A clear distinction is drawn between the pain itself (regarded as primary) and one's reaction to it, which includes all responses such as anger, fear, anxiety, depression, avoidance and catastrophizing (seen as secondary). The client is urged to accept the primary pain and to reduce the secondary which he does through strategies such as breath and body awareness. It is a technique which helps the client to live with the pain. Evaluation of the Breathworks Programme revealed a clinically significant change in the health status of affected individuals, with effect sizes ranging between 0.84 and 0.52 (Burch et al 2006).

Chronic pain characterizes the condition of fibromyalgia for which a meditation procedure might have something to offer. Astin and colleagues (2003) combined mindfulness meditation with qigong and tested their efficacy in the treatment of this condition. Their randomized controlled trial used an education and support group as control. They found that both groups made statistically significant improvements during training and these were maintained at follow-up 6 months later. However, there was no evidence that mindfulness meditation offered any advantage over education and support.

Some researchers have explored the effects of this kind of meditation on the immune system. Davidson et al (2003) trained 25 healthy participants in mindfulness meditation over an 8-week period and found significant increases in antibody titres to influenza vaccine. The authors concluded that brain and immune function may be changed in positive ways by this practice.

It has also been suggested that mindfulness meditation might be a useful strategy in smoking cessation. Davis et al (2007) gave a programme of MBSR to 18 participants who expressed a wish to quit. All had a smoking history of 20 cigarettes a day for 26 years. After 6 weeks, 10 of the 18 were no longer smoking and reported a reduction in stress and affective distress. The authors suggest that mindfulness training may help some people to give up smoking.

Reviewing the literature on anxiety and depression, Tonneatto & Nguyen (2007) were, however, less convinced of the effectiveness of mindfulness approaches and find the evidence equivocal.

Thus, while evidence is growing in a number of areas to support the effectiveness of mindfulness, a cautious optimism is advocated.

Mindfulness-based cognitive therapy

In recent years mindfulness has been combined with cognitive therapy to form an approach called mindfulness-based cognitive therapy (MBCT). It differs from cognitive therapy proper (with its focus on *content* of thoughts) by emphasizing *awareness* of and *relationship* to thoughts (Segal et al 2004, p 54). MBCT teaches the individual to separate himself from these thoughts and to regard them as passing events of little importance rather than decisive events which must be closely inspected.

The programme was originally designed as a preventive intervention for patients experiencing unipolar major depression in periods of remission and it aims to teach such people to become more aware of and to relate differently to their thoughts. Clients are taught how to disengage from thought patterns which feed their depression and are encouraged to see their reactions as separate mental events.

A principal feature of both MBSM and MBCT is the idea of acceptance, an idea which frees the client from the kind of self-scrutiny that tries to judge his efforts. Mindfulness in all its forms is thus essentially non-judgemental and as such, is based on experience rather than knowledge.

However, mindfulness approaches do have differences and this makes some authors reluctant to credit the notion of combining an acceptance-based approach, such as meditation, with a change-based strategy, such as cognitive therapy, viewing them as direct opposites, the first being noted for its absence of a goal while the second may have a particular goal in mind. In defence of MBCT, Segal et al (2004) suggest that the idea of acceptance should be seen as the primary principle and cognitive considerations viewed as secondary. These authors speak of bringing 'a kindly awareness' to the matter in hand, rather than an active determination to modify the thoughts. It is an approach which may help the individual to understand herself at a deeper level.

The approach is underpinned not only by Buddhist principles of awareness and meditation, but also by cognitive theory.

Procedure for mindfulness-based cognitive therapy

The MBCT programme is similar to the MBSR one except that it has a stronger cognitive element (see Chs 1 and 16). Both place emphasis on an attitude of acceptance, an awareness of the reality of the present moment and the relationship of the individual to his thoughts. MBCT, however, includes a cognitive component which, among other things, seeks to show the patient how to disengage from dysfunctional automatic thoughts. Also featured are diary keeping and various forms of cognitive and physiological relaxation. Daily home practice is essential.

Evidence of effectiveness of mindfulness-based cognitive therapy

An early investigation into the combined effect of mindfulness meditation and cognitive approaches was conducted by Teasdale and colleagues (2000). This randomized, three-centre controlled trial compared the combined intervention with treatment as usual. Participants were a group of severely depressed people whose symptoms were in remission. The trial ran for 8 weeks. In the treatment period it was found that a fall in relapse rate which was statistically significant occurred in those participants who had had three or more episodes of severe depression, prior to the study, compared with participants who had treatment as usual. Participants who had had only one or two previous episodes experienced no such fall in relapse rate. Thus, people with multiple episodes of severe depression derived benefit from a course in MBCT which was not shared by those with a history of fewer relapses. This study was supported by further work which resulted in similar findings (Ma & Teasdale 2003).

MBCT has also been used in the treatment of substance abuse with co-occurring mood disorders. Early findings suggest that this approach may be useful in reducing the likelihood of relapse (Hoppes 2006).

Lau et al (2005) reviewed studies which integrated mindfulness meditation and cognitive therapy and found that the combination created efficacious treatments.

A recent trial attempted to tease out the relative benefits of the component parts of MBCT by comparing the effects of MBSR with those of cognitive–behaviour therapy. Koszicki et al (2007) randomly divided 53 patients with social anxiety disorder into two groups. One received an 8-week cognitive–behaviour course, the other, 12 sessions of MBSR. The researchers found that the cognitive–behaviour group rated significantly higher on response, remission rate, mood and quality of life than the MBSR group although improvement occurred in both groups.

Critically reviewing the topic, Segal and colleagues (2004) consider MBCT to be 'one of the most potentially productive avenues' of future development in psychotherapy. This view is endorsed by Whitfield (2006) who points to a growing body of empirical evidence demonstrating effectiveness of the approach in certain disorders.

Final remarks

Some readers may feel that mindfulness meditation has religious overtones which do not accord with their beliefs. The way in which it is presented here, however, is in the form of a secular practice.

Others may feel that mindfulness sits unhappily in a book of techniques, since the approach is more a way of life than a skill; therefore it should not be considered a technique. The key question, however, is whether mindfulness meditation induces relaxation. To answer that question, one returns to the notion of acceptance which is central to mindfulness approaches. It can be argued that relaxation also is, in essence, a state of acceptance. Such a view suggests a similarity which clearly warrants the inclusion of mindfulness meditation in a handbook of relaxation methods.

KEY MESSAGES

- Mindfulness-based meditation is an ancient practice which has been adopted by therapists wishing to reduce stress levels in their clients.
- Its central principle is the awareness of each moment as it passes.
- The meditator adopts an attitude of non-judgemental acceptance. This allows him to separate himself from his thoughts and emotions. He is aware of them without responding to them.
- The approach is sometimes combined with cognitive therapy where it has particular relevance in the treatment of severe depression and anxiety.

Further reading

Kabat-Zinn, J., 2006. Mindfulness for beginners (CD). Sounds True: soundstrue.com. ISBN: 1-59179-464-1

Chapter Twenty Four

24

Brief techniques

Introduction

The goal of most methods described in previous chapters has been the induction of deep relaxation, a slowly induced state which allows the individual to lose all tension. In order to achieve this, she must detach herself from environmental stimuli and focus all her attention on the method. This approach is appropriate where total relaxation is required and where the environment is making no current demands on her.

The individual may, however, be looking for a shorter technique which works fast, a strategy to lighten the effect of a stressor suddenly imposed upon her. The aim here is not to release all tension but to lose superfluous tension. Far from being detached from the environment, the individual wants to be fully alert to deal with its challenges. Instead of eliminating stressors, she wants to increase her tolerance of them. What she needs is a technique which can be implemented at a moment's notice and still allow her to carry on with the task, whatever it might be.

Shortened forms of techniques have already been referred to. The rapid relaxation of Öst (1987) is one example (see Ch. 9 , p85), where the individual recites a cue word on exhalation while scanning the body for tension. Mitchell's (1987) 'key movements', which are capable of unlocking the body from tense postures (see Ch. 11, p102), are another example.

Although the aim of brief techniques is to lose excess tension, retaining only what is necessary for the task, these techniques are not the same as differential relaxation. Differential relaxation is a principle to be applied throughout the day, regardless of activity. By contrast, brief techniques are designed to exert a momentary effect in the face of sudden threat.

A variety of methods for inducing relaxation at short notice are presented in this chapter. They are derived from methods already described, being, for the most part, abbreviated versions of them. They work best in individuals who have given the parent method many hours of practice. It is practice that enables the individual to switch on the full effect at short notice. Thus, brief techniques are shorthand versions of lengthier methods previously learned.

Characteristics of brief techniques

In essence, brief techniques should be:

- portable: short enough and convenient enough to be used in most situations
- unobtrusive: not attracting attention or interrupting ongoing work
- capable of inducing moderate levels of relaxation. The object is not to induce deep relaxation but to enable the individual to carry on with the task, in as relaxed a state as possible.

Factors affecting the success of brief techniques

Not every strategy is going to succeed every time. A number of factors may influence the outcome.

1. *Situation.* The degree of inherent threat in a situation may vary. Situations of high threat tend to reduce the effectiveness of the technique.

2. *Sensitivity to internal cues.* A person's ability to recognize her own physiological and psychological cues is important. As stress levels rise, the cues become more pronounced. The earlier she is able to pick them up, the more effective will be the relaxation device that she applies.

3. *Level of skill attained by previous practice.* The capacity to 'switch on' relaxation whenever the individual feels under stress depends to a great extent on the level of skill attained in any one technique. This in turn depends on the amount of home practice that has been carried out.

4. *Personal preference in choice of technique.* Individuals have preferences for some methods over others. The method in which a person feels most at ease will be likely to induce greater relaxation than a method which feels alien to her.

5. *Diversionary content of the technique.* Diversion, such as the reciting of a mantra, is said to contribute to the effect of a relaxation device. The stronger the diversionary

element, the greater the power of the technique. It is a useful feature where all that is required is a reduction in stress levels, as in the condition of panic. Where successful coping relies on intellectual and verbal skills, distraction is less useful, and a technique which leaves the mind free to focus on the issue is more appropriate.

The exercises

A technique may be picked from any of the following approaches:

- physical actions
- scanning
- breathing
- cognitive strategies.

Physical actions

When under stress, the individual tends to close up physically. It is an unconscious reaction to any kind of threat and has the effect of making her feel less exposed. Although the action may not be observable, the muscles involved may nevertheless be minutely contracting. To help release that tension, one of the following manoeuvres could be adopted:

- key changes
- posture
- shaking a sleeve down
- stretchings.

Key changes

Certain physical actions may serve as keys to unlock body patterns of tension (Mitchell 1987) (see Ch. 11, p102). The individual may find her personal key in one of the following four actions.

1. *Spreading the fingers.* The order is: fingers and thumbs long ... hold them there for a moment ... then stop ... let them recoil into a gently curved position.

2. *Separating your teeth.* The order is: drag your jaw downwards ... feel your jaw hanging down inside your mouth ... then stop ... feel your throat slack, your tongue loose and your lips gently touching.

3. *Pulling the shoulders towards the feet.* Feel a distance growing between your shoulders and your ears … and, stop pulling … let your shoulders rest where they are.

4. *Pushing the head back.* With your shoulders pulled down, lift your head; carry it up and back, keeping your chin pointing towards your feet. Stop. The resulting position should feel comfortable.

Posture

A mental impression of being at one's full height promotes a sense of ease and confidence. Reminders are contained in phrases such as:

- think 'tall'
- think 'up'.

The second item is drawn from the Alexander technique (see Ch. 12, p106).

Shaking a sleeve down

This action loosens the muscles in the arm and shoulder and has the added advantage of appearing a quite natural thing to do.

Stretchings

Musculoskeletal benefit is derived from stretchings (see Ch. 14, p117). In the context of brief relaxation, they are aimed at structures which have been held in one position for some length of time, such as the spinal joints during long-distance motoring. A few examples appear below:

- trunk twisting (Fig. 14.15)
- back arching (Fig. 14.16)
- crouching (Fig. 14.17).

Other stretching exercises may be found in Chapter 14, p117.

Scanning

Scanning is a shortened version of passive relaxation. It involves a brief tour of the body during which the participant checks for unnecessary tension. Four approaches are described:

1. relaxation by recall with counting

2. behavioural relaxation checklist

3. sweeping the body

4. the ripple.

Relaxation by recall with counting

Bernstein & Borkovec (1973) condensed their progressive relaxation training programme into a release-only format for four groups of muscles: the arms, the head and neck, the trunk and the legs. In its most summarized form, it consists of a counting procedure: two counts are allotted to each body part as attention is focused on it and tension released (see Ch. 8, p73).

> *One … two (arms relax) … three … four (head and neck relax) … five … six (trunk relax) … seven … eight (legs relax) … nine … ten (whole body relax) …*

Behavioural relaxation checklist

This is based on the assumption that if an individual looks relaxed, to some extent he will feel relaxed. A checklist (see Table 10.1), which can be memorized, covers 10 postures characteristic of relaxation (Poppen 1988).

- Feet … resting with toes lying free
- Hands … fingers gently curled
- Body … without movement
- Shoulders … dropped and level
- Head … still, and facing forwards
- Mouth … teeth separated, lips unpursed
- Throat … loose
- Breathing … slow and gentle
- Voice … no sound
- Eyes … lightly closed behind smooth eyelids.

Sweeping the body

Kermani (1990) describes a routine used for releasing body tension. It involves sweeping the surface of the body with an imaginary large, soft paintbrush (see Ch. 8, p77).

> *Starting at your feet, sweep the brush, in your mind's eye, up your legs and the front of your body as far as your shoulders … then down your arms to your fingertips … then, a long sweep up the full length of the back … continuing into the*

neck and scalp ... over the brow ... and down to the face and jaw.

The ripple

This is a single wave of relaxation which begins at the head and rolls down the body to the feet (Priest & Schott 1991) (see Ch. 8, p74).

Starting at the top of your head, feel the relaxation rolling down your body in one continuous wave ... feel it releasing tension as it descends ... relaxing each part of your body in turn ... until it reaches the tips of your toes. Try synchronizing the ripple with a slow breath out.

Breathing

Stress is associated with physiological arousal. This arousal is brought about by the action of the sympathetic nervous system, and includes an increase in the respiratory rate. Slowed breathing is associated with parasympathetic activity. Thus, by consciously slowing the breathing rate, it may be possible to counteract the effects of the sympathetic nervous system and generally check the symptoms of arousal.

Three techniques are described. Each one has a greater chance of success if it is introduced before the state of stress becomes established.

1. Abdominal breathing
2. Using words as cues
3. A breathing cycle

Abdominal breathing

Since sudden stress is associated with apical (upper costal) respiratory movements, and relaxation with abdominal respiratory movements, breathing which is focused on the abdomen will tend to have a quietening effect (see Ch. 4, p38).

Let your attention focus on your abdomen. Feel it swelling as you breathe in and sinking as you breathe out. Keep the breathing light, gentle and slow.

Using words as cues (cue-controlled relaxation)

Repeated past associations of a word such as 'relax' with the relaxed state give the word the status of a cue. When subsequently recited on the outbreath, this word tends to bring about a state of relaxation (Öst 1987) (see Ch 9, p87).

Let your breathing be as natural as possible ... just before you begin to breathe out, think the word 'relax' ... slowly release the air as you focus on the word ... breathe in ... and, repeat the sequence ... keep the rhythm as gentle as you can ... avoid deliberately deepening the breaths ... continue for a few moments ...

A short version might run:

In ... relax and out slowly ... in ... relax and out slowly ...

or simply:

Relax

A breathing cycle

A single breath cycle can be useful for helping to relieve stress in a crisis situation. It consists of a deeper than usual breath in, which is held for a few seconds before being slowly exhaled. Lichstein (1988) points out how each component of the exercise has value: the inbreath diverts attention from the distressing thoughts; the breath retention raises the PCO_2 level, inducing mild lethargy, and the slow outbreath helps to reduce muscle tension. The cycle begins with an outbreath in the exercise below.

Breathe out a little more fully than usual. Let the air flow in to fill your lungs. Hold it for 5 seconds. Then exhale slowly. As you let the air out, feel the tension going with it. Then, let your breathing recover its normal rhythm.

Since deep breathing can increase the possibility of hyperventilation, immediate repetition of this exercise is not recommended.

Cognitive strategies

These are methods which deal with stress by changing our thoughts. They include the following approaches:

1. self-talk
2. autogenic phrases
3. imagery
4. attention switching
5. thought stopping
6. thinking of a smile
7. environmental markers
8. additional strategies.

Self-talk

Since thoughts influence feelings, positive thoughts will tend to generate positive feelings. Phrases affirming the value of the self, repeated often, colour our view of ourselves, and in a positive direction (see Ch.19, p163). Feeling in control and feeling relaxed will tend to increase coping powers whatever the source of the stress.

Phrases tending to promote a sense of control over the situation include:

* I am competent
* I can deal with this
* I am in control
* My coping powers are good.

Phrases tending to induce a relaxed state of mind include:

* I feel at peace
* I am relaxed
* I am calm
* My thoughts are peaceful ones.

The above phrases provide examples of positive self-talk; however, the most effective phrases are those which the individual has composed for herself.

Autogenic phrases

Training in autogenics (see Ch. 20, p171) can result in relaxation occurring after recitation of a single phrase. It could be a heaviness phrase, a warmth phrase or one relating to feelings of peace. When recited, it can act as a key to switch on autogenic effects.

Imagery

Both single images and transformations can promote relaxation. Two examples of the former are the rag doll and the piece of seaweed (see Ch.18, p154). Identifying with the characteristics of an inert image can help to mitigate feelings of stress. Anger, panic and frustration may all respond to this kind of imagery.

Transformations refer to the mutation of one substance into another (see Ch.18, p155). The first substance is harsh, the second smooth and they are linked by some sensory quality as in the following items (Fanning 1988):

* sandpaper … to … silk
* chalk squeaking on the blackboard … to … high musical notes
* burnt toast fumes … to … baking bread
* fluorescent orange … to … soft peach
* sour gooseberries … to … sweet raspberries.

The individual focuses attention on the harsh image which she then resolves into the smooth one. The transformation becomes a metaphor for her own feelings which are thereby helped to undergo a change from negative to positive.

Thought stopping

Thought stopping (Quick & Quick 1984) intercepts stress-inducing thoughts and substitutes stress-neutralizing ones. The technique involves the word 'STOP', spoken or imagined, but in such a way that it momentarily blots out the disturbing thought. This is immediately replaced with an idea or an activity which diverts and holds the attention, such as counting games, puzzles or physical exercise.

Thinking of a smile

Facial expression has been found to influence emotions. A positive expression tends to induce a positive feeling in that individual (see Ch. 10, p87). Thus, if a person smiles, her feelings of stress will tend to be diminished. However, as it is not always appropriate to smile, it is enough to stay with the thought of it and simply to imagine the smile.

The environmental marker

Several writers suggest placing a mark on appliances which are potential sources of stress (Öst 1987,

Mitchell 1987) (see Chs 9 and 11). Coloured dots stuck, for instance, on to the telephone, wristwatch or steering wheel serve to remind the individual to maintain low levels of tension. Öst suggests changing the colour of the markers frequently since their effect dwindles as the eye gets habituated to the dot.

Additional strategies

A range of techniques can be used to distract the attention, including images of strong light and memorized telephone numbers. In the case of 'strong light', the trainee can be asked to imagine an intensely bright light beamed into his eyes from a dark background. With regard to the 'telephone number', he can be asked to look at a new number, concentrating so hard that he memorizes it, then closes his eyes and recites it several times.

Section **Four**

Working towards best practice

Chapter Twenty Five

Measurement

25

CHAPTER CONTENTS

This chapter is devoted to the topic of measurement and includes discussion on patient assessment and clinical audit. Measurement, in this context, is the process of observing and recording the outcomes resulting from treatment intervention. Measurement, however, is not finite; errors and uncertainties can arise, undermining accuracy. To minimize this effect, assessment tools need to be reliable and valid.

Selecting the most appropriate tool can be challenging as there are many kinds of measuring tools,

including questionnaires, self-assessment inventories, sweat sensors, heart rate monitors and biofeedback monitors. Before deciding on the measuring tool, some basic questions should be considered such as: What is likely to change as a result of applying the treatment intervention? What is it I am trying to measure? Is there a validated tool that I can use? Is it applicable for this population, with regard to age, gender, culture and condition? Do I need training to be able to use it? Is it freely available or do I need to purchase it? How often should I use it?

Knowledge and experience of the topic may help to suggest a suitable tool. If not, the Centre for Evidence-Based Physiotherapy in Maastricht can provide a wide range of validated outcome measuring devices. Box 25.1 contains contact information about this and other sources of information. As some tools are designed for particular diseases or certain population groups (such as children or older people), it is necessary to check that the selected tool is an appropriate one.

Box 25.1

Databases providing information regarding outcome measures

National Centre for Health Outcomes Development. http://phi.uhce.ox.ac.uk
National Institute forHealth & Clinical Excellence. www.nice.org.uk
Centre for Evidence-Based Physiotherapy in Maastricht. www.cebp.nl

In this chapter the reader is taken through the process of assessment and provided with a few examples of assessment tools which could be used in the context of relaxation. A section on measuring exercise intensity is also included to illustrate how assessment can be applied to physical activity (see Ch. 15).

Patient assessment

Assessment means 'estimating' or 'judging' (*Harraps Chambers Concise Dictionary* 2004), in this case estimating the degree of stress, anxiety or relaxation present in an individual. Two types of information are found during assessment: objective and subjective. *Objective* information is factual and measurable. *Subjective* information relates to the personal experience of the individual, her interpretation of events and other thoughts and feelings. Both areas of information are equally important in gaining an understanding of the problem (Table 25.1). Assessment is ongoing and the health care professional will constantly monitor, reassess and update the information gathered.

Assessment tools

The most commonly used tool for initial assessment is the clinical interview. In the course of this and in a relatively short time, relevant information will emerge. This will refer to previous medical history, current signs and symptoms, reason for referral and information specific to the client's

Table 25.1 Examples of objective and subjective information

Objective information	Subjective information
• Blood pressure • Pulse • Respiration rate • Temperature • Distance that can be walked in a given time • Ability to follow relaxation instruction • Ability to complete exercise diary • Quality of sleep – ability to record hours of sleep	• The person's interpretation of her stress • How well (or unwell) she feels • Degree to which she likes a particular relaxation method • Her belief in the usefulness of relaxation and or exercise as an intervention for stress • Types of physical activity she finds most satisfying

sense of current well-being. The findings from this interview will be written up in case notes. Other assessments may also be undertaken at this time or on subsequent visits.

The data collected can be broadly grouped into three categories: nominal, functional and attitudinal. *Nominal* data describe people by their ethnic origin, place of residence and the type of work they do. Such data give some idea of the person's identity and allow the health care professional to make a few assumptions such as the ability to attend weekly classes. They may also provide some clues about stress levels.

Functional data are items of information which reflect the overall functional ability of the individual, such as her inclination to learn from and apply knowledge, her ability to cope with general tasks or demands and her willingness to discuss health and well-being. Functional data include the readiness of the client to take part in relaxation, exercise or other physical activity, a feature which is highlighted by the World Health Organization (2001).

Attitudinal data are gathered by taking account of the client's opinions, mindset and cultural beliefs. By asking questions, the health care professional can elicit information which will be helpful when analysing the data and in selecting an appropriate intervention.

Assessment findings should be reviewed with the client, checking that she understands the findings and giving her time to ask questions. The proposed intervention is then discussed with the client, together with its likely time-scale. It is important to gain her agreement before proceeding any further. Where function is limited, measurement is accompanied by a standardized assessment. This is a tool with a clearly defined scope, designed to identify a particular aspect of a condition. It has typically been through a process to check its reliability and validity. Such standard measures usually carry instructions regarding method of scoring and interpretation of results (Burlingame & Blaschko 2002). They will also indicate the type of professional for whom they are designed.

Why give assessments?

With regard to relaxation training, assessment is needed for the following reasons.

1. To obtain a profile of the individual's problems as they are observed and expressed

by the individual and communicated to the health care practitioner. It is likely that the relaxation training will be part of a wider programme of anxiety management, in which case the activities of the relevant professionals will need to be integrated.

2. To measure existing indicators of stress, for example heart rate, blood pressure, anxiety levels. One or more of these measures can provide a baseline when evaluating progress. The assessment should be carried out after a short period of rest to allow for the relaxation effects which occur, in the absence of any relaxation technique, as part of the process of adapting to a restful environment.

3. To inform decisions regarding the selection of interventions: for example, where there are high levels of worrying intrusive thoughts, cognitive–behavioural approaches may be recommended.

4. To measure the benefits of the relaxation training in terms of key outcomes over time. A key outcome could be muscle tension, heart rate, mood state or sense of well-being. This can be assessed prior to and immediately after a relaxation session and/or 1 week and up to 6 months following relaxation training. Alternatively, assessment may focus on symptoms such as tension headache or hypertension and the degree to which these have been relieved by the relaxation training.

5. To evaluate the success of the intervention and provide feedback to both the health care professional and the participant. Positive feedback acts as a reinforcer, negative feedback indicates the need for corrective action.

6. To gather quantifiable data for the purpose of retrospective research or where data are being collected as part of an intervention study, for example, measuring the effectiveness of relaxation in reducing tension headaches.

Although patient assessment is time-consuming, it is an essential process with clear benefits.

For those who wish to manage their own stress and anxiety, and who are using this book as a self-help guide, self-monitoring is also important. (See below for ways in which the reader can measure her own progress.)

Ways of measuring relaxation

Relaxation has psychological, physiological and behavioural components, so a test which is restricted to only one of these cannot claim to be comprehensive. To give an accurate measure of the degree of relaxation present, standardized assessment should cover all three components. Only an assessment which takes account of these multiple dimensions can reflect the complexity of the relaxation state.

Since there is no test which covers all three, the components must be measured separately.

Psychological assessment

Measurement covers a wide range of psychosocial factors including mood state, anxiety and depression, mental well-being and quality of life. This type of assessment is generally undertaken by questionnaires and self-rating scales. Where these indicate moderate to severe depression or anxiety, referral to the general practitioner or other specialist within the health care team should be considered. Previous medical history is also an important factor.

Questionnaires

A questionnaire is a list of questions requiring 'yes/no' or similar answers, which can be converted into numerical scores. Its purpose is to obtain information about a specific topic. A standardized questionnaire is the instrument of choice as it will have been tested on different groups of people and average scores will have been established, against which the individual's scores can be compared. As a validated assessment tool, this kind of questionnaire is the only kind that can be used for quantitative assessment and research. In the case of relaxation, such a questionnaire could be used to obtain information both at the start and at the end of a course of treatment, in order to see how people progress and to compare them with groups diagnosed as 'anxious' or 'normal', for example.

The advantages of questionnaires are that they are quick, cheap and easy to complete. It is also easy to collate the results. Their disadvantages include the possibility of inaccuracy if the questions are misunderstood or of missing out information, if forcing responses into 'yes/no' categories should fail to express the complexity of a person's position.

The interview schedule

An alternative and more sensitive approach is to use an interview schedule. Here, the interviewer guides the individual through the questions, making sure those questions have been understood and drawing fuller answers than are possible in a questionnaire. Thus, the interview schedule provides more detailed and more complete information than the questionnaire. Quantifying the additional information, however, is more difficult and the interview schedule is subject to variability between interviewers, each of whom may have different ways of interviewing people. The value of the interview depends to a great extent on the clinical experience and judgement of the interviewer.

Examples of questionnaires

There is available a wide range of standardized questionnaires, each designed to measure specific or generic aspects of mental distress. The following are examples of questionnaires that may be considered for measuring anxiety, depression and mental health.

- *State Trait Anxiety Inventory Y (STAI Y)* (Spielberger 1980). This contains 40 questions in two 20-item scales with a range of four possible responses to each. The measure differentiates between the temporary condition of 'state anxiety' and the more general and long-standing 'trait anxiety'. The scale measures feelings of apprehension, tension and nervousness. It is the most widely used instrument for measuring anxiety and is available in 40 languages. The inventory takes 10 minutes to complete. This tool has been found to be sensitive to measuring change in state anxiety following relaxation training. An example of the questions is provided in Figure 25.1.
- *The Hospital Anxiety and Depression Scale (HAD)* (Zigmond & Snaith 1983). This contains 14 items, seven relating to anxiety

1	2	3	4
Not at all	Somewhat	Moderately so	Very much so

			1	2	3	4
A	I feel at ease		1	2	3	4
B	I feel upset		1	2	3	4

(a)

1	2	3	4
Almost never	Sometimes	Often	Almost always

			1	2	3	4
A	I am a steady person		1	2	3	4
B	I lack self-confidence		1	2	3	4

(b)

Figure 25.1 • (a) The State Anxiety Scale consists of 20 statements that evaluate how respondents feel 'right now, at this moment'. (b) The Trait Anxiety Scale consists of 20 statements that assess how respondents feel 'generally'.

and seven to depression. The score gives an indication of the degree to which the individual is suffering from either condition. The scale is also able to pick up alterations over time.

- *The Short Form 36 (SF-36)* (Ware & Sherbourne 1992). This measure consists of 36 questions and is designed to provide information regarding a person's current physical and emotional health, including the ability to participate in daily activities and work . The questions were designed to be easy to understand and relevant to most people's lives. It was originally developed in the USA and is now one of the most commonly used measures of quality of life. It has been translated into many languages and has been used as an outcome measure in over 2000 studies. (For further information on the SF-36 version 2, see Wade et al 2000.)
- *The Beck Depression Inventory* (Beck 1988, Beck et al 1961). Measures of the level of depression can be obtained from this questionnaire which can be used at different stages of illness and recovery.
- *The Cognitive Anxiety Questionnaire* (Lindsay & Hood 1982). This contains 12 items and reflects some of the most common thoughts associated with anxiety. It measures the tendency of the individual to engage in such thoughts.

These are all simple screening devices for use with individuals. The results, when obtained at the beginning and end of a training course, give an indication of change over time in the individual concerned. The results can also be used to assess the effectiveness of relaxation training on groups of people and can be used in clinical trials under controlled conditions.

The Hospital Anxiety and Depression Scale is shown in Figure 25.2. It has been picked as an example because of its widespread use and general applicability. Questions 1, 4, 5, 8, 9, 12 and 13 relate to anxiety, and questions 2, 3, 6, 7, 10, 11 and 14 relate to depression. Scoring instructions are attached to the assessment sheet but not included here. A score of 8–10 in either section indicates a mild degree of the condition, while a score of 11 or above suggests the advisability of referral to a specialist agency. Although the scale is seen as a screening tool, it is, in the present context, used primarily to measure tendencies to states of distress which may change over the period in which relaxation is practised. Any resulting change should not, however, be totally

attributed to relaxation, since other factors such as changing environmental circumstances may be contributing to alterations in scores.

Tests show that the HAD possesses a considerable degree of validity and reliability although, as with most scales, further testing is required before confident judgements on its performance can be made. The scale is also easy to understand and has been found acceptable to patients, taking only 5 minutes to complete (Bowling 1997).

The Centre for Evidence-Based Physiotherapy in Maastricht provides a helpful link to a wide range of validated measures and is accessible through the internet (see Box 25.1). Some of these tools, such as the State Trait Anxiety Inventory, need to be purchased. Others, like the Hospital Anxiety and Depression Scale, are freely available.

Self-rating

Related to the questionnaire is the self-rating scale, i.e. the rating an individual gives herself. It often takes the form of a visual analogue. Though it is a highly subjective assessment, it nevertheless has value since relaxation is an internal state with a strong subjective component. The self-rating scale is particularly useful for recording levels of pain and anxiety. Two forms are described here.

- A rating scale in the form of a line calibrated from 0 to 10 where 0 represents total relaxation and 10 maximum tension. The intervening numbers refer to intermediate states. The participant rings the appropriate number.
- A rating scale which consists of numbered descriptors signifying different degrees of relaxation and tension, as in Poppen's (1998) self-rating scale (see Ch. 10, p91). Again, the participant rings the appropriate number.

These may be used before and after the relaxation session. Marking scales in this way gives a measure of the effect of the treatment.

Another form of self-monitoring is the diary, seen as a useful way of logging feelings of tension and situations of high anxiety. The diary can be used to record immediate change after a relaxation ession and also change over a longer period. It provides feedback and can act as an extrinsic motivator, helping to ensure that practice is carried out.

A record sheet is another way of logging the occurrence and intensity of anxious feelings. Figure 9.2 (p81) illustrates this approach and contains a

SECTION 1

NAME: DATE: AGE:

This section is designed to help identify how you feel. Read each item and place a tick in the box opposite the reply which comes closest to how you have been feeling in the past few weeks. Don't take too long over your replies: your immediate reaction to each item will probably be more accurate than a long thought-out response.

Tick only one box in each section

(1) I feel tense or 'wound up':
- Most of the time
- A lot of the time
- Time to time. Occasionally
- Not at all

(2) I feel as if I am slowed down:
- Nearly all the time
- Very often
- Sometimes
- Not at all

(3) I still enjoy the things I used to enjoy:
- Definitely as much
- Not quite so much
- Only a little
- Hardly at all

(4) I get a sort of frightened feeling like 'butterflies' in the stomach:
- Not at all
- Occasionally
- Quite often
- Very often

(5) I get a sort of frightened feeling as if something awful is about to happen:
- Very definitely and quite badly
- Yes, but not too badly
- A little, but it doesn't worry me
- Not at all

(6) I have lost interest in my appearance:
- Definitely
- I don't take so much care as I should
- I may not take quite as much care
- I take just as much care as ever

(7) I can laugh and see the funny side of things:
- As much as I always could
- Not quite so much now
- Definitely not so much now
- Not at all

(8) I feel restless as if I have to be on the move:
- Very much indeed
- Quite a lot
- Not very much
- Not at all

(9) Worrying thoughts go through my mind:
- A great deal of the time
- A lot of the time
- From time to time but not too often
- Only occasionally

(10) I look forward with enjoyment to things:
- As much as ever I did
- Rather less than I used to
- Definitely less than I used to
- Hardly at all

(11) I feel cheerful:
- Not at all
- Not often
- Sometimes
- Most of the time

(12) I get sudden feelings of panic:
- Very often indeed
- Quite often
- Not very often
- Not at all

(13) I can sit at ease and feel relaxed:
- Definitely
- Usually
- Not often
- Not at all

(14) I can enjoy a good book or radio or TV programme:
- Often
- Sometimes
- Not often
- Very seldom

Figure 25.2 • The Hospital Anxiety and Depression Scale. (Adapted from Zigmond & Snaith 1983 Acta Psychiatrica Scandinavica 67:361-370 with permission from the authors. Reproduced from Powell and Enright 1990, Fig. 3.3, with permission from Routledge, Taylor & Francis Books Ltd.)

numbered scale relating to feelings, together with details of the particular coping strategy adopted.

Homework can be recorded on a form such as that in Figure 9.3 (p82). This is a useful method of ensuring that practice is carried out, as well as providing an indication of the degree of benefit obtained.

Written self-reports have the advantage of being quick, easy, cheap and non-threatening to the participant. They are an essential part of the process in dealing with varying levels of stress and anxiety. Monitoring relaxation sessions, i.e. writing down feelings and behaviours immediately before and after the session and then at other key points throughout the day, provides an element of control over situations of stress/anxiety, where feelings of helplessness or limited control might otherwise prevail.

The value of self-rating lies particularly on an individual level, where it helps the client to check her own progress. It is less useful in research, where two or more groups are being compared and where a validated questionnaire would be the tool of choice. A range of self-report measures can be found in Johnstone et al (1995).

Physiological assessment

Assessing the effect of relaxation training on body systems provides an objective measurement. A variety of indicators are in current use, including pulse rate, blood pressure, respiratory rate, muscle tension, peripheral blood flow, palmar sweating and electrical activity in the brain. Most of these can easily be measured and machines are available for the purpose. The results show the level of physiological arousal in an individual, and the test or tests are carried out before and after relaxation sessions. The baseline is established before training begins and, in common with all pretreatment measures, should be recorded after a short period of rest.

It might be supposed that this approach offered the perfect solution. The field of physiological assessment, however, is not as straightforward as it appears. Keable (1997) discusses certain points.

- Physiological measures can be distorted by circumstances. The individual may have eaten prior to a relaxation session, which would result in artificially low arousal scores; she may have taken exercise immediately before, which would raise her scores; emotional distress would also raise them and drugs would distort them.

Tests therefore need to be conducted under controlled conditions.

- Since the physiological response of individuals is to some extent idiosyncratic, a single measure may not include relevant information. To gain an accurate picture, therefore, a system which provides multiple measurements is needed.

Poppen (1998) adds the following point.

- Even in the case of specific symptoms, it is not always clear how their measurement should be approached. In tension headache, for example, it might be thought that electromyography of the surrounding muscles would be appropriate; however, exactly which muscles should be measured is less clear. Or again, instead of measuring the electrical activity, it might be more constructive to measure the blood flow through the surrounding muscles (Olton & Noonberg 1980). Researchers hold different views.

Furthermore, while measurement of the pulse and breathing rate are simple procedures, most other physiological measures require equipment and expertise, neither of which may be available. In spite of these difficulties, however, physiological measurement is an important part of general assessment.

Measuring change through goal setting

All stress-reducing programmes have a goal. It may be getting to the supermarket without experiencing feelings of panic; it may be facing an audience without shaking with fright. These goals can seem insurmountable to the individual who has high levels of stress. One solution is to break them down into short-term goals as these will appear more manageable than the main goal while yet leading in the desired direction (see Fig. 19.1). The concept of a goal can be compared to a staircase where the main goal is to reach the landing above; the easiest way of doing this is by travelling through the intervening steps. Goal setting is a useful way of measuring behaviour change.

What is a long-term goal?

Goals that produce a desired outcome are called long-term goals, such as reducing the number of panic attacks. Short-term goals are daily actions which lead to the long-term goal and include, for example, attending a weekly relaxation class and keeping a diary. Both activities focus on specific targets which can be documented, such as the number of relaxation sessions attended, the level of anxiety experienced or the type of benefit obtained. Feedback for the individual is thereby provided and, for the health care professional, a means of reviewing progress.

Goal setting is jointly decided between the client and the therapist which means that the client retains ownership of the goal. Consequently she is more likely to give it priority status.

Setting goals

A useful acronym relating to goal setting, SMART, is explained in Box 25.2, which lists ways in which the goals can be made more powerful, and itemizes the following.

Specific: a defined target such as 'I want to attend a weekly class and learn how to relax' is easier to follow than a vague aspiration such as 'I'd like to be more relaxed'. Specific short-term goals can be set up, and these are effective because they enable people to know whether they are moving in the right direction; if they are not, those goals can be adjusted. The process provides a continuous assessment. Where goals have not been met, a commentary on the supposed reason should be included in the report.

Measurable: it is important that goals should be measurable. This is made possible by careful

record keeping with the use of diaries and/or tabulated sheets which reflect the work done at home. Reading back entries provides the client with feedback which helps to maintain motivation. It also enables the healthcare professional to review progress or chart setbacks.

Attainable: all goals must be realistic. The possibility of achievement must exist in the mind of both client and therapist; otherwise the goals are doomed to failure and loss of confidence. Information gathered in the clinical interview will enable the healthcare professional to judge whether or not the client's goal is attainable.

Relevant: any goal must relate to the individual's life as she wishes to lead it. It is for this reason that the goals are set jointly.

Time bound: effective treatment in the domain of relaxation training needs to be limited by a time span. It helps the client to focus on the process. A time-restricted treatment scheme should be agreed at the start.

Why is goal setting important?

Stress and anxiety can prevent people from fulfilling their hopes. Goal setting can help to reduce that stress by offering a step-by-step approach in the form of short-term goals. As each one is achieved, the possibility of reaching the desired outcome increases. Thus, by setting a goal and defining the steps needed to reach it, a difficult challenge is transformed into a series of routine daily behaviours. Advice on setting up the goals can be provided by health care professionals; however, the success of the programme depends largely on the strength of the client's personal desire and her determination to work for the outcome of her choice.

Measuring progress in the self-help context

For people using this book as a self-help approach, progress can be monitored by setting short- and long-term goals following the SMART principles. Keeping a diary to monitor feelings of tension and mood change allows the individual to track her own progress. Printed forms, as illustrated in Figures 9.2 and 9.3, can also be used for this purpose. The measurement of physiological outcomes is relatively easy: pulse rate and blood pressure can

---

Box 25.2

SMART goals

A useful way of making goals more powerful is to use the SMART mnemonic. SMART, in this context, stands for:

- **S** Specific
- **M** Measurable
- **A** Attainable
- **R** Relevant
- **T** Time bound.

A long-term goal, such as 'I want to stop having panic attacks when I go shopping', is less powerful than 'In 6 months' time I want to have stopped having panic attacks every time I go shopping'. The second statement requires that a number of short-term goals are successfully completed.

be monitored using one of the electronic devices available from a local pharmacy. Electronic heart rate monitors are also widely available at retail outlets and consist of a simple device worn as a chest strap, plus a wrist watch.

The placebo effect

The belief in a treatment and the benefit felt to be derived from that treatment is important for a positive outcome. Faith in the remedy will aid recovery (Kaptchuk et al 2008). This is called the placebo effect and it is separate from the procedure's intrinsic value. Simply believing in the treatment creates benefit, and this contributes to the total effect. The placebo response, however, is not the same as spontaneous improvement. It may produce the same result but whereas spontaneous improvement is unrelated to treatment, the placebo response is an essential feature of treatment. When conducting randomized controlled trials to investigate the efficacy of a relaxation intervention, it is therefore necessary to have a placebo control as well as a waiting list control.

Since recovery, to a large extent, depends on the client's belief in the efficacy of the intervention, without it, recovery may be delayed or hindered; harm may even arise. This is called the nocebo effect (Benson & Stark 1996). To reduce the likelihood of the nocebo effect, it is important that participants are involved in the choice of appropriate relaxation technique.

Tools for measuring exercise intensity

A standard measure of exercise intensity is the percentage of maximum oxygen uptake ($\dot{V}O_2max$). This requires skills and apparatus which may not always be available. Simpler to measure is the percentage of maximum heart rate (HRmax) and since the two scales bear a linear relationship to each other, the HRmax is the method commonly employed (Smeaton 1995).

HRmax is estimated by subtracting the person's age from the figure 220. In the case of a 40-year-old individual this would be 180, representing his hypothetical maximum. If the programme requires a 60–65% HRmax level of intensity, then the pulse rate for this individual should be kept within the range of 108–117 during exercise.

This figure is appropriate for healthy individuals. People who are less fit, however, can take the figure of 200 instead of 220 as their starting point, and those under medical supervision should seek the advice of their doctor.

Criticisms of this method include the possibility of error within the age categories and difficulty in palpating the pulse for those unfamiliar with the practice (Birk & Birk 1987). An alternative method for determining exercise intensity has been developed by Borg (1970, 1998). This researcher considers that the single best indicator of physical strain is the individual's own perception of exertion. This entails the integration of signals from all parts of the body including muscles, joints, pulmonary and cardiac organs and the central nervous system. For the novice, this means concentrating on what Morgan (1981) has called the 'total inner feeling of exertion'.

Borg, a psychologist from Stockholm, devised a scale for rating this perceived exertion. It consists of descriptive phrases indicating the subjective response to different levels of exercise intensity (Fig. 25.3). The perceived exertion rating of 13–14 is seen as corresponding to 70% HRmax and the rating of 10–11 as corresponding to 60% HRmax. Thus, a glance at the scale helps the exerciser to judge the degree of effort required. Its sheer simplicity makes the scale attractive. Validity has been repeatedly demonstrated and high coefficients obtained (Borg 1998). Burke & Collins (1984) have found that the scale correlates strongly with

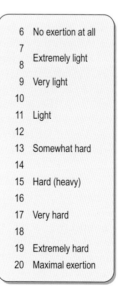

6	No exertion at all
7	
8	Extremely light
9	Very light
10	
11	Light
12	
13	Somewhat hard
14	
15	Hard (heavy)
16	
17	Very hard
18	
19	Extremely hard
20	Maximal exertion

Figure 25.3 • The Borg Scale.

oxygen consumption. Reliability has also been shown but although coefficients have often been high, Bowling (2001) considers that more work still needs to be done. Negative criticisms include the possibility of discrepancies between subjective reports and physiological effects.

Regarding targets of distance and energy expenditure, electronic devices can be purchased. For example, a device which counts steps and converts them into calorific values can be used to monitor progress in walking. Measures can be taken before and after physical activity to estimate immediate effect, on the one hand, and longer term (over periods up to 6 months) on the other.

Clinical audit

Clinical audit consists of the systematic analysis of procedures used for diagnosis, care and treatment (Department of Health 1994). It poses questions such as:

- To what extent do these procedures benefit the patient?
- Do these procedures make the best use of resources?
- Can this service be improved?

Clinical audit was introduced into the NHS in the early 1990s and it has continued to be developed since that time. A practical handbook on clinical audit, published by the NHS and accessible on line, provides useful guidance for healthcare professionals (Copeland 2005). The handbook aims to provide guidance through the processes and structures necessary to deliver clinical audit.

Audit assesses the effectiveness of a particular intervention in a particular context or location and acts as a guide in the planning of services. Interventions result in outcomes of different kinds: they may be measures of access to care (e.g. time to first appointment) or results of care (blood pressure reduction in response to a relaxation programme). The audit can be undertaken either retrospectively (involving the analysis of data such as medical case notes) or prospectively. One advantage of prospective audit is that it can be planned with regard to the selection of an appropriate timescale and outcome measure(s). In addition, prospective audit allows time for clinical staff to be allocated in a more fruitful way (Copeland 2005).

As well as measuring the effects of clinical practice, audit is concerned with issues such as resource allocation and may be used to highlight a need for departmental funding. This distinguishes it from research whose aim is to generate new knowledge or to test old knowledge and methods of treatment, seeking to identify the most effective intervention. Put another way, audit examines existing practice and looks for examples of good practice while research defines best practice (Sealey 1999). However, there is an interaction between audit and research in that the standards by which clinical practice is measured are established mainly from the research literature (Barnard & Hartigan 1998, Bury & Mead 1998). This relationship underlies the principles of evidence-based practice.

If the set standards are not met by current practice, changes are discussed and introduced, followed by further evaluation to assess the quality of the changes. The result of this process is called the outcome, which has been defined as 'that part of the output of a process which can be attributed to the process' (Long et al 1993). In the context of healthcare, outcome can be seen as change in the health of an individual which is likely to be due to the therapeutic intervention.

Outcome is measured by an instrument, which might be a questionnaire or other measuring tool, and the results then undergo analysis in order to determine the degree to which the intervention was responsible for any change in the health status of the individual.

Outcome measures can be objective or subjective. Objective measures include quantifiable factors such as blood pressure; subjective measures include, on the one hand, the level of pain experienced by the patient and on the other, observational judgements made by the therapist (Barnard & Hartigan 1998).

Tools for measuring outcome are designed for different purposes. They may also vary in their range of concern, i.e. be multidimensional or condition specific. An example of a multidimensional outcome measure is the Short Form 36 (Ware & Sherbourne 1992); an example of a condition-specific outcome measure is the Beck Depression Inventory (Beck 1988) which focuses on one particular area of mental health. Since a treatment outcome can have several aspects, the question can be answered more fully if a variety of measures are used.

It can be seen that the same devices may be used for assessing the patient's progress as for auditing the service or conducting research. For example, an instrument such as the Beck Depression Inventory can be useful in all three contexts. To make outcome measurement as accurate as possible, certain criteria must be fulfilled (Donaghy 2001). The measuring device should be:

- appropriate, i.e. suitable for the purpose and contain relevant items
- valid, i.e. shown to be measuring what it claims to measure
- reliable, i.e. capable of providing the same answer when the test is repeated by other therapists or by the same therapist on different occasions
- responsive, i.e. sensitive to change, able to detect small variations over time and sensitive to individual differences
- specific, i.e. able to isolate particular characteristics, for example, to focus on depressive symptoms as opposed to general symptoms of ill health
- acceptable, i.e. presented in such a way that the clients feel comfortable with the questions and fully understand what is being asked
- feasible, in the sense of the equipment being available and within budget costs.

Clinical audit is thus concerned with the ability to demonstrate effectiveness, which, together with efficiency, form the basis of Cochrane's philosophy (Cochrane 1972). Its essential feature is measurement, as it is in patient assessment. However, in seeking to make therapeutic care more effective for all clients, audit goes beyond the treatment outcome of the individual patient to encompass wider issues.

National clinical audit topics are published and regularly reviewed. Their selection at a local level should be informed by the usual service criteria of high volume, high risk, high profile and high cost, that is to say, high levels of those factors indicate areas to be focused on. Clinical audit should include as many members of the multidisciplinary team delivering care as possible. Copeland (2005) recommends that, as a minimum, 10% of audits should be across service providers, 30% of audit should be multiservice and 50% should be multiprofessional.

Further discussion of audit is beyond the scope of this book but the interested reader is referred to the works of Copeland (2005).

KEY MESSAGES

- Measurement is an essential part of monitoring outcomes from treatment interventions.
- Measurement tools need to be reliable, valid and appropriate for the selected outcome.
- Assessment of relaxation interventions covers physiological, psychological and behavioural outcomes.
- The clinical assessment should include nominal, functional and attitudinal data.
- Goals should be agreed, recorded and regularly reviewed.
- Personal activity goals should be developed using SMART principles.
- The placebo effect should be considered in relaxation training and in the design of clinical trials.
- Clinical audit is integral to the improvement of patient care in the NHS.

Further reading

Copeland, G., 2005. A Practical Handbook for Clinical Audit. NHS Clinical Governance Support Team, Leicester.

Chapter Twenty Six

26

Evidence from research

Introduction

There is a pressing need for therapists to demonstrate the effectiveness of their treatments, not only to serve the client in the best way but also to validate their work. Carefully designed and rigorously executed studies, repeated many times, help to build a robust foundation of effective treatments which contribute to current best practice.

Much work has been done to measure the effect of different methods or to weigh up relaxation training against other approaches such as cognitive interventions, exercise or pharmacology. This work is, however, beset by frequent methodological shortcomings; moreover, the diversity of methodologies makes it difficult to compare one study with another (Donaghy & Morss 2000).

This chapter draws on systematic reviews and clinical studies, most of which have been published in the last 5 years. It explores the effectiveness of relaxation techniques in the context of 35 specified conditions. The range of conditions discussed is by no means comprehensive. Many other conditions have been investigated which are not included. The chapter simply offers a selection to give the reader a glimpse of the kind of work that is being carried out in the field of relaxation training. A table suggesting applications for the various relaxation techniques may be found in Appendix 1. In some cases relaxation treatment is provided on its own, as a monotherapy; in others it is used adjunctively, alongside other approaches such as pharmacology or exercise, according to the requirements of the condition.

Although the choice of technique is based on information from research, it is intended only as a guide.

What is the evidence?

Of the areas which attract research interest, the following are discussed in this chapter:

- addiction – illicit drugs
- alcohol dependence
- anxiety
- arthritis
- asthma
- athletic injury
- cancer
- cardiac rehabilitation
- childbirth
- chronic fatigue syndrome
- depression
- diabetes
- dysmenorrhoea
- eating disorders
- fibromyalgia
- headache and migraine
- HIV/AIDS
- hypertension
- irritable bowel syndrome
- low back pain
- menopause
- multiple sclerosis
- musculoskeletal problems

- obsessive compulsive disorder
- occupational stress
- pain
- panic
- Parkinson's disease
- post-traumatic stress disorder
- pre- and postoperative states
- psoriasis
- schizophrenia
- sleep disorders
- tinnitus
- weight problems.

Addiction – illicit drugs

The use of illegal drugs for recreational purposes has increased over the last two decades. Substance misuse is becoming one of the most prevalent psychiatric disorders in modern society, with addiction to opiates, crack cocaine, heroin and tranquillizers creating problems of addiction worldwide. Addictions are linked to multifactorial psychosocial and cultural factors; however, in some situations drugs may be taken to reduce stress. Cannabis smoking is the most common recreational drug used in the UK. Hoppes (2006) reviewed the evidence regarding the use of mindfulness-based cognitive therapy in addictive disorders. He discussed the theory underpinning it and the effectiveness of its application and proposed that prolonged use of addictive substances impairs the brain pathways which help to control the emotions and offered a structured protocol for the treatment of co-occurring addictive and mood disorders (see Ch. 23).

Of the many treatments which have been applied to drug addiction, cognitive–behavioural therapy has often been found to be successful (Denis et al 2006). In their systematic review these researchers found extended individual cognitive–behavioural therapy to be more effective than brief individual motivational therapy.

Participation in structured exercise programmes can also bring benefits. Six studies published between 1991 and 2002 provide some support for the use of a structured programme of exercise for people in drug rehabilitation. Such a programme may be useful in reducing withdrawal symptoms; it could also increase physical fitness levels and self-esteem (Donaghy & Ussher 2005).

Smith (2006) undertook a multiple baseline design study with 21 participants in a 10-week structured exercise programme. While adherence to the programme was a problem, qualitative data gathered in the study indicated that it helped participants to feel fitter and improved their feelings of mental well-being. Biddle & Mutrie (2008) suggest that for those who find it difficult to maintain regular exercise class attendance, home-based exercise, through a video or DVD, may be useful, backed up by regular phone call support.

Alcohol dependence

There is a substantial body of evidence to support the use of cognitive–behavioural approaches as a treatment in alcohol dependence (Donaghy 2008a). These approaches are primarily effective in developing new coping strategies for dealing with addictive inclinations; for example, social skills training may help to strengthen the client's motivation to abstain or cut down. Practising these skills helps to develop self-efficacy which leads to greater confidence, while the cognitive restructuring helps the client to see herself in a new light.

Alcohol dependence is a condition which is often accompanied by high levels of depression and anxiety, where exercise is shown to have more to offer than relaxation. Exercise regimens lead to improved aerobic fitness and strength which help people to view themselves more favourably. Such links with self-esteem help to increase the client's confidence in his capacity to change his behaviour. Exercise is thus a useful adjunct to other treatments (Donaghy & Ussher 2005).

Anxiety

Most diseases and conditions are accompanied by some degree of fear: fear of pain, fear of deterioration and doubts about recovery. The notion of relaxation as a useful intervention would therefore be logical. Anxiety conditions themselves have been found to respond to this training. Manzoni et al (2008) carried out a systematic review investigating the effects of relaxation in the context of different forms of anxiety. Results indicated an efficacy which was both consistent and significant although the component trials were not tested for their rigour (see Ch. 1, p15). Conrad & Roth (2007) studied the efficacy of muscular relaxation

techniques in this context but found their work hampered by inadequate evidence and were unable to support a theory which suggested that decreased physiological activation took place when patients reported feeling less anxious. Self-reporting of muscle tension does not always match that of the physiological recording.

Generalized anxiety disorder (GAD) is common, affecting 7% of the general population. In a systematic review of this condition, Hunot (2007) found that symptoms were alleviated by cognitive–behavioural approaches and that these were more effective than usual treatment. Other systematic reviews suggest that both applied relaxation and cognitive–behavioural training (CBT) are effective in the treatment of GAD (Gorman 2003, Siev & Chambless 2007). These approaches were often effective whether used as monotherapies or adjunctive treatments.

Transcendental meditation has been shown to reduce anxiety but its effect was no greater than that of other relaxation therapies, including yoga (Krisanaprakornkit et al 2006). Mindfulness meditation produced results which were equivocal when applied to anxiety and mood symptoms (Toneatto & Nguyen 2007); however, the authors in this case found the results had low reliability because adherence to the programme in the trials was not always assessed.

Social anxiety disorder, another commonly reported condition, has been shown to benefit from cognitive–behavioural therapy in a number of investigations. For example, Clark et al (2006) conducted a randomized controlled trial which compared cognitive therapy with a combination of applied relaxation and exposure in the context of public speaking. Their conclusions pointed to a greater effectiveness of cognitive therapy over applied relaxation and exposure.

CBT has been shown to provide benefit in most systematic reviews of psychotherapeutic approaches to anxiety disorders (Gorman 2003, Hambrick et al 2003, Hunot et al 2007, Rodebaugh et al 2004, Siev & Chambless 2007). Many researchers find it the treatment of choice. However, exercise and relaxation have also been found to make valuable contributions. Relaxation training is frequently used as part of cognitive–behavioural interventions to reduce anxiety (Ralston 2008).

In the case of exercise, Jorm et al (2004) found that, together with relaxation training, it was an effective procedure for treating GAD. However, the paucity of evidence suggested to Larun et al (2006) that the effect of exercise might be quite modest.

Some reviews have focused on different age groups. For example, Ayers et al (2007) studied the effect of relaxation training and CBT in different forms of late-life anxiety. Here, CBT was found to be particularly effective. An earlier work had produced a similar finding, while also indicating the benefit of relaxation training for subjective anxiety symptoms (Wetherell et al 2005).

Other researchers have concentrated on children and adolescents with anxiety disorders and found CBT more effective than waiting list or attention control (James et al 2005). This finding applied to more than half the participants.

Conclusions drawn from systematic reviews can vary according to not only the results of their component trials but also the quality of the research. This is particularly so where evidence is sparse.

Arthritis: rheumatoid and osteo

Psychological interventions such as relaxation training and CBT have been investigated for their effectiveness in the pain management of rheumatoid arthritis (Astin et al 2002). These authors suggest that such interventions are useful as adjunctive therapies alongside medical management of the condition, adding that efficacy is likely to be greater in the early stages of the disease.

Bagheri-Nesami et al (2006) conducted a study to investigate the effect of Benson's relaxation technique on rheumatoid arthritis. Their results suggested that the approach might help to slow down the disease process (see Ch. 22, p189).

Osteoarthritis has been shown to benefit from a programme of combined progressive relaxation and guided imagery in a longitudinal randomized controlled study (Baird & Sands 2004). Twenty-eight older women with osteoarthritis participated. At the end of the course they reported significantly reduced pain and a significant reduction in difficulties associated with mobility. No differences in pain or mobility were reported in the control group.

Asthma

Breathing retraining has received considerable attention from researchers, as a way of helping to relieve symptoms of asthma. A systematic review was set up to assess the value of breathing exercises in this area. However, the authors, Holloway & Ram (2004), were unable to draw conclusions because treatment interventions and outcome measurements varied so much. On the whole, studies looking into relaxation therapies for asthma find a lack of evidence for their efficacy. The systematic review of Huntley and colleagues (2002), hampered by poor methodology and the problems inherent in this field, did, however, find some evidence that muscular relaxation might improve lung function in an adjunctive role. This benefit was not observed with other relaxation techniques.

In a paper discussing the effectiveness of progressive relaxation in adult asthma, Ritz (2001) suggests a possible mechanism for its effects. Contrary to popular belief, he proposes that the *tensing* component is the one which might be useful in relieving asthma since tensing is associated with excitation of the sympathetic nervous system, one of whose functions is to open the airways. By contrast, the release component is associated with parasympathetic dominance and a relative constriction of the airways.

It is believed that some asthma is triggered by psychological factors; however, on the basis of the current literature, this hypothesis cannot be supported. Yorke et al (2005) reviewed the role of psychological factors as they affect children and concluded that, while they might play an important part in the aetiology of asthma, the evidence to support their involvement in subsequent attacks was lacking.

Mental imagery has also been put forward as a possible means of relieving symptoms of asthma. Epstein et al (2004) explored this idea but were unable to draw conclusions regarding efficacy.

It is suggested that asthma is associated with overbreathing. The theory underpinning the claim suggests that asthma is exacerbated by hyperventilation with resulting hypocapnia and bronchoconstriction. Two approaches are based on this assumption: the Buteyko and the Papworth methods. Evidence for these approaches is reported in Ch. 4 (p44).

Athletic injury

Athletic injury carries with it a number of stresses. In addition to the fear of pain and the fear of non-recovery, there is the fear of reinjury when play is resumed. Cupal & Brewer (2001) studied the effects of muscular relaxation and guided imagery in 30 participants undergoing rehabilitation following anterior cruciate ligament reconstruction. Among the positive effects demonstrated at 6-month follow-up was a significantly reduced level of reinjury anxiety and a decreased level of pain.

Long-term injuries are known to lower the mood of injured athletes. In an attempt to find a way of raising that mood, Johnson (2000) studied the effect of different short-term interventions such as stress management, goal setting and relaxation training with guided imagery. Of the three interventions, the only one to show statistical differences of benefit was relaxation training with guided imagery. In a further study Johnson et al (2005) found that psychologically based intervention programmes significantly reduced the number of injuries, critical incidents and stress among 32 soccer players. The interventions employed were somatic and cognitive relaxation, stress management, goal setting training, attribution and self-confidence training. This work was supported by that of Maddison & Prapavessis (2005) who, in a controlled study of 48 rugby players, found that psychological interventions resulted in less time lost in recovery from injuries than in control conditions.

Donaghy (2008b) reviewed the sports literature on the use of relaxation techniques (within stress management packages) to reduce risk of injury but found the evidence for efficacy of prevention limited by the small number of randomized controlled trials, most of which had methodological weaknesses. Evidence which supported the use of stress management techniques in the mental preparation of athletes for competition was more convincing.

Imagery is widely used in sport and particularly by athletes in training and competition. Sordoni et al (2002) defined three kinds: motivational, cognitive and healing. All three types are used by athletes, whether in recreational or competitive situations; however, competitive athletes use more cognitive imagery than do their recreational counterparts. When athletes are injured they also use healing imagery which has been found to be associated with a variety of benefits such as decreased pain, anxiety and distress, accelerated healing and improved immune responses. Healing imagery is also related to self-efficacy; that is to say, athletes with a strong sense of self-efficacy tend to use more healing imagery than those with a weaker sense (see Ch. 19, p170).

Cancer

There is a large body of research focusing on the pain and distress associated with different forms of cancer. Patients with cancer frequently develop anxiety and depression for which psychological treatments are prescribed. Sloman (2002) measured the effects of progressive muscle relaxation and guided imagery on the psychological health of 56 people with advanced cancer and accompanying anxiety and depression and found that, whereas there were significant positive changes for depression, no significant improvement occurred for anxiety. Guided imagery is a psychological technique commonly used with cancer patients. Roffe et al (2005) conducted a systematic review to test its effectiveness as a sole adjuvant cancer therapy but found it had little to offer in the relief of nausea and vomiting associated with chemotherapy. However, there were indications that it might help to increase comfort and provide psychological support.

Mindfulness meditation has been found to be supportive to patients experiencing cancer care. In their systematic review, Smith et al (2005) found improvements in mood, reduction in stress and better sleep quality following a course of mindfulness-based stress reduction although a number of the included studies had methodological defects. The authors concluded that mindfulness-based stress reduction may have clinically valuable potential. As a further advantage, it could be self-administered. A meditation programme designed for patients with cancer was proposed in an article by Tacon (2003).

Negative thought intrusions can add to the pain experienced by cancer sufferers. Antoni et al (2006) set up a stress reduction programme consisting of relaxation training, cognitive restructuring and coping skills in a controlled trial of 200 women newly treated for stage 0–III breast cancer. Significant benefit was derived in the form of reduced thought intrusion and reduced anxiety and distress over the year following recruitment. The conclusion drawn from this trial was that group-based cognitive–behavioural stress management was a helpful adjunct to medical treatment in this context.

Ernst et al (2006) conducted a systematic review of randomized controlled trials investigating the effect of psychological interventions for breast cancer. Among the mind–body techniques tested were CBT, group support and a combination of progressive muscle relaxation and imagery. However, the authors were unable to draw conclusions on account of the poor quality of much of the methodology.

The value of increased activity for people with cancer has been emerging over the last decade and is linked to survival rates. Benefits of this increased activity include a measure of relief in their symptoms of nausea and fatigue (Stricker et al 2004). Recent research looking at breast cancer survivors has indicated that those who are regularly active have a 50% reduction in mortality when compared to those who are inactive (Holmes et al 2005). The large study by Mutrie and colleagues (2007), looking at women with breast cancer who participated in a 12-week exercise programme, found they had significant improvements in functional and psychological outcomes compared to women who received care as usual. These benefits, alongside the findings that women with breast cancer who exercise have an improvement in quality of life up to 1 year following their cancer treatment (Daley et al 2004, 2007), make this an area worthy of promotion in cancer treatment programmes. Knols and colleagues (2005), in a systematic review of exercise trials with cancer patients, conclude that benefit may be derived from exercise, particularly where patients are ambulant and their limitations allow it.

There are special considerations for this population related to muscle weakness following chemotherapy and the time required to recover from surgery and chemotherapy. There may also be embarrassment due to obvious signs of treatment such as hair loss or scarring following surgical intervention.

Cardiac conditions

This section addresses a variety of cardiac problems including post infarction, ischaemic heart disease and cardiac failure. In their systematic review and meta-analysis, van Dixhoorn & White (2005) studied the effects of muscular relaxation therapy on recovery from a cardiac ischaemic event. Various forms of progressive relaxation were employed. Findings included a reduction in resting heart rate, improved exercise tolerance and increased high-density lipoprotein cholesterol. There was no effect on low-density cholesterol or blood pressure. State anxiety and depression were reduced, attacks of angina became less frequent and arrhythmia and exercise-induced ischaemia less of

a problem. Cardiac events and death became less frequent. These effects, however, tended to be quite small in those studies which used abbreviated methods of relaxation. The authors concluded that intensive supervised muscular relaxation practice can play a valuable role in the rehabilitation of people recovering from an ischaemic heart event, making an important contribution to secondary prevention. This approach is best combined with a programme of appropriate exercise.

Secondary prevention was an area of concern to Walton et al (2002) in their review of randomized controlled trials exploring the effectiveness of transcendental meditation in the area of cardiovascular disease. Earlier work had shown that this approach might help to reduce risk factors and slow down the pathological changes which lead to or exacerbate this disease. However, they found that transcendental meditation had similar effects to those of conventional practices. A further review in 2004 resulted in a strengthening of these views (Walton et al 2004).

Childbirth

Relaxation training has for long been associated with childbirth. Simkin & Boulding (2004) conducted a review of non-pharmacological methods of pain relief and found evidence in favour of continuous support in labour, maternal movement and positioning, baths, and nerve blocks. Other methods may confer similar benefit but require further study before conclusions can be drawn. User satisfaction, however, was high among all methods.

The psychological and emotional benefits of physical activity during pregnancy are emerging. In a well-controlled study, Rankin (2002) assigned 157 women to antenatal classes with and without exercise. They were assessed at early and late stages of pregnancy and following childbirth. The study found that adding exercise to routine antenatal care prevented a decline in the women's perceptions of their well-being which is often seen during pregnancy. These findings led to local service changes, with exercise being included in antenatal classes and training provided for leaders of these classes.

Chronic fatigue syndrome

Chronic fatigue syndrome (also known as myalgic encephalomyelitis) is a condition in which the predominating symptom is tiredness in the absence of previous exertion. Dysfunction is present in the neurological, endocrine and immune systems and this gives rise to a wide range of symptoms in addition to fatigue. The aetiology is unknown. Tested therapies include graded exercise, CBT and relaxation.

Graded exercise, carried out in a flexible manner to suit the capacity of the client, has been shown in an audit to result in significant improvement (White & Naish 2001). Walking, swimming, cycling and tai chi were the activities featured in a programme where exercise was gentle and individually tailored.

The value of this approach was endorsed in a randomized controlled trial published in 2005. Its authors, Stulemeijer et al, gave 10 sessions of activity (appropriate to the participant's condition) to 71 adolescent patients in a cognitive–behavioural framework. The results indicated a significantly greater decrease in fatigue severity as reported by the intervention group than was reported by the controls. This echoed the findings of Price & Couper (2003) whose systematic review of adults had previously found cognitive techniques to be not only effective but significantly more effective than orthodox medical management. Cognitive techniques were also shown to be more effective than relaxation.

Depression

Depression is characterized by a lack of interest and a loss of pleasure in usual concerns. It is described as clinical when symptoms become marked enough to interfere with normal activities and to persist for 2 weeks or longer (Peveler et al 2002). Depression can be a primary disorder, as in the case of major depression, or it may be secondary to the experience of an already existing disorder such as cancer (Craft & Landers 1998). CBT has been found to be effective in the treatment of depression either as a non-pharmacological sole treatment or as an adjunct to medication (Davidson 2008).

In a recent review of exercise and mental health, Donaghy (2007) highlights the efficacy of structured exercise for reducing symptoms of clinical depression as well as for mild to moderate depression, where exercise is advocated either as a treatment in its own right or as an adjunct to other forms (see Ch. 15).

With regard to relaxation training, potential benefit has been found in a Cochrane review which suggests that relaxation techniques may make a useful first-line psychological treatment (Jorm et al 2008). The study is reported in Chapter 1 (p15).

Most research has focused on adults. However, a few studies have been on children. Larun et al (2006) systematically reviewed these studies to determine the effect of exercise on children and adolescents who were depressed. However, the authors found the evidence base too small at this stage to draw conclusions.

Paucity of good-quality evidence also precludes the drawing of conclusions in the field of post-partum depression. A wide variety of non-biological methods (relaxation training, CBT, psychotherapy, counselling, massage, maternal exercise) have been tested, only to find no difference between them in terms of efficacy (Dennis 2004).

Diabetes mellitus types 1 and 2

Physical activity forms part of the treatment of diabetes mellitus, along with medication, dietary control and monitoring of glucose levels. This holds for both type 1 (insulin dependent) and type 2 (non-insulin dependent) diabetes and is now well established. A diabetic patient, however, needs to be carefully prepared for exercise and for this reason, a comprehensive set of guidelines has been produced describing the effects on the cardiovascular, peripheral arterial and metabolic systems (American College of Sports Medicine 1997). People with type 1 diabetes need to maintain a critical balance between insulin control, glucose levels and exercise (its amount and timing). It is essential that patients are guided to monitor blood glucose before and after exercise and are helped by an appropriate healthcare professional in making decisions about frequency, duration and intensity of exercise.

Type 2 diabetes is spreading, particularly in the developing world, and is linked to lifestyles. Changes in diet and activity have contributed to its prevalence. People with type 2 diabetes have needs which are different from those in type 1 and which may be linked to motivation and obesity. The work of Marsden and Kirk (Kirk et al 2008, Marsden & Kirk 2005) provides a comprehensive guide for healthcare professionals and exercise consultants when constructing exercise regimens for people in both type 1 and type 2 diabetes categories.

While the role of exercise is now established, there is also an indication that relaxation can provide benefits. One study found that relaxation was as useful as exercise in controlling blood glucose levels. Van Rooijen et al (2004) conducted a randomized trial to compare the effect of exercise with that of relaxation, using the Hb A_1c as the outcome measure (a high reading indicates an uncontrolled diabetes). These two groups consisted of South African females with type 2 diabetes mellitus. The trial ran for 12 weeks after which time significant improvement was seen in both groups but with no significant difference between them.

Dysmenorrhoea

As period pain is related to uterine cramps it has been suggested that relaxation techniques may help to relieve it. Proctor et al (2007) reviewed behavioural interventions for this condition. The reviewers found some evidence to suggest that progressive relaxation with or without imagery may be a useful strategy for relieving cramping pain; however, methodological deficiencies in some of the component studies made it necessary to view these results with caution.

Eating disorders

Eating disorders are common in Western society. One of these is bulimia nervosa, a disorder characterized by bingeing followed by self-induced vomiting or starvation. Hay et al (2004) carried out a systematic review of psychotherapies for this condition but found that the sample sizes were generally small and the quality of the research variable, making it difficult to have confidence in the results. From the more rigorous of the studies, however, it emerged that benefit could be gained from cognitive–behavioural approaches which were found to be significantly better than no treatment and more effective than other strategies at reducing binge eating.

The reverse disorder, anorexia nervosa, can be life-threatening and requires specialist treatment not covered in this work.

Fibromyalgia

This is a chronic condition which displays a variety of symptoms. Pain is the most evident but there is a degree of chronic fatigue and long-term functional impairment. Stress seems to play a part. The defining criteria, however, reflect medical opinion rather than hard science (Skelly 2008) so it is best seen as a syndrome, not a disease. In many respects it resembles chronic fatigue syndrome with which it is often confused.

Research into fibromyalgia has been systematically reviewed by Sim & Adams (2002). The review indicates an absence of strong evidence for any single non-pharmacological intervention in the treatment of this condition, although there was some preliminary support for moderate aerobic exercise. Williams (2003) suggests that greatest benefit is derived from a combination of exercise and cognitive–behavioural techniques used adjunctively with medical treatment. Guided imagery has also been investigated as a therapeutic intervention in the randomized controlled trial of Fors and colleagues (2002) in which it was suggested that fibromyalgic pain could be reduced by pleasant visualizations.

Headache and migraine

These are conditions in which psychological treatments are widely used and in a variety of populations ranging from children to the elderly. Tension-type headache is characterized by pain on both sides of the head and a feeling of pressure as if a tight band is encircling the head. The headache can last for hours or days.

In their overview, Rains and colleagues (2005) report that behavioural interventions produce benefit which is significantly greater than that provided by control conditions. This benefit has been shown to vary in magnitude between 35% and 55%. Among the behavioural interventions employed were relaxation training, CBT and stress management training. Loder & Rizzoli (2008), in their evaluation of treatment for tension-type headache, found evidence for the effectiveness of a combination of amitriptyline and biofeedback-assisted relaxation training.

In the case of school children, Eccleston and colleagues (2003) report that there is good evidence for the effectiveness of relaxation and cognitive–behaviour training in children and adolescents with chronic headache; both severity and frequency of attack have been shown to fall. Other researchers working in this context, however, have pointed out methodological deficiencies which reduce the confidence that can be placed in these results (Verhagen et al 2005). Larsson et al (2005) found that relaxation techniques were more effective when administered by a trained therapist rather than an untrained adult or the patient himself.

It has been suggested that autogenic training is effective in preventing tension-type headaches. Kanji and colleagues (2006) conducted a systematic review to determine its efficacy but they found no consistent evidence that autogenic training was superior to other psychological or behavioural interventions.

In contrast with tension-type headache, migraine is characterized by one-sided throbbing pain which results from spasm and overdilation of certain arteries. It is sometimes preceded by visual disturbance described as an aura. Nausea and vomiting are frequently experienced. Much of the investigatory work on migraine has been done with children and adolescents where it has focused on prophylaxis. A systematic review of non-pharmacological trials suggested that relaxation was effective in this area. It also found evidence to suggest that relaxation plus behaviour therapy was more effective than placebo or waiting list controls (Damen et al 2006).

Many treatments for this condition consist of multiple approaches. In order to determine which component of treatment was responsible for the effects, Kaushik and colleagues (2005) carried out a randomized test to compare the effects of relaxation with those of propranolol. Results showed that the relaxation training had a long-term prophylactic effect that significantly exceeded that of the drug. The relaxation techniques used in the study were diaphragmatic breathing and muscular relaxation accompanied by daily home practice for 6 months.

HIV/AIDS

Alongside pharmacological approaches to treatment for HIV/AIDS are mind–body techniques such as mindfulness, which has been associated with improved management of the stress which accompanies this condition (Logsdon-Conradsen 2002).

Ampunsiriratana et al (2005) combined mindfulness meditation with Watson's caring theory in an 8-week programme to develop a model for self-care. Sixteen selected patients took part. Researchers found that participants were able to cultivate self-healing in a number of physical and

psychological dimensions of pain. This programme was found to be particularly helpful during the later stages of the disease.

Mindfulness is seen by some researchers as the antithesis of impulsivity: a state of mind which promotes action without thought as to its consequences. Impulsive behaviour, in the case of AIDS, carries risks of interpersonal contamination and tendencies to seek intoxication. Lower levels of impulsivity are likely to lead to reduced risk behaviour and drug use.

In a randomized clinical trial with a sample of 38 HIV-positive drug users, the effects of mindfulness were compared with those of standard care. Patients' reports showed that greater reductions in impulsivity and intoxicant use were found among the mindfulness group than in the standard care group. The authors, Margolin et al (2007), regard this work as a first step in the examination of the role of mindfulness in this context.

Cognitive-behavioural interventions are sometimes used in the treatment of HIV/AIDS. Brown & Carlos (2003) used a psycho-educational module as a means of reducing the symptoms of anxiety and depression in people testing positive for HIV/AIDS. The intervention did not, however, result in a statistically significant outcome.

Hypertension

Non-pharmacological methods, for example, relaxation training, have been extensively studied with respect to their effectiveness in reducing blood pressure. Much of this work has supported the use of relaxation techniques. Muscular techniques, autogenic training and meditation have repeatedly been associated with a lowering of blood pressure (both systolic and diastolic) in hypertensive patients, often by a significant margin (Stefano & Esch 2005).

The review of King and colleagues (2002) looked at the research on transcendental meditation in the treatment of hypertension and coronary heart disease. In their conclusions they also found an association between transcendental meditation and lowered blood pressure, together with indications that the method showed promise as a preventive strategy.

In the management of essential hypertension it has been shown that the risk factor with the strongest and most consistent correlation (apart from age) is being overweight (Anand 1999). A cognitive–behavioural approach with an exercise component would seem an appropriate way to address this problem. Although a wealth of research supports the use of exercise in helping to reduce blood pressure, previous studies have chiefly focused on aerobic exercise, resistance training having conventionally been avoided. However, Cornelissen & Fagard (2005) conducted a meta-analysis of nine randomized controlled trials in which resistance training was the sole intervention and concluded that moderate resistance training should not be contraindicated.

As the strongest risk factor in hypertension is age, it would be useful to know how effective behavioural interventions can be for this group of people. Schneider and colleagues (2005) reviewed randomized controlled trials in which transcendental meditation and other stress-reducing interventions had been employed. Results indicated that transcendental meditation may well contribute to a decrease in mortality in older people with systemic hypertension.

Lifestyle has attracted the attention of some researchers working in the field of hypertension. Dickinson et al (2006) tested the role of lifestyle interventions which were believed to reduce blood pressure. The most effective approaches were found to be weight reduction, regular exercise, restricted alcohol and reduced salt intake (see Ch. 15 for role of exercise). There was less support for stress reduction. Relaxation therapy had a significant effect when compared with non-intervention controls but this was not as great as that provided by lifestyle changes.

Irritable bowel syndrome

A small body of research, much of it flawed, has tested the commonly held belief that psychological treatments are useful in cases of irritable bowel syndrome. One such study compared the effects of relaxation training with those of CBT, using a control of standard care. Improvement occurred in all three groups in equal measure, suggesting that participants were not gaining added benefit from the psychological treatments and that the standard care was adequate (Boyce et al 2003).

More recently, Levy and colleagues (2007) reviewed work in respect of the illness behaviour associated with inflammatory bowel disease. They found that client reactions became more positive following psychological therapies such as relaxation training, CBT and social learning. Benefit was also shown to occur from body awareness therapy (see Glossary, p255).

Low back pain

Pain is a complex phenomenon with biological, psychological and cultural dimensions. In recent years these strands have come together to inform the treatment of chronic low back pain. From a wide array of approaches, the most frequently used is CBT, i.e. the modification of the patient's cognitive processes and environmental contingencies. It is administered either in place of or in combination with usual treatment, i.e. physiotherapy, back education and medical treatment (Martin & McLeod 2008).

Multidisciplinary group rehabilitation for women with chronic low back pain was evaluated in a randomized trial to determine whether this approach was more effective than individual physiotherapy. The groupwork consisted of back school, physical training, relaxation training, workplace interventions and cognitive–behavioural stress management. The individual physiotherapy consisted of physical exercise and mobilization. In both interventions the before-and-after measurements showed favourable effects which were maintained at 2-year follow-up. No statistically significant differences were found between the two treatment approaches and the authors concluded that multidisciplinary group rehabilitation and individual physiotherapy seemed equally effective in the treatment of women with chronic low back pain (Kaapa et al 2006).

Chou & Huffman (2007) conducted a systematic review of non-pharmacological therapies for acute and chronic low back pain, They found that, for chronic low back pain, the use of CBT, exercise, spinal manipulation and interdisciplinary rehabilitation was supported by good evidence of moderate efficacy. For acute low back pain, superficial heat was the only intervention that was effective. However, the evidence from systematic reviews is not consistent. Ostelo and colleagues (2005), reviewing 21 studies, found that when CBT with a progressive relaxation component was compared with usual treatment, no significant differences were found. There was some benefit when compared to a waiting list control but this was not maintained. Thus, it is suggested that cognitive-behavioural approaches may be no more effective than usual treatment.

Menopause

A review of non-pharmacological treatments for the adverse symptoms of menopause, such as hot flushes, was carried out by McKee & Warber (2005). They found that exercise and a range of relaxation techniques (progressive relaxation and abdominal slow breathing) may help some women to reduce these symptoms. The evidence to support the benefits of regular physical activity to alleviate symptoms other than bone loss has mostly been gathered from surveys.

In a large UK survey, Daley et al (2007) reported better health-related quality of life scores for women who were physically active, suggesting that menopausal women who participated in regular physical activity benefited psychologically. The psychological benefits of physical activity, however, extend to women at all stages of life. This includes the elderly. A study in a large cohort of Australian women in their 70s across a 3-year period demonstrated an association between physical activity and emotional well-being (Lee & Russell 2003).

Multiple sclerosis

Psychological interventions include the process of helping people adjust to and cope with their condition. This is nowhere more relevant than in multiple sclerosis. The systematic review of Thomas and colleagues (2006) has suggested that cognitive–behavioural approaches can go some way towards achieving a better adjustment. CBT has also been found to alleviate the anxiety and depression which often accompany the knowledge that one has developed multiple sclerosis.

Musculoskeletal disorders

Certain occupations give rise to repetitive strain injuries. These can be very painful and can interfere with output. A form of rehabilitation which takes account of the patients's social and psychological life is believed to augment the benefits of a physical approach. Karjalainen and colleagues (2007) reviewed the research in biopsychosocial rehabilitation for upper limb repetitive strain injuries in working-age adults but were unable to form any conclusion owing to a lack of high-quality trials in this field.

Psychosocial aspects of musculoskeletal disorders are particularly relevant in the world of the performing arts. De Greef and colleagues (2003) reported on a programme addressed to professional musicians in situations where there was a high rate of absenteeism owing to musculoskeletal disorders. Its aim was to change the playing habits of the musicians and reduce the effects of physical overload which interfere with perceived physical competence. The programme consisted of relaxation procedures, postural exercises for the shoulder, neck and lower back and exercises to cope with mental stress. Researchers found that the programme significantly decreased playing-related musculoskeletal disorders. At the same time it increased perceived physical competence.

Obsessive compulsive disorder

O'Kearney and colleagues (2006), in their systematic review, evaluated the effects of cognitive–behavioural approaches in the treatment of obsessive compulsive disorder (OCD). Findings showed that CBT had favourable effects in the treatment of this condition. There is no evidence to suggest that the psychological approach is better than medication, or medication better than the psychological approach, but when the two treatments are combined the outcome is better than when medication is administered on its own. Their combined effect is not, however, any different from the effect of CBT on its own. These findings suggest that CBT has potential value in the treatment of OCD and might serve as a useful adjunct to conventional treatment.

Occupational stress

In the case of healthcare workers, stress may arise for a variety of reasons including high expectations, time constraints, inadequate work skills and ineffective social support.

A systematic review found that both person-directed and work-directed interventions could be effective in relieving work stress. Cognitive–behavioural approaches with relaxation techniques were found to ease the situation for individuals while visible management modifications were found useful for institutions. Benefits derived from well-designed stress reduction programmes were found to survive long after closure of the programme, i.e. for 6–24 months. However, results should be interpreted with caution owing to a mixed quality of research evidence (Marine et al 2006).

Pain

A widely adopted view sees the perception of pain as governed by a neural 'gate' in the spinal cord (Melzack & Wall 1965). When this gate is open it allows signals from the pain receptors on the skin to pass to the brain, exposing the individual to the full experience of the pain. However, signals sent down from the cortex can help to 'close' the gate, thereby reducing the perceived intensity of the pain. For example, if you are enjoying a film you will be less inclined to notice bodily irritations that might otherwise claim your attention. Most non-pharmacological pain relief can be explained by the gate theory.

There exists a body of research relating to non-pharmacological methods which are said to 'close' the gate. Their effectiveness has been the subject of several literature reviews. Kwekkeboom & Gretarsdottir (2006) systematically reviewed randomized trials of relaxation interventions for pain in adults. Findings showed support for these interventions in eight out of 15 studies. Progressive muscle relaxation stood out as the most frequently supported technique, particularly for arthritis, but jaw relaxation and passive muscular relaxation were found effective for the relief of postoperative pain. There was little support for autogenic training and none for rhythmic breathing. Researchers call for more well-designed trials to test all relaxation techniques.

Kessler et al (2003) reviewed work featuring relaxation and hypnosis, both of which were found to significantly reduce different indices of pain. Of the two interventions, the evidence for hypnosis is stronger, being effective in acute and chronic pain. In the case of relaxation, the evidence is modest for acute pain, although more convincing for chronic. The authors add that neither hypnosis nor relaxation was found to be consistently more effective than other self-regulation methods. They suggest that these approaches might form useful adjunctive therapies in various conditions of pain.

Evidence for mind–body therapies has also been reviewed by Astin (2004). He looked at muscular relaxation, meditation, imagery and CBT in the treatment of pain. Based on his findings, he made the following recommendations.

1. *Low back pain*: this may respond favourably to a combination of relaxation training, coping skills, stress management and cognitive restructuring.

2. *Arthritis, rheumatoid and osteo*: these seemed to benefit from a combination of CBT and education administered adjunctively to conventional treatment.

3. *Tension headache*: this appeared to benefit from relaxation and muscle biofeedback, while migraine seemed to respond to relaxation training and thermal biofeedback.

4. *Perioperative states*: postoperative recovery time may be reduced when techniques are taught preoperatively. Suggested methods include muscular relaxation, imagery and hypnosis.

5. *Invasive medical procedures*: the pain that accompanies some of these procedures can be ameliorated by mind–body approaches used adjunctively.

Schaffer & Yucha (2004) investigated the role of Benson's relaxation response in the management of chronic and acute pain (see Ch. 22, p189) and Weydert (2006) reported on the effects of imagery in children with abdominal pain (see Ch. 18, p158).

Panic disorder

Cognitive–behaviour therapy stands out as being the treatment of choice for panic disorder (Carlbring et al 2003, Siev & Chambless 2007, Wetherell et al 2005). Studies in the area of anxiety and panic disorder tend to show specific treatment effects; for example, relaxation training and cognitive therapy show equivalent effects in generalized anxiety disorder while for panic disorder, cognitive therapy provides greater benefit (Siev & Chambless 2007). Or again, in a review of psychological interventions, relaxation training showed particular effectiveness in cases of subjective anxiety whereas for generalized anxiety disorder and panic, the treatment of choice was CBT (Wetherell et al 2005).

Many people with panic disorder also experience agoraphobia which makes it difficult for them to travel to treatment locations. A solution has been created in the form of Internet-Administered Self-Help whose effectiveness was tested by Carlbring et al (2003, 2007). These studies are reported in Chapter 9, p86.

Parkinson's disease

Stallibrass et al (2002) conducted a randomized controlled trial to investigate whether the Alexander technique benefited people with idiopathic Parkinson's disease. They found that motor symptoms in the Alexander group improved significantly compared to no treatment (see Ch. 12, p111).

Post-traumatic stress disorder (PTSD)

Traumatic events can give rise to this condition with accompanying distress and reduced functioning. Psychological interventions are therefore commonly employed in the treatment of this disorder. Bisson & Andrew (2007) conducted a systematic review to determine their effectiveness. Results showed that individual trauma-focused CBT and eye movement desensitization and reprocessing (see Glossary) offer significant benefit. Stress management and group trauma-focused CBT are also useful. Trauma-focused approaches were more effective than non-trauma focused ones and treatment was best started within 3 months of the event. Drug treatment was second line.

Post-traumatic stress disorder may occur in childhood where a single incident has been experienced (Adler-Nevo & Manassis 2005). In this review, the same forms of treatment as above were in use, with the addition of play therapy. Most of the studies showed statistically significant improvement. However, the methodology was not always sound enough for conclusions about best treatment to be drawn.

Pre- and postoperative states

A programme of mixed relaxation techniques was carried out in a randomized controlled trial on 102 adults following abdominal surgery in a large hospital in Thailand. It resulted in reports of decreased pain sensation and distress in the intervention group compared with the control. State anxiety reduction did not quite reach significance but the trend was noticeably in that direction. Most participants reported

that their pain had been reduced by the intervention and fewer participants asked for opioids. They liked the sense of control which the relaxation techniques had offered them (Roykulcharoen & Good 2004).

Laurion & Fetzer (2003) tested the effect of guided imagery and music on gynaecological laparoscopy outcomes such as pain levels. Results showed a significant reduction of reported pain among the intervention participants compared with controls. The mechanism is unclear but the authors suggest that the distraction inherent in the treatment reduces the reporting of negative outcomes.

Psoriasis

This is a skin disorder estimated to affect 2% of the population. It is characterized by a proliferation of the epidermal layers of the skin creating red raised patches covered with white scales. In plaque psoriasis, these appear typically on the knees, elbows and scalp. The condition is commonly treated with ultraviolet light which promotes clearing of the lesions.

The role of stress has been tested by Picardi et al (2005). These researchers investigated the relationship between stress, perceived social support, emotional awareness and diffuse plaque psoriasis. Stress was assessed by the impact of negative life events experienced by the individual, using Paykel's Interview for Recent Life Events (Paykel 1997). The researchers found a correlation between psychological distress and the length of time it took for phototherapy to clear the plaque. They also found that a mindfulness-based approach significantly reduced the healing time. In their conclusions they suggested that increased emotional awareness and greater social support might help to reduce susceptibility to exacerbations of psoriasis.

Life events as a measure of perceived stress were also employed by Payne et al (1985) in a controlled study which compared the effect of such events on plaque psoriasis with their effect on three other skin disorders: viral warts, fungal infections and new growths. Thirty two patients with varying degrees of plaque psoriasis participated in a matched pair design. However, in this small study no significant difference between the groups was found and results suggested that exacerbations of psoriasis were no more affected by life events than were warts, fungal infections and new growths.

Schizophrenia

For some years now the suggested psychological treatment for schizophrenia has been CBT. This approach addresses the problem by linking feelings with thinking patterns. In their systematic review of the effectiveness of CBT, Jones and colleagues (2004) found that this treatment holds promise, particularly in the short term.

Hallucinations experienced by people with schizophrenia are frequently treated with distraction techniques. As a coping strategy within a cognitive–behavioural framework, these techniques are applied adjunctively. Crawford-Walker and colleagues (2005) systematically reviewed studies in this area but no clear effect emerged owing partly to a paucity of good evidence.

Exercise has been shown in a review to have potential benefits, both in reducing negative symptoms and as a coping strategy for the positive symptoms of schizophrenia (Faulkner & Biddle 1999). These findings are supported in a study investigating the patient experience: people with schizophrenia who participated in a 3-month programme of exercise in a community care setting in Melbourne indicated through focus groups that they enjoyed the graduated, individualized programme and took pleasure in feeling fitter. They also enjoyed participating in group exercise and they all indicated their intention to continue with the exercise programme (Fogarty & Happel 2005).

Sleep disorders

Without sleep, we can hardly be said to enjoy psychological well-being. Interventions for the relief of insomnia have typically been pharmacological. However, a wide range of non-pharmacological treatments exist in the form of sleep health techniques, stimulus control instruction, sleep restriction, relaxation therapy, cognitive therapy, paradoxical intention and others. These approaches are popular with people who fear the possibility of drug side effects and dependency which can occur with many pharmacological remedies. Side effects include daytime sedation, increased risk of motor accidents, falls, and cognitive impairment.

A review of the above treatments was authorized by the American Academy of Sleep Medicine. Reporting on its findings, Morgenthaler and colleagues (2006) showed that psychological and behavioural interventions were effective in the treatment of both primary and secondary insomnia. The most effective treatments for chronic insomnia were stimulus control therapy, relaxation training and CBT.

Sleep problems often increase with age but because of the high risk of falls in older age groups, there has been a need to search for effective alternatives to drug treatment. A review conducted by Montgomery & Dennis (2003) focused on cognitive-behavioural interventions among adults over 60 years of age. Sleep quality and duration were examined. However, in the absence of an adequate research base, the authors could not draw conclusions beyond suggesting a mild benefit derived from CBT.

A meta-analysis of behavioural interventions for insomnia was carried out by Irwin and colleagues (2006). They were looking at the effect of relaxation training, behavioural and CBT on quality, latency and duration of sleep for people in the second half of life. All three methods showed robust and similar improvement for middle-aged and older participants. These results suggest that mature adults with insomnia benefit from a wide range of non-pharmacological treatments.

Insomnia accompanies many conditions, one of which is post-traumatic stress disorder. A critical review sees CBT as a promising treatment option (Lamarche & de Koninck 2007). Health care professionals faced with this condition are advised to collaborate with mental health professionals or sleep medicine specialists.

Recent work has focused on the combination of pharmacological and non-pharmacological therapies for insomnia. The author (Mendelson 2007) considered the way in which these two approaches might interact with each other and decided there was a possibility of the one potentiating the other. However, he found the research base too small to draw firm conclusions.

Tinnitus

Tinnitus is a condition characterized by ringing or buzzing in the ears, in the absence of external accoustic stimulation. In recent years it has been treated with CBT which has included applied relaxation, distraction, imagery, restructuring of beliefs and thoughts and management of sleep. Andersson (2002), in his overview, found that CBT showed promise of being effective, but at present there is no specific therapy that suits all patients.

In a recent review by Martinez and colleagues (2007) the researchers looked for differences between the subjective loudness of the tinnitus before CBT and its perceived loudness after treatment. They found no significant difference between the two. Neither was there any difference in the degree of associated depression experienced by the patients before and after treatment. However, the researchers did find a significant improvement in the reported quality of life and this was important because it suggested that patients found it easier to cope with the tinnitus after a course of CBT.

Some authors have suggested that tinnitus is associated with psychophysiological overactivation of the head and shoulder muscles. Rief et al (2005) conducted a randomized controlled trial to test this hypothesis. Psychological outcome measures were self-ratings, questionnaires and diary data while physiological outcome measures were muscle activity of the head and shoulders and electrodermal activity. After seven treatment sessions, participants in the intervention group had improved significantly more than their counterparts on the waiting list. The authors concluded that these results appeared to support the hypothesis that tinnitus is associated with overactive head and shoulder muscles.

Weight problems

Proposals to lose weight are associated with psychological factors such as motivation, compliance and self-control. Shaw and colleagues (2005) reviewed the area where 36 studies met the inclusion criteria. They found that behavioural and cognitive–behavioural strategies were effective and particularly so when combined with exercise and dietary changes. A small number of studies investigated the influence of relaxation techniques to enhance weight loss but there was not enough evidence to reach a conclusion. However, the authors pointed to research which, though slender, suggested a possible role for relaxation training.

Different forms of research

While research is not the only source of evidence for the value of relaxation training, it is the principal one, enabling the healthcare professional to provide the best treatment. Other sources include clinical experience, expert consensus, reflective practice, patient assessment and patient preferences (Bury & Mead 1998).

Evidence of effectiveness is most valued in the form of the review, which collects and scrutinizes relevant studies. Reviews may vary in terms of scientific rigour, the most respected one being the Cochrane systematic review. Here, strict criteria are laid down, i.e. the databases employed must be cited, the years which relate to the search stated, the number and quality of papers involved recorded, the basis on which the selection was made stated and the key words listed. Meta-analysis is another way of presenting reviewed work: here, the data from the studies included in the review are reanalysed using statistical techniques; this allows the pooling of a number of studies to obtain an effect size which can be stated as an overall conclusion.

A critical review is also a useful document. It is often described as a narrative review and tends to express the opinion of the researcher. Critical reviews can vary in quality. Another type of review is the overview which is a description of key findings.

Individual studies can also be classified in terms of scientific rigour. Here, the most highly respected form is the randomized controlled trial (RCT). A hypothesis is first formulated and tested, then the data are analysed for statistical significance. A well-designed RCT will fulfil the following criteria. It will:

- contain a control group which does not receive the intervention and acts as a baseline
- adopt a randomized process , both for the selection of participants and their assignment to particular groups
- allow for blinding of study participants and, where appropriate, also the researcher
- be designed so that the results can be statistically analysed
- consist of a sample large enough to have a chance of reaching statistical significance
- carry a precise description of the intervention so that the study can be replicated
- be free of bias and order effects which may confound the results
- follow intention-to-treat analysis of data.

When these criteria are not met the study is said to be methodologically flawed, which means that the results lose some of their credibility. However, it is not always ethical or appropriate to use the randomized controlled trial as a design and in these situations other forms of trial may be adopted such as non-randomized controlled studies and single-system studies.

The experiment, however, is not the only way to answer a question in research: a qualitative approach, in which descriptive data are collected, can also provide useful information and may be the method of choice where the function of research is one of exploration (Sim 1999). Interviews can be employed here.

Wherever subtleties in the therapeutic situation are being studied, the qualitative approach has much to offer. It reflects the lived experience of clients (Gibson & Martin 2003). Qualitative methods can also be used to complement the findings of experimental work, thereby building up a more complete picture.

KEY MESSAGES

- Most stress-related conditions seem to benefit in some degree from relaxation training.

- Cognitive-behavioural therapy and exercise have also been shown to play a part in the relief of stress.
- In some instances relaxation is presented as sole treatment; in others, the relaxation forms part of a wider approach.
- Results of scientific investigation indicate to the therapist which technique is likely to bring benefit in a particular condition.
- Therapists should seek out guidelines where they are available. These may be obtained from organizations such as the National Institute for Clinical Excellence (NICE) and the Scottish Intercollegiate Guidelines Network (SIGN) which have used panels of reviewers to provide evidence statements and best practice guidance. As new evidence emerges, the healthcare worker may be directed to different approaches.
- Although relaxation has been around for many years, the research base is relatively small. For this reason, findings may need to be interpreted with caution. This leaves many questions unanswered.

27

Drawing the threads together

CHAPTER CONTENTS

This chapter addresses a few topics not so far covered. It begins with a discussion of the similarities among the methods. This is followed by a consideration of the ways in which techniques can be combined and leads into a script which illustrates this approach.

Similarities among approaches

In an enterprise such as relaxation training where many approaches all lead to the same goal, there are likely to be wide areas of overlap; for example, dwelling on the breath (as in meditation), reciting phrases (as in autogenic training) and concentrating on muscle sensations (as in progressive relaxation) are activities which resemble one another in that they all involve attention focusing and the reduction of motor activity. Moreover, all three methods are characterized by a monotonous, repetitive stimulus equivalent to the mantra. Thus, the differences between the methods might be more apparent than real, their similarities concealed by their terminology. This might help to explain why the different methods are so often shown to be equally effective when compared with each other.

Combining approaches

It is not suggested in this book that attention should be systematically given to each of the methods in turn. The health care professional may take up any method she feels comfortable with. She may, however, wish to take up more than one method and to present them in a single tuition period. This can have advantages. Combinations of different relaxation and stress reduction techniques seem to be more effective than single techniques (Davis et al 2000).

Ways of combining techniques may be found in *The relaxation and stress reduction workbook* (Davis et al 2000) from which the following two combinations are drawn. The first is for mental stress, the second is for physical tension.

1. 'Changing channels':

    a. thought-stopping (Ch. 24, p201)

    b. guided imagery (Ch. 18, p157)

    c. coping mantra, e.g. 'I am at peace' (Ch. 21, p184).

2. 'Stretch and relax':

    a. stretchings (Ch. 14)

    b. abdominal breathing (Ch. 4, p38)

    c. Mitchell's method (Ch. 11).

For groups of people with varied kinds of stress, more general combined programmes can be constructed. A few examples from the present authors are given below.

1 Abdominal breathing (Ch. 4 , p38), tense–release (Ch. 7) and guided imagery (Ch. 18, p157).

2 Passive relaxation (Ch. 8), goal-directed visualizations using receptive and programmed components (Ch. 19) and self-statements (Ch. 19, p166).

3 Abdominal breathing (Ch. 4, p38), warmth and heaviness phrases (Ch. 20) and differential relaxation (Ch. 13).

4 Passive relaxation (Ch. 8), Benson's meditation (Ch. 22) and self-awareness exercises (Ch. 17).

5 Behavioural relaxation training (Ch. 10, p87), breathing meditation (Ch. 4, p39) and guided imagery (Ch. 18, p157).

6 Breathing pouch (Ch. 4, p39), eye and tongue muscle work (Ch. 5, p53) and meditation on a visual object (Ch. 21, p181).

Set patterns will not suit everyone since the needs and preferences of each person are different. Davis et al (2000) urge people to construct their own combination of techniques.

Although client preferences cannot be predicted, it is clear that they exist (Davis et al 2000, Payne 1989) and that they may be important (McPherson 2009). In the authors' experience it is useful to ask the client which techniques best suit her. Involving the client in the choice of technique, as in other aspects of therapy, enriches the treatment. All this, of course, means that therapists may need to learn several methods if they are to respond to the client's needs.

Example of a script containing a variety of approaches

As well as grouping different techniques together, several techniques can be worked into a single passage, as shown here.

Please lie down. Get yourself comfortable. Allow your eyelids to grow heavy and eventually to close.

Feel the rest of your body also growing heavy … feel it sinking into the rug or the upholstery … compressing the fibres … sinking down so that more body area comes in contact with it … let your weight flow out … feel your body totally freed from its responsibility to hold you up …

Turn your attention to your breathing … without attempting to alter its rhythm, become aware of the movement of your chest and abdomen … notice the passage of the air … the coolness of the air entering your nostrils … travelling through your nose and down the back of your throat … notice also the warm, moist air being exhaled … next time you breathe out, think the word 'relax' … continue slowly …

Now, I'd like you to scan your muscle groups one by one, checking them for tension … adjust your position if you are uncomfortable … starting with the feet, notice how they rest heavily on the floor … heavy as lead … now your legs, imagine them too heavy to lift … your hips too are lying heavily … and your shoulders, feel how they are dropped down … with your arms resting heavily by your sides …

Now, your head, let it sink back, giving its weight to the pillow, making a dent in it … feel your brow smoothed and your jaw relaxed … feel your whole body heavy, warm and relaxed … if tension returns, just let it go … let it flow out through your fingertips and toes …

Transfer yourself in your mind's eye to a sandy beach … see yourself lying in the soft sand … run your fingers through the dry grains … smell the sea air … feel the hot sun on your skin … listen to the waves breaking on the shore … enjoy the peace … if disturbing thoughts intrude, accept that they exist … then let them drift away like clouds passing across the sky … you'll attend to them later …

When you are ready, let the scene fade … gradually bring your attention back to the room in which you are lying … count one … two … three … and slowly open your eyes … then give your arms and legs a gentle stretch …

However, not all researchers support the notion of combining techniques. For example, Manzoni et al (2008), in their systematic review and meta-analysis, suggest that some clients may find it easier to respond to a single-method programme than one which involves a variety of methods. Again, this is a matter of client preference.

Concluding comments

Relaxation training is part of the growing trend to view health in terms of the whole person. Its techniques are designed to have a global effect whether they are targeting the healthy individual with difficulty 'switching off' or the person with a chronic condition trying to self-manage her disease.

The book is not comprehensive; many relaxation methods are not included. The reader will find only a selected range in these chapters (see Introduction, p4) but they are presented with enough detail to be used by someone previously unfamiliar with them. Such a work can be regarded as a toolkit, a collection of techniques from which the healthcare professional can choose whatever seems appropriate for the task in hand. The book does not profess to turn people into experts. Training courses exist for that purpose. Perhaps the book is best described as a professional starter.

After reading Chapter 26, the reader may feel the evidence to support the use of relaxation techniques is not compelling. Such an impression may be gained because relaxation therapy is a new science with a comparatively small research base. Many of its studies contain methodological flaws. Moreover, scientific investigation in this area is beset by intrinsic problems which means it is not easy to draw conclusions. No clear picture regarding the effectiveness of the different methods has yet emerged. Techniques where research is currently prominent include mindfulness, cognitive–behavioural therapy and physical activity; however, more research is needed before we can confidently present best relaxation techniques, which are themselves likely to vary with each condition. Much also depends on psychosocial aspects of the client's life. Lack of evidence, however, is not the same as lack of effect and findings do paint a general picture of benefit.

Health care professionals are well placed to deliver relaxation techniques since the topic features in their own training. It is one of the areas where they share common ground, where resources can be pooled to create a functioning interdisciplinary service.

Training courses are widely available for health care professionals who wish to extend their knowledge (see Appendix 02). The authors suggest that therapists consider including relaxation training among their professional skills. Readers of this book may themselves derive benefit from the regular use of relaxation techniques, as part of a healthy lifestyle.

Section **Five**

Appendices, glossary, references and index

Appendix 1

Table of methods and some suggested applications

Method	Major principles	Suggested applications	Relevant chapters
Progressive relaxation	• relaxed musculature is reflected in a relaxed mind • underpinned by unitary theory • physiological principles predominate but there are cognitive elements	anxiety, psychiatric conditions, hypertension, tension headache, asthma, insomnia, chronic pain, ulcerative colitis, before and after surgery, epilepsy, athletic injury, HIV/AIDS, chronic obstructive pulmonary disease, panic, migraine	Chapters 5, 26
Progressive relaxation training	• similar to progressive relaxation except that the cognitive element is stronger because of the use of suggestion	similar to progressive relaxation	Chapters 6, 26
Applied relaxation	• built around a core technique of progressive relaxation • addresses the concept of anxiety from cognitive and behavioural as well as physiological standpoints	anxiety, panic attacks, phobia, headache, tinnitus, epilepsy, chronic pain	Chapters 9, 26
Behavioural relaxation training	• underpinned by behaviourist principles of reinforcement and corrective adjustment • contains physical and cognitive elements	learning difficulties, ataxic tremor	Chapters 10, 26
Mitchell's method	• based on physiological principles of reciprocal inhibition • has a weak cognitive element	childbirth, hypertension, rheumatoid arthritis	Chapters 11, 26
Alexander technique	• underpinned by principles of body positioning • is atheoretical	performance stress, motor problems, Parkinson's disease	Chapters 12, 26
Stretchings	• these link into physiological principles • the process of stretching entails a relaxation of the muscles being stretched	physical and psychological stress, generalized anxiety, chronic neck tension	Chapters 14, 26

Method	Major principles	Suggested applications	Relevant chapters
Exercise	• essentially a physical approach to relaxation • linked to neurobiological changes, it is underpinned by physiological principles	cardiovascular problems, osteopenia, osteoporosis, depression, chronic fatigue syndrome, drug and alcohol dependence, eating disorders, low self-esteem	Chapters 15, 26
Breathing	• based on physiological principles which link the method to the autonomic nervous system • slow breathing is associated with parasympathetic dominance • a cognitive feature is represented by the imagery which accompanies some breathing sequences	coronary heart disease, hypertension, panic attacks, chronic pain, occupational stress	Chapters 4, 26
Self-awareness	• a cognitive approach concerned with the thoughts one has about the self	low self-esteem	Chapters 17, 26
Imagery	• cognitive principles underlie this approach • image making is thought to be governed by the right cerebral hemisphere	chronic pain, anxiety, before and after surgery, athletic injury, occupational stress	Chapters 18, 26
Goal-directed visualizations	• a cognitive approach which uses techniques of imagery and self-suggestion • based on the belief that the body cannot distinguish between the event as imagined and the event as experienced	performance stress, alcohol and substance misuse, eating disorders, smoking abstinence, chronic pain, sport and athletics, phobia and panic attack	Chapters 19, 26
Autogenics	• based on principles of suggestion, which create a light trance • primarily a cognitive approach, although the sensations of warmth generated by the phrases provide a physiological element • is atheoretical	anxiety, depression, insomnia, drug and alcohol misuse, eating disorders, tension headache, hypertension, coronary heart disease, injury rehabilitation, asthma, HIV/AIDS, different kinds of pain	Chapters 20, 26
Meditation	• a cognitive activity involving what is considered to be a shift in cerebral hemispherical dominance from left to right	hypertension, coronary heart disease, menopausal symptoms, insomnia, occupational stress, HIV/AIDS	Chapters 21, 26
Benson's method	• underpinned by unitary theory • cognitive principles predominate in the focusing of attention on the mantra • in diminishing the activity in the sympathetic nervous system, it draws on physiological principles	hypertension, coronary heart disease, psychological stress, irritable bowel syndrome, menopausal problems	Chapters 22, 26

Method	Major principles	Suggested applications	Relevant chapters
Cognitive behavioural approaches	• these use a variety of techniques drawn from cognitive principles on the one hand and behavioural principles on the other • the client is encouraged to adopt a collaborative role in the management of her condition	anxiety, depression, eating disorders, panic disorder, drug and alcohol dependence, hypertension, chronic fatigue syndrome, insomnia, HIV/AIDS, psychiatric disorders, chronic pain	Chapters 16, 26
Mindfulness meditation	• based on principles of meditation with an emphasis on the moment, accepting it as it occurs without judgement or criticism	Cancer, chronic pain, fibromyalgia, smoking cessation, addictive practices, stress, depression	Chapters 23, 26

Training courses and contact information

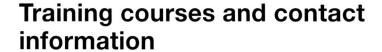

The authors are not in a position to endorse all the following training courses but include them for information. The training courses mentioned here are all in the UK. People reading this book in other countries should consult their in-country register which is available on the Internet.

British Autogenic Society
The Royal London Homeopathic Hospital
60 Great Ormond Street
London WC1N 3HR
Telephone: 0207 391 8908
Website: www.autogenic-therapy.org.uk
Email: admin@autogenic-therapy.org.uk

Training in this approach is offered to those who already hold a qualification in the field of medical, psychological, nursing, therapy or counselling professions.

Research Council for Complementary Medicine
The Royal London Homeopathic Hospital
UCLH NHS Foundation Trust
60 Great Ormond Street
London WC1N 3HR
Website: www.rccm.org.uk
Email: info@rccm.org.uk

This organization provides information on university courses that offer training in complementary and alternative medicine to healthcare professionals.

Alexander Technique
Anthony Kingsley
The Alexander Studio

16 Balderton Street
London W1K 6TN
Telephone: 0207 629 1808
Website: www.alexanderteacher.co.uk
Email: enquiries@alexanderteacher.co.uk

This is one of the registered schools which offers training in the technique.

British Association for Behavioural and Cognitive Psychotherapies (BABCP)
Victoria Buildings
9–13 Silver Street
Bury BL9 0EU
Telephone: 0161 797 4484
Website: www.babcp.com
Email: babcp@babcp.com or comms@babcp.com

BABCP can provide information regarding cognitive-behavioural courses run by universities and other educational establishments. The Internet is a useful source of information. Students are advised to contact the course providers to determine their entry requirements.

Breathworks
16–20 Turner Street
Manchester M4 1DZ
Email: info@breathworks.co.uk
Website: www.breathworks-mindfulness

This organization runs courses in mindfulness meditation for healthcare professionals who wish to become trainers.

Appendix 3

Events and 1995 life change unit (LCU) values for the Recent Life Changes Questionnaire

Reprinted from Miller MA, Rahe RH 1997 Life changes scaling for the 1990s. Journal of Psychosomatic Research 43(3):291-292, with permission from Elsevier.

Life change event	LCU
Health	
An injury or illness which:	
kept you in bed a week or more, or sent you to the hospital	74
was less serious than above	44
Major dental work	26
Major change in eating habits	27
Major change in sleeping habits	26
Major change in your usual type and/or amount of recreation	28
Work	
Change to a new type of work	51
Change in your work hours or conditions	35
Change in your responsibilities at work:	
more responsibilities	29
fewer responsibilities	21
promotion	31
demotion	42
transfer	32
Troubles at work:	
with your boss	29

Life change event	LCU
with co-workers	35
with persons under your supervision	35
other work troubles	28
Major business adjustment	60
Retirement	52
Loss of job:	
laid off from work	68
fired from work	79
Correspondence course to help you in your work	18
Home and family	
Major change in living conditions	42
Change in residence:	
move within the same town or city	25
move to a different town, city or state	47
Change in family get-togethers	25
Major change in health or behaviour of family member	55
Marriage	50
Pregnancy	67
Miscarriage or abortion	65
Gain of a new family member:	
birth of a child	66
adoption of a child	65
a relative moving in with you	59
Spouse beginning or ending work	46

Life change event	LCU
Child leaving home:	
to attend college	41
due to marriage	41
for other reasons	45
Change in arguments with spouse	50
In-law problems	38
Change in the marital status of your parents:	
divorce	59
remarriage	50
Separation from spouse:	
due to work	53
due to marital problems	76
Divorce	96
Birth of grandchild	43
Death of spouse	119
Death of other family member:	
child	123
brother or sister	102
parent	100
Personal and social	
Change in personal habits	26
Beginning or ending school or college	38
Change of school or college	35
Change in political beliefs	24

Life change event	LCU
Change in religious beliefs	29
Change in social activities	27
Vacation	24
New, close, personal relationship	37
Engagement to marry	45
Girlfriend or boyfriend problems	39
Sexual difficulties	44
'Falling out' of a close personal relationship	47
An accident	48
Minor violation of the law	20
Being held in jail	75
Death of a close friend	70
Major decision regarding your immediate future	51
Major personal achievement	36
Financial	
Major change in finances:	
increased income	38
decreased income	60
investment and/or credit difficulties	56
Loss or damage of personal property	43
Moderate purchase	20
Major purchase	37
Foreclosure on a mortgage or loan	58

Appendix 4

PAR-Q Physical Activity Readiness Questionnaire

Physical Activity Readiness
Questionnaire - PAR-Q
(revised 2002)

PAR-Q & YOU

(A Questionnaire for People Aged 15 to 69)

Regular physical activity is fun and healthy, and increasingly more people are starting to become more active every day. Being more active is very safe for most people. However, some people should check with their doctor before they start becoming much more physically active.

If you are planning to become much more physically active than you are now, start by answering the seven questions in the box below. If you are between the ages of 15 and 69, the PAR-Q will tell you if you should check with your doctor before you start. If you are over 69 years of age, and you are not used to being very active, check with your doctor.

Common sense is your best guide when you answer these questions. Please read the questions carefully and answer each one honestly: check YES or NO.

YES	NO	
☐	☐	**1. Has your doctor ever said that you have a heart condition <u>and</u> that you should only do physical activity recommended by a doctor?**
☐	☐	**2. Do you feel pain in your chest when you do physical activity?**
☐	☐	**3. In the past month, have you had chest pain when you were not doing physical activity?**
☐	☐	**4. Do you lose your balance because of dizziness or do you ever lose consciousness?**
☐	☐	**5. Do you have a bone or joint problem (for example, back, knee or hip) that could be made worse by a change in your physical activity?**
☐	☐	**6. Is your doctor currently prescribing drugs (for example, water pills) for your blood pressure or heart condition?**
☐	☐	**7. Do you know of <u>any other reason</u> why you should not do physical activity?**

If you answered

YES to one or more questions

Talk with your doctor by phone or in person BEFORE you start becoming much more physically active or BEFORE you have a fitness appraisal. Tell your doctor about the PAR-Q and which questions you answered YES.

- You may be able to do any activity you want — as long as you start slowly and build up gradually. Or, you may need to restrict your activities to those which are safe for you. Talk with your doctor about the kinds of activities you wish to participate in and follow his/her advice.
- Find out which community programs are safe and helpful for you.

NO to all questions

If you answered NO honestly to <u>all</u> PAR-Q questions, you can be reasonably sure that you can:
- start becoming much more physically active — begin slowly and build up gradually. This is the safest and easiest way to go.
- take part in a fitness appraisal — this is an excellent way to determine your basic fitness so that you can plan the best way for you to live actively. It is also highly recommended that you have your blood pressure evaluated. If your reading is over 144/94, talk with your doctor before you start becoming much more physically active.

DELAY BECOMING MUCH MORE ACTIVE:
- if you are not feeling well because of a temporary illness such as a cold or a fever — wait until you feel better; or
- if you are or may be pregnant — talk to your doctor before you start becoming more active.

PLEASE NOTE: If your health changes so that you then answer YES to any of the above questions, tell your fitness or health professional. Ask whether you should change your physical activity plan.

<u>Informed Use of the PAR-Q</u>: The Canadian Society for Exercise Physiology, Health Canada, and their agents assume no liability for persons who undertake physical activity, and if in doubt after completing this questionnaire, consult your doctor prior to physical activity.

© Canadian Society for Exercise Physiology, **www.csep.ca**. Reproduced with permission..

Source: *Physical Activity Readiness Questionnaire (PAR-Q)* © 2002. Used with permission from the Canadian Society for Exercise Physiology www.csep.ca.

Glossary

Aerobic Exercise Sustained, rhythmic activity. It involves large muscle groups contracting in a repetitive manner at low-to-moderate levels of energy expenditure for long periods of time. Examples include walking, jogging, distance running, swimming, dancing and cycling.

Blinding This is a condition built into the study design whereby participants are kept in ignorance of the group they are in: experimental or control. When the researchers are also in ignorance of this fact, the situation is called double blind. Single and double blinding are techniques for reducing the risk of bias in the results.

Biopsychosocial This approach gives weight to psychosocial aspects as well as biological ones.

Body Awareness Therapy A therapy based on the notion that human movement has a psychological dimension. Movements carried out by the body are recognized as part of the self and therefore, part of a person's identity.

Catecholamines These include adrenaline, noradrenaline and dopamine. They play an important role as neurotransmitters in the functioning of the autonomic and central nervous systems.

Catharsis In psychoanalytic theory, this refers to the release of tension which occurs when repressed thoughts are brought into consciousness.

Centring Refers to the focusing of attention on the interior of the self. To achieve this state all external stimuli must be disregarded. The purpose is to find and make contact with the essence of the self.

Clinical Depression Diagnosed by a cluster of symptoms that persist for weeks or months. Symptoms include feelings of hopelessness, sadness, guilt. They are accompanied by physical symptoms such as loss of energy, appetite, sleeplessness and a lack of concentration. Diagnosis of depression is usually undertaken by clinical interview. In research studies depression may be measured by using standardized screening devices such as the Beck Depression Inventory in which the severity of the condition can be classified into mild, medium and severe.

Cognitive–behavioural Therapy An approach concerned with helping the patient to identify and correct faulty patterns of thinking. It can lead to improved clinical outcomes. Patient and therapist are engaged in a collaborative effort to address and solve or alleviate the patient's problem. The therapy is of predetermined and short duration and is focused on the patient's current circumstances.

Cognitive Restructuring This involves a re-evaluation of a person's perception of danger or vulnerability and a questioning of the beliefs which underlie it. The technique consists of three stages: identifying negative thoughts, challenging their accuracy and replacing them with constructive alternatives based upon new judgements about the degree of risk.

Confidence Interval The distance between an upper and a lower point between which the true value lies with a probability of 95%. Presented in this way, the result assumes a range of possibilities. A narrow range will indicate a more precise result than a wide one.

Control Group The basic scientific study consists of two groups, resembling each other in as many ways as possible. One of these groups is the experimental group which receives the intervention; the other group is the control which does not receive the intervention. The control thus provides a baseline against which to measure the effects of the intervention.

Effect Size This refers either to the strength of the association or to the effect of the intervention and is expressed as a percentage of the total possible effect.

Epidemiology The study of diseases in populations and concerned with the cause of the disease and the way the disease is distributed within a given population.

Evidence-based Practice Practice informed by research findings. It consists of procedures which current evidence shows to be the most effective. Thus, it may be referred to as best practice.

Exposure Techniques These are introduced to help individuals face situations which they find stress inducing such as, for example, public speaking. Exposure generally involves a hierarchy of low-to-high-threat versions of this event. The individual is first presented with the item of lowest threat. With the help of a relaxation technique, she works to overcome her fear at that level. When she succeeds, she moves on to the next level of threat, dealing with it in the same way.

Eye Movement Desensitization and Reprocessing This is a treatment employed in post-traumatic stress disorder: the client focuses on the traumatic event while receiving bilateral stimulation, usually in the form of eye movements.

Fear Avoidance This is behaviour which the individual adopts to avoid situations which give rise to fear. However, by avoiding the situation, the fear attached to it mounts. Avoidance may result in an immediate sense of relief but creates an increase in anxiety levels on the next occasion of threat. The solution is to face the feared situation.

Generalized Anxiety Disorder Characterized by excessive worry, overtense muscles and impairment of function, all of which have persisted for at least 6 months and are not confined to any specific circumstances.

Homeostasis The process whereby a balanced state is maintained in body systems throughout varying external conditions. An example can be found in the regulation of body temperature during extreme heat and cold.

Hypothesis This is a statement which acts as a provisional explanation. In science a hypothesis must undergo a test, the findings of which will tell the researcher whether the hypothesis has been supported or whether it should be rejected. The conclusion reached, however, will only apply within the context of the particular piece of research.

Locus of Control This refers to the source of control of the behaviour of an individual. If he tends to take responsibility for his actions, he is said to have an internal locus; if he tends to attribute events to chance effects or external factors, he is said to have an external locus. In practice, people tend to display both forms; this places the individual's locus of control on a continuum, where it exhibits varying levels, internal and external, at different times.

Meta-analysis A statistical technique which collates and analyses the findings of many different studies and identifies trends in outcome.

Mind–body Approaches These are defined by the National Institutes of Health as 'interventions designed to facilitate the mind's capacity to affect bodily function and symptoms'. In a word, holistic.

Mindfulness This refers to awareness and acceptance of the moment as it occurs; cherishing it, whatever we happen to be doing.

Motor Skill Refers to a skill which involves physical movement.

Number Needed to Treat (NNT) This represents the number of people who would need to receive the intervention before one specific outcome occurred or one specific adverse outcome was avoided. For example, in an experimental group of elderly women wearing hip protectors, the NNT is an estimate of how many participants would be necessary before one hip fracture was prevented. The NNT is a way of presenting the usefulness of a treatment.

Outcome Measures The products of measurement used to determine the results of interventions. A range of tools are specifically designed for this purpose.

Pacing Refers to the way a learning programme is structured to allow for the varying level of skill in the performer. New material is introduced in a gradual and controlled way, alternating with periods of rest.

Pre-experimental Studies Here, a single system such as a cohort is studied to explore an idea. The exercise helps in formulating a hypothesis which may later be tested.

Psychogenic This adjective is applied to symptoms which are brought about by faulty patterns of thinking or overemotional reactions.

Psychosocial The word encompasses both psychological and social aspects of a person's life. The 'psychological' includes a person's beliefs and attitudes while the 'social' refers to environmental influences, including the influence of other people.

Quasi-experimental Studies These bear some characteristics of a true experiment but lack the full requirements of a randomized controlled trial. They feature, for example, in research where randomization is not possible.

Randomization A process by which researchers allocate people into different groups. An example of this process is the use of numbered sealed envelopes; computer-aided lists are another. Randomization allows all study participants to have an equal chance of being selected for the active experimental intervention. The process helps to ensure that the groups are similar at the start of the study.

Randomized Controlled Trials These are studies which carry the full rigour of a scientific experiment. Participants are selected by a random process and divided into two or more groups, one of which receives the intervention. The presence of a control is essential but it can take different forms.

Reflective Practice Refers to thinking about knowledge gained from one's experience in the past and the creative application of it in unfamiliar situations.

Reinforcement Positive reinforcement refers to action which increases the likelihood of a certain behaviour; for example, giving a dog a biscuit every time it brings back a ball makes it more likely the dog will bring back the ball next time it is thrown.

Reliability Refers to the consistency of results when the test is repeated, either by the same researcher on different occasions or by different researchers on the same occasion.

Repression A psychoanalytical concept in which anxiety-inducing thoughts are prevented from reaching conscious awareness.

Reviews Scientific reviews collate the results of all studies in a particular field. They are the result of extensive literature searches and provide the health care professional with the kind of information needed to form a view of the best treatment.

Schizophrenia This condition is characterized by symptoms such as hallucinations and thought disturbances. It may also be accompanied by social withdrawal, low self-esteem, reduced motivation, emotional and attentional deficits and other symptoms of depression.

Self-efficacy The ability of an individual to predict her success in achieving a particular task in a given situation. Efficacy is effectiveness; self-efficacy is the belief in one's effectiveness.

Skill This enables a person to achieve a goal with a high level of certainty and an economy of time and energy.

Somatization This is said to occur when an individual complains of symptoms, such as pain, which cannot be explained in terms of organic disease. It differs from hypochondriasis where the individual is constantly in fear of developing a disease.

States of Altered Consciousness These are states of mental functioning which are different from the ordinary pattern. Examples are dreaming, drug-induced states, hypnotism, meditation, day-dreaming, deep relaxation, guided imagery.

Statistical Significance Means that there is a 95% likelihood that the result of the experiment is due to the manipulations of the experimenter and not to chance factors. Expressed another way, the result achieved in the experiment could only have occurred by chance in fewer than 5 out of 100 cases.

Stimulus-control Behaviour This is behaviour which is triggered and maintained by environmental stimuli.

Trait Anxiety An inherent tendency to interpret circumstances as more dangerous than they are and to respond with a disproportionate degree of anxiety. It contrasts with *state anxiety* which reflects the normal level of anxiety attached to particular events and situations perceived as threatening.

Validity A test is valid when it measures what it claims to measure. It has internal validity when it is devoid of bias, and external validity when its results can be generalized to other situations. It has content validity when its components are representative of the item to be measured and face validity when it *seems* valid after superficial appraisal.

References

Achterberg, J., 1985. Imagery in Healing: Shamanism and Modern Medicine. New Science Library, Boston.

Ackerman, C.J., Turkoski, B., 2000. Using guided imagery to reduce pain and anxiety. Home and Healthcare. Nurse 18 (8), 524–530.

Adams, M.A., Hutton, W.C., 1985. The effect of posture on the lumbar spine. J. Bone. Joint. Surg. 67B, 625–629.

Adams, M.A., McNally, D.S., Chinn, H., Dolan, P., 1994. Posture and the compressive strength of the lumbar spine. Clin. Biomech. 9, 5–14.

Adler-Nevo, G., Manassis, K., 2005. Psychological treatment of pediatric post-traumatic stress disorder: the neglected field of single-incident trauma. Depress. Anxiety 22 (4), 177–189.

Alberti, R., Emmons, M., 1982. Your Perfect Right: A Guide to Assertive Living, fourth ed. Impact, San Luis Obispo, California.

Alexander, F.N., 1932. The Use of the Self. Dutton, New York.

Allied Dunbar National Fitness Survey, 1992. Activity and Health Research: A Report on Activity Patterns and Fitness Levels. Sports Council and Health Education Authority, London.

American College of Sports Medicine 1997. American College of Sports Medicine and American Diabetes Association joint position statement: diabetes mellitus and exercise Med. Sci. Sports Exerc. 22, 265–274.

American Psychiatric Association, 1994. Diagnostic and Statistical Manual of Disorders, fourth ed. American Psychiatric Association, Washington, DC.

Ampunsiriratana, A., Triamchaisri, S., Nontasorn, T., et al., 2005. A palliated-suffering model for HIV infected patients: a combination of the foundations of mindfulness meditation and Watson's Caring. Thai. J. Nurs. Res. 9 (4), 268–280.

Anand, M.P., 1999. Non-pharmacological management of essential hypertension. J. Indian Med. Assoc. 97 (6), 220–225.

Anderson, B., 1983. Stretching and sports. In: Appenzeller, O., Atkinson, R. (Eds.) Sports Medicine, second ed. Urban and Schwarzenberg, Baltimore.

Andersson, G., 2002. Psychological aspects of tinnitus and the application of cognitive-behavioural therapy. Clin. Psychol. Rev. 22 (7), 977–990.

Antoni, M.H., Wimberly, S.R., Lechner, S.C., et al., 2006. Reduction of cancer-specific thought intrusions and anxiety symptoms with a stress management intervention among women undergoing treatment for breast cancer. Am. J. Psychiatry 163 (10), 1791–1797.

Apter, M., 2003. On a certain blindness in modern psychology. The Psychol. 16 (9), 474–475.

Argyle, M., 1978. The Psychology of Interpersonal Behaviour, third ed. Pelican, Harmondsworth, Middlesex.

Arias, A.J., Steinberg, K., Banga, A., et al., 2006. Systematic review of the efficacy of meditation techniques as treatments for medical illness. J. Altern. Complement. Med 12 (8), 817–832.

Aspinwall, L.G., Taylor, S.E., 1997. A stitch in time: self-regulation and proactive coping. Psychol. Bull. 121, 417–436.

Assagioli, R., 1965. Psychosynthesis. Turnstone Books, London.

Astin, J.A., 2004. Mind-body therapies for the management of pain. Clin. J. Pain 20 (1), 27–32.

Astin, J.A., Beckner, W., Soeken, K., et al., 2002. Psychological interventions for rheumatoid arthritis: a meta-analysis of randomized controlled trials. Arthritis Rheum. 47 (3), 291–302.

Astin, J.A., Berman, B.M., Bausell, B., et al., 2003. The efficacy of mindfulness meditation plus qigong movement therapy in the treatmant of fibromyalgia: a randomized controlled trial. J. Rheumatol. 30 (10), 2257–2262.

Atkinson, R.L., Atkinson, R.C., Smith, E.E., Bem, D.J., Nolen-Hoeksema, S., 1999. Hilgard's Introduction to Psychology, thirteen ed. Harcourt Brace, Fort Worth.

Ayers, C.R., Sorrell, J.T., Thorp, S.R., et al., 2007. Evidence-based psychological treatments for late-life anxiety. Psychol. Aging 22 (1), 8–17.

Babyak, M., Blumenthal, J.A., Herman, S., et al., 2000. Exercise treatment for major depression: maintenance of therapeutic benefit at 10 months. Psychosom. Med. 62, 633–638.

Bach, L.J., David, A.S., 2006. Self-awareness after acquired and traumatic brain injury. Neuropsychol. Rehabil. 16 (4), 397–414.

Bagheri-Nesami, M., Mohseni-Bandpei, M.A., Shayesteh-Azar, M., 2006. The effect of Benson's relaxation technique on rheumatoid arthritis patients: extended report. Int. J. Nurs. Pract. 12 (4), 214–219.

Baird, C.L., Sands, L., 2004. A pilot study of the effectiveness of guided imagery with progressive muscle relaxation to reduce chronic pain and mobility difficulties of osteoarthritis. Pain Manag. Nurs. 5 (3), 97–104.

Bandura, A., 1977. Self-efficacy: towards a unifying theory of behaviour change. Psychol. Rev. 84, 191–215.

Bandura, A., 1986. Social Foundations of Thought and Action: A Social Cognitive Theory. Prentice-Hall, Englewood Cliffs, NY.

Bandura, A., 1997. Self-efficacy: The Exercise of Control. W H Freeman, San Francisco, CA.

Banquet, J., 1973. Spectral analysis of the EEG in meditation. Electroencephalogr. Clin. Neurophysiol. 35, 143–151.

Barber, T.X., 1969. Hypnosis: A Scientific Approach. Van Nostrand-Reinhold, New York.

Barber, T.X., 1970. LSD, Marijuana, Yoga and Hypnosis. Aldine, Chicago.

Barber, T.X., 1984. Hypnosis, deep relaxation and active relaxation: data, theory and clinical applications. In: Woolfolk, R.L., Lehrer, P.M. (Eds.) Principles and Practice of Stress Management. Guilford Press, New York.

Barber, T.X., Chauncey, H.M., Winer, R.A., 1964. The effect of hypnotic and non-hypnotic suggestion on parotid gland response to gustatory stimuli. Psychosom. Med. 26, 374–380.

Barlow, W., 1975. The Alexander principle. Arrow, London.

Barnard, S., Hartigan, G., 1998. Clinical Audit in Physiotherapy: From Theory into Practice. Butterworth-Heinemann, Oxford.

Barnes, V.A., Treiber, F.A., Davis, H., 2001. Impact of transcendental meditation on cardiovascular function at rest and during acute stress in adolescents with high normal blood pressure. J. Psychosom. Res. 51 (4), 597–605.

Batson, G., 1996. Conscious use of the human body in movement: the peripheral neuro-anatomic basis of the Alexander Technique. Med. Probl. Perform. Art. 11 (1), 3–11.

Beauregard, M., O'Leary, D., 2008. Believing can make it so: The Neuroscience of the Placebo Effect: Advances Ch 25, Simon & Schuster, London.

Beck, A.T., 1976. Cognitive Therapy and the Emotional Disorders. International Universities Press, New York.

Beck, A.T., 1984. Cognitive approaches to stress management. In: Woolfolk, R.L., Lehrer, P.M. (Eds.) Principles and Practice of Stress Management. Guilford Press, New York.

Beck, A.T., 1988. The Beck Depression Inventory. Psychological Corporation, Sidcup.

Beck, A.T., Ward, C.H., Mendelson, M., Mock, J.E., Erbaugh, J.K., 1961. An inventory for measuring depression. Arch. Gen. Psychiatry 4, 53–63.

Bell, J.A., Saltikov, J.B., 2000. Mitchell's relaxation technique: is it effective? Physiotherapy 86 (9), 473–478.

Benson, H., 1976. The Relaxation Response. Collins, London.

Benson, H., Stark, M., 1996. Timeless Healing: The Power and Biology of Belief. Scribner, New York.

Bernaards, C.M., Jans, M.P., van den Heuvel, S.G., Hendriksen, I.J., Houtman, I.L., Bongers, P.M., 2006. Can strenuous leisure time physical activity prevent psychological complaints in a working population? Occup. Environ. Med. 63, 10–16.

Bernstein, D.A., Borkovec, T.D., 1973. Progressive Relaxation Training: A Manual for the Helping Professions. Research Press, Champaign, IL.

Bernstein, D.A., Given, B.A., 1984. Progressive relaxation: abbreviated methods. In: Woolfolk, R.L., Lehrer, P.M. (Eds.) Principles and Practice of Stress Management. Guilford Press, New York.

Bernstein, D.A., Borkovec, T.D., Hazlett-Stevens, H., 2000. New Directions in Progressive Relaxation Training: A Guide Book for Helping Professionals. Praeger, Westport, CT.

Biddle, S.J.H., Mutrie, N., 2008. Psychology of Physical Activity: Determinants, Well-Being and Interventions, second ed. Routledge, New York.

Biddle, S.J.H., Fox, K.R., Boucher, S.H. (Eds.), 2000. Physical Activity and Psychological Well-Being. Routledge, London, pp. 63–88.

Bird, J., Pinch, C., 2002. Autogenic therapy: Self-Help for Mind and Body. Newleaf, Dublin.

Birk, T.J., Birk, C.A., 1987. Use of ratings of perceived exertion for exercise prescription. Sports Med. 4, 1–8.

Bishop, S.R., 2002. What do we really know about mindfulness-based stress reduction? Psychosom. Med. 64, 71–83.

Bisson, J., Andrew, M., 2007. Psychological treatment of post-traumatic stress disorder (update). Cochrane Database Syst. Rev. Issue 3. CD003388.

Blackburn, I.M., Twaddle, V., 1996. Cognitive Therapy in Action. Souvenir Press, London.

Blaine, B., Crocker, J., 1993. Self-esteem and self-serving biases in reactions to positive and negative events: an integrative review. In: Baumeister, R.F. (Ed.), Self-Esteem: The Puzzle of Low Self-Regard. Plenum, New York, pp. 55–86.

Blair, S.N., 1995. Exercise prescription for health. Quest 47, 338–353.

Blair, S.N., Kohl, H.W., Gordon, N.F., Paffenbarger, R.S., Jr. 1992. How much physical activity is good for health? Ann. Rev. Public Health 13, 99–126.

Blumenthal, J.A., Babyak, M.A., Moore, K.A., Craighead, W.E., Herman, S., Khatri, P., 1999. Effects of exercise training on older patients with major depression. Arch. Intern. Med. 159, 2349–2356.

Blumenthal, J.A., Babyak, M.A., Doraiswamy, M., et al., 2007. Exercise and pharmacology in the treatment of major depressive disorder. Psychosom. Medicime 69, 587–596.

Bootzin, R.R., Perlis, M.L., 1992. Non-pharmacological treatments of insomnia. J. Clin. Psychiatry 53 (Suppl), 37–41.

Borg, G.A.V., 1970. Perceived exertion as an indicator of somatic stress. Scanda. J. Rehabil. Med. 2, 92–98.

Borg, G.A.V., 1998. Borg's Perceived Exertion and Pain Scales. Human Kinetics, Europe.

Borkovec, T.D., Mathews, A., 1988. Treatment of non-phobic anxiety disorders: a comparison of non-directive cognitive and coping desensitization therapy. J. Consult. Clin. Psychol. 56 (6), 877–884.

Borkovec, T.D., Newman, M.G., Pincus, A., Lytle, R., 2002. A component analysis of cognitive behavioural therapy for general anxiety disorder and the role of interpersonal problems. J. Consult. Clin. Psychol. 70, 288–298.

Bowler, S.D., Green, A., Mitchell, C.A., 1998. Buteyko breathing techniques in asthma: a blinded randomized controlled trial. Med. J. Aust. 169, 575–578.

Bowling, A., 1997. Measuring Health: A Review of Quality of Life Measurement Scales, second ed. Open University Press, Buckingham.

Bowling, A., 2001. Measuring Disease: A Review of Disease-Specific Quality of Life Measurement Scales, second ed. Open University Press, Buckingham.

Boyce, P.M., Telley, N.J., Balaam, B., et al., 2003. A randomized controlled trial of cognitive behaviour therapy, relaxation training and routine clinical care for the iritable bowel syndrome. Am. J. Gastroenterol. 98 (10), 2209–2218.

Bricklin, M., 1990. Meditation: the healing silence. In: Bricklin, M. (Ed.), Positive Living and Health. Rodale Press, Emmaus, PA.

Brion, M., 2003. Autogenic Therapy and Neurolinguistic Psychotherapy. British Autogenic Society, London.

Broocks, A., Bandelow, B., Pekrun, G., et al., 1998. Comparison of aerobic exercise, clomipramine and placebo in the treatment of panic disorder. Am. J. Psychiatry 155 (5), 603–609.

Brown, T.A., Campbell, L.A., Lehman, C.L., et al., 2001. Current and life-time co-morbidity of the DSMIV anxiety and mood disorders in a large clinical sample. J. Abnorm. Psychol. 110, 585–599.

Brown, W.H., Carlos, A., 2003. A cogitive behavioural intervention to decrease symptoms of depression, anxiety and somatic complaints in adults diagnosed with human immunodeficiency virus (HIV) and acquired immunodeficiency syndrome (AIDS). Diss. Abstr. Int. Sci. Eng. 64 (5B), 2412.

Bruton, A., Lewith, G.T., 2005. The Buteyko breathing technique for asthma: a review. Complement. Ther. Med. 13 (1), 41–46.

Bruton, A., Armstrong, M., Chadwick, C., Gibson, D., Gahr, K., 2006. Preliminary investigations into the effects of end-tidal CO_2 measures in patients with asthma and healthy volunteers during a single treatment session. Physiotherapy 93 (1), 30–36.

Bulley, C., Donaghy, M.E., Payne, A., Mutrie, N., 2007. A critical review of the validity of measuring stages of change in relation to exercise and moderate physical activity. Crit. Public Health 17 (1), 17–30.

Burch, V., Hennessy, G., Fricker, S., 2006. Exploring How Different Management and Treatment Approaches Affect the Subjective Experience of Long-Term Back Pain Sufferers: A Qualitative Analysis. Breathworks, Manchester.

Burke, E.J., Collins, M.S., 1984. Using perceived exertion for the prescription of exercise in healthy adults.

In: Cantu, R.C. (Ed.), Clinical Sports Medicine. Collamore Press, Lexington, VA.

Burlingame, J., Blaschko, T., 2002. Assessment Tools for Recreational Therapy and Related Fields, third ed. Idyll Arbor, USA.

Burnard, P., 1991. Coping with Stress in the Health Professions: A Practical Guide. Chapman and Hall, London.

Burnard, P., 1992. Know Yourself! Self-Awareness Activities for Nurses. Scutari Press, London.

Bury, T.J., Mead, J.M. (Eds.), 1998. Evidence-Based Health Care: A Practical Guide for Therapists. Butterworth-Heinemann, Oxford.

Butler, A.C., Chapmen, J.E., Forman, E.M., et al., 2006. The empirical status of cognitive-behavioural therapy: a review of meta-analyses. Clin. Psychol. Rev., Ch 26, 17–31.

Canter, P.H., 2003. The therapeutic effects of meditation (leading article). Br. Med. J. 326, 1049–1050.

Canter, P.H., Ernst, E., 2003. The cumulative effect of transcendental meditation on cognitive function: a systematic review of randomized controlled trials. Wien. Klin. Wochenschr. 115 (21–22), 758–766.

Canter, P.H., Ernst, E., 2004. Insufficient evidence to conclude whether or not transcendental meditation decreases blood pressure: results of a systematic review of randomized clinical trials. J. Hypertens. 22 (11), 2049–2054.

Carlbring, P., Ekselius, L., Andersson, G., 2003. Treatment of panic disorder via the Internet: a randomized controlled trial of cognitive behavioural therapy versus applied relaxation. J. Behav. Ther. Exp. Psychiatry 34 (2), 129–140.

Carlbring, P., Gunnarsdóttir, M., Hedensjö, L., Andersson, G., Ekselius, L., Furmark, T., 2007. Treatment of social phobia: randomised trial of internet-delivered cognitive-behavioural therapy with telephone support. Br. J. Psychiatry 190, 123–128.

Carless, D., Fox, K.R., 2003. The physical self. In: Everett, T., Donaghy, M., Feaver, S. (Eds.) Interventions in Mental Health. Butterworth-Heinemann, Oxford.

Carlson, C.R., Hoyle, R.H., 1993. Efficacy of abbreviated progressive muscle relaxation training: a quantitative review of behavioural medicine research. J. Consult. Clin. Psychol. 61 (6), 1059–1067.

Carlson, C.R., Collins, F.L., Nitz, A.J., Sturgis, E.T., Rogers, J.L., 1990. Muscle stretching as an alternative relaxation training procedure. J. Behav. Ther. Exp. Psychiatry 21 (1), 29–38.

Carlson, L.E., Garland, S.N., 2005. The inpact of mindfulness-based stress reduction on sleep, mood, stress and fatigue symptoms in cancer outpatients. Int. J. Behav. Med. 12 (4), 278–285.

Carlson, L.E., Speca, M., Faris, P., et al., 2007. One year pre-post intervention follow-up of psychological, immune, endocrine and blood pressure outcomes of mindfulness-based stress reduction in breast and prostate cancer outpatients. Brain, Behav. Immun. 21 (8), 1038–1049.

Carrington, P., 1984. Modern forms of meditation. In: Woolfolk, R.L., Lehrer, P.M. (Eds.) Principles and Practice of Stress Management. Guilford Press, New York.

Carroll, D., Seers, K., 1998. Relaxation for the relief of chronic pain: a systematic review. J. Adv. Nurs. 27 (3), 476–487.

Cassidy, T., 1999. Stress, Cognition and Health. Routledge, London.

Chang, B.H., Jones, D., Hendricks, A., et al., 2004. Relaxation response for veterans with congestive heart failure: results from a qualitative study within a clinical trial. Prev. Cardiol. 7 (2), 64–70.

Chaouloff, F., 1997. The serotonin hypothesis. In: Morgan, W.P. (Ed.), Physical Activity and Mental Health. Taylor and Francis, Washington, DC, pp. 179–198.

Cheung, Y.L., Molassiotis, A., Chang, A.M., 2003. The effect of progressive muscle relaxation training on anxiety and quality of life after stoma surgery in colorectal cancer patients. Psycho-Oncol. 12 (3), 254–266.

Chou, R., Huffman, L.H., 2007. Non-pharmacologic therapies for acute and chronic low back pain: a review of the evidence for an American Pain Society/American College of Physicians' clinical practice guideline. Ann. Intern. Med. 147 (7), 492–504.

Clark, D.M., 1986. A cognitive approach to panic. Behav. Res. Ther. 24, 461–470.

Clark, D.M., Salkovskis, P.M., Chalkley, A.J., 1985. Respiratory control as a treatment for panic attacks. J. Behav. Ther. Exp. Psychiatry 16, 23–30.

Clark, D.M., Ehlers, A., Hackmann, A., et al., 2006. Cognitive therapy versus exposure and applied relaxation in social phobia: a randomized controlled trial. J. Consult. Clin. Psychol. 74 (3), 568–578.

Cochrane, A.L., 1972. Effectiveness and Efficiency: Random Reflections on Health Services. Nuffield Provincial Hospitals Trust, London.

Cohen, S., Wills, T.A., 1985. Stress, social support and the buffering hypothesis. Psychol. Bull. 98, 310–357.

Conrad, A., Roth, W.T., 2007. Muscle relaxation therapy for anxiety disorders: it works, but how? J. Anxiety Disord. 21 (3), 243–264.

Cooper, C.L., 1981. The Stress Check. Prentice-Hall, New Jersey.

Cooper-Patrick, L., Ford, D.E., Mead, L.A., Chang, P.P., Klag, M.J., 1997. Exercise and depression in midlife: a prospective study. Am. J. Public Health 87 (4), 670–673.

Copeland, G., 2005. A Practical Handbook for Clinical Audit. NHS Clinical Governance Support Team, Leicester. www.cgsupport.nhs.uk/downloads/practical.

Cornelissen, V.A., Fagard, R.H., 2005. Effect of resistence training on resting blood pressure: a meta-analysis of randomized controlled trials. J. Hypertens. 23 (2), 251–259.

Cowie, R.L., Conley, D.P., Underwood, M.F., Reader, P.G., 2008. A randomized controlled trial of the Buteiko method technique as an adjunct to conventional management of asthma. Respir. Med. 102 (5), 726–732.

Cowley, D.S., 1987. Hyperventilation and panic disorder. Am. J. Med. 83, 929–937.

Cox, T., 1978. Stress. Macmillan, London.

Cox, T., Mackay, C.J., 1976. A Psychological Model of Occupational Stress. Paper presented to the Medical Research Council. Mental Health in Industry, London, November.

Craft, L.L., Landers, D.M., 1998. The effect of exercise on clinical depression and depression resulting from mental illness: a meta-analysis. J. Sport Exerc. Psychol. 20, 357–399.

Crawford-Walker, C.J., King, A., Chan, S., 2005. Distraction techniques for schizophrenia. Cochrane Database of Syst. Rev. CD004717.

Crist, D.A., Rickard, H.C., 1993. A 'fair' comparison of progressive and imaginal relaxation. Percept. Mot. Skills 76, 691–700.

CSP Interactive, 2008. Respiratory Care. Chartered Society of Physiotherapy, London.

Cupal, D.D., Brewer, B.W., 2001. Effects of relaxation and guided imagery on knee strength, reinjury anxiety and pain following anterior cruciate ligament reconstruction. Rehabil. Psychol. 46 (1), 28–43.

Daley, A.J., Mutrie, N., Crank, H., Coleman, R., Saxton, J., 2004. Exercise therapy in women who have had breast cancer: design of the Sheffield women's exercise and well-being project. Health Educ. Res. 19 (6), 686–697.

Daley, A.J., Crank, H., Saxton, J., Mutrie, N., Coleman, R., Roalfe, A., 2007. A randomized trial of exercise therapy in women treated for breast cancer. J. Clin. Oncol. 25 (13), 1713–1721.

Dalloway, M., 1992. Visualization: The Master Skill in Mental Training. Optimal Performance Institute, Phoenix, AZ.

Damen, L., Bruijen, J., Koes, B.W., et al., 2006. Prophylactic treatment of migraine in children. Part 1: a systematic review of non-pharmacological trials. Cephalalgia 26 (4), 373–383.

Davidson, K., 2008. Cognitive-behavioural therapy: origins and developments. In: Donaghy, M., Nicol, M., Davidson, K. (Eds.) Cognitive-Behavioural Interventions in Physiotherapy and Occupational Therapy. Butterworth-Heinemann, Edinburgh, pp. 3–18.

Davidson, R.J., Kabat-Zinn, J., Schumacher, J., et al., 2003. Alterations in brain and immune function produced by mindfulness meditation. Psychosom. Med. 65, 564–570.

Davis, J.M., Fleming, M.F., Bonus, K.A., Baker, T.B., 2007. A pilot study on mindfulness-based stress reduction for smokers. BMC Complement. Altern. Med. 7, 2.

Davis, M., Eshelman, E., McKay, M., 1988. The Relaxation and Stress Reduction Workbook, third ed. New Harbinger, Oakland, CA.

Davis, M., Shellman, E., McKay, M., 2000. The Relaxation and Stress Reduction Workbook, fifth ed. New Harbinger, Oakland, CA.

Dawes, R.M., 1994. House of Cards: Psychology and Psychotherapy Built on Myth. Free Press, New York.

Degotardi, P.J., Klass, E.S., Rosenberg, B.S., Fox, D.G., Gallelli, K.A., Gottlieb, B.S., 2006. Development and evaluation of a cognitive-behavioural intervention for juvenile fibromyalgia. J. Paediatr. Psychol. 37, 714–723.

de Greef, M., van Wijck, R., Reynders, K., et al., 2003. Impact of the Groningen Exercise Therapy for Symphony Orchestra Musicians program on perceived physical competence and playing-related musculoskeletal disorders of professional musicians. Med. Probl. Perform. Art. 18 (4), 156–160.

de Leon, D., 1999. The relaxation response in the treatment of chronic pain. In: Micozzi, M.S., Bacchus, A.N. (Eds.) The Physician's Guide to Alternative Medicine. American Health Consultants, Atlanta, GA, pp. 335–337.

Denis. C., Lavie, E., Fatseas, M., Auriacombe, M., 2006. Psychotherapeutic interventions for cannabis abuse and/or dependence in outpatient settings. Cochrane Database Syst. Rev. Issue 3. Art. No.: CD005336. DOI: 10.1002/14651858.CD005336.pub2.

Dennis, C.L., 2004. Treatment of postpartum depression part 2: a critical review of non-biological interventions. J. Clin. Psychiatry 65 (9), 1252–1265.

Department of Health, 2004. At Least Five a Week: Evidence on the Impact of Physical Activity and its Relationship to Health A report from the Chief Medical Officer. HMSO, London.

Dickinson, H.O., Mason, J.M., Nicolson, D.J., et al., 2006. Lifestyle interventions to reduce raised blood pessure: a systematic review of randomized controlled trials. J. Hypertens. 24 (2), 215–233.

DiClemente, C.C., Prochaska, J.O., Gibertini, M., 1985. Self-efficacy and the stages of self-change of smoking. Cognit. Ther. Res. 9, 181–200.

Donaghy, M.E., 2001. A Critical Approach to Physiotherapy in Mental Health. Workshop pack. Queen Margaret University College, Edinburgh.

Donaghy, M.E., 2007. Exercise can seriously improve your mental health: fact or fiction? Adv. Physiother. 9 (2), 76–89.

Donaghy, M.E., 2008a. Cognitive-behavioural approaches in the treatment of alcohol addiction. In: Donaghy, M., Nicol, M., Davidson, K. (Eds.) Cognitive-Behavioural Interventions in Physiotherapy and Occupational Therapy. Butterworth-Heimemann Elsevier, Edinburgh, pp. 105–120.

Donaghy, M.E., 2008b. The importance of psychological preparation in injury prevention. The 13th European Conference in Sports Science, Estoril.

Donaghy, M.E., Durward, B., 2000. A Report on the Clinical Effectiveness of Physiotherapy in Mental Health. Chartered Society of Physiotherapy, London.

Donaghy, M.E., Morss, K., 2000. Guided reflection: a framework to facilitate and assess reflective practice within the discipline of physiotherapy. Physiother. Theory Pract. 16, 3–14.

Donaghy, M.E., Ussher, M., 2005. Exercise interventions in drug and alcohol rehabilitation. In: Faulkner, G., Taylor, A.H. (Eds.) Exercise Health and Mental Health: Emerging Relationships. Routledge, London, pp. 46–89.

Donaghy, M.E., Nicol, M., Davidson, K., 2008. Cognitive Behavioural Interventions in Physiotherapy and Occupational Therapy. Butterworth-Heinemann Elsevier, Edinburgh.

Dossey, B.M., 1988. Imagery: awakening the inner healer. In: Dossey, B.M., Keagan, L., Guzzetta, C.E., Kolkmeier, L.G. (Eds.) Holistic Nursing: A Handbook for Practice. Aspen, Rockville, MD.

Duncan, E.A.S., 2003. Cognitive-behavioural therapy in physiotherapy and occupational therapy Ch.10. In: Everett, T., Donaghy, M.E., Feaver, S. (Eds.) Interventions for Mental Health: An Evidence-Based Approach for Physiotherapists and Occupational Therapists. Butterworth-Heinemann, Oxford.

Dunn, A., Trivedi, M.H., Kampert, J., Clark, C.G., Chambliss, H.O., 2005. Exercise treatment for depression: efficacy and dose response. Am. J. Prev. Med. 28, 1–8.

Eccleston, C., Yorke, L., Morley, S., Williams, A.C.deC., Mastroyannopoulou, K., 2003. Psychological therapies for the management of chronic and recurrent pain in children and adolescents. Cochrane Database Syst. Rev. Issue 1. Art. No.: CD003968. DOI: 10.1002/14651858. CD003968.

Elkin, I., Shea, M.T., Watkins, J.T., et al., 1989. General effectiveness of treatments. Arch. Gen. Psychiatry 46, 971–982.

Ellis, A., 1962. Reason and Emotion in Psychotherapy. Lyle Stuart, New York.

Ellis, A., 1976. The biological basis of human irrationality. J. Individ. Psychol. 32, 145–168.

Epstein, G.N., Halper, J.P., Barret, E.A.M., 2004. A pilot study of mind–body changes in adults with asthma who practise mental imagery. Altern. Ther. Health Med. 10 (4), 66–71.

Erickson, M., Rossi, E., 1979. Hypnotherapy: An Exploratory Casebook. Irvington, New York.

Ernst, E., Canter, P.H., 2003. The Alexander Technique: a systematic review of controlled clinical trials. Forsch. Komplementarmed. Klass. Naturheilkd. 10 (6), 325–329.

Ernst, E., Schmidt, K., Baum, M., 2006. Complementary/ alternative therapies for the treatment of breast cancer: a systematic review of randomized clinical trials and a critique of current terminology. Breast J. 12 (6), 526–530.

Ernst, S., Goodison, L., 1981. In Our Own Hands: A Book of Self-Help Therapy. Women's Press, London.

Everett, T., 2003. Chronic fatigue syndrome. In: Everett, T., Donaghy, M.E., Feaver, S. (Eds.) Interventions for Mental Health. Butterworth-Heinemann, Oxford, p. 257.

Everly, G.S., Rosenfeld, R., 1981. The Nature and Treatment of the Stress Response. Plenum Press, New York.

Fahrni, W.H., Trueman, G.E., 1965. Comparative radiological study of the spines of a primitive population with North Americans and Northern Europeans. J. Bone. Joint. Surg. 47B, 552–555.

Fanning, P., 1988. Visualization for Change. New Harbinger, Oakland, CA.

Farmer, K.U., 1995. Biofeedback and visualization for peak performance. J. Sport. Rehabil. 4, 59–64.

Farmer, M., Locke, B., Moscicki, E., Dannenberg, A., Larson, D., Radloff, L., 1988. Physical activity and depressive symptoms: The NHANES-1 epidemiological follow-up study. Am. J. Epidemiol. 128, 1340–1351.

Farrell, P., Ebert, T., Kampine, J., 1991. Naloxone augments muscle sympathetic nerve activity during isometric exercise in humans. Am. J. Physiol. 260, E379–E388.

Faulkner, G., Biddle, S., 1999. Exercise as an adjunct treatment for schizophrenia: a review of the literature. J. Ment. Health 8 (5), 441–457.

Ferrucci, P., 1982. What we May be. Mandala, London.

Finke, R.A., 1989. Principles of Mental Imagery. Massachusetts Institute of Technology, Cambridge, MA.

Fogarty, M., Happel, B., 2005. Exploring the benefits of an exercise programme for people with schizophrenia: a qualitative study. Issues Ment. Health Nurs. 26, 341–351.

Folkman, S., Moscovitz, J.T., 2004. Coping: pitfalls and promise. Ann. Rev. Psychol. 55, 745–774.

Fontana, D., 1991. The Elements of Meditation. Element, Shaftesbury.

Fontana, D., 1992. The Meditator's Handbook: A Comprehensive Guide to Eastern and Western Meditation Techniques. Element, Shaftesbury.

Fordham, F., 1966. An Introduction to Jung's Psychology, second ed. Pelican, London.

Fors, E.A., Sexton, H., Gotestam, K.G., 2002. The effect of guided imagery and amitriptyline on daily fibromyalgic pain: a prospective randomized controlled trial. J. Psychiatr. Res. 36 (3), 179–187.

Fox, K.R. (Ed.), 1997. The Physical Self: From Motivation to Well-Being. Human Kinetics, Leeds.

Fremont, J., Craighead, L.W., 1987. Aerobic exercise and cognitive therapy in the treatment of dysphoric moods. Cognit. Ther. Res. 11, 241–251.

Freud, S., 1973. Introductory lectures on psychoanalysis (trans Strachey J). Penguin, Harmondsworth.

Friedman, M., Rosenman, R.H., 1974. Type A Behaviour and Your Heart. Knopf, New York.

Ganster, D.C., Victor, B., 1988. The impact of social support on mental and physical health. Br. J. Med. Psychol. 61, 3–17.

Gardner, W.N., 1992. Hyperventilation syndromes. Respir. Med. 86, 273–275.

Gardner, W.N., Bass, C., 1989. Hyperventilation in clinical practice. Br. J. Hosp. Med. 41, 73–81.

Garssen, B., de Ruiter, C., van Dyke, R., 1992. Breathing retraining: a rational placebo? Clin. Psychol. Rev. 12, 141–153.

Gauvin, L., Spence, J.C., 1996. Physical activity and psychological well-being: knowledge base, current issues and caveats. Nutr. Rev. 54 (4), S53–S65.

Gibson, B.E., Martin, D.K., 2003. Qualitative research and evidence-based physiotherapy practice. Physiotherapy 89 (6), 350–358.

Gift, A.G., Moore, T., Soeken, K., 1992. Relaxation to reduce dyspnoea and anxiety in chronic obstructive pulmonary disease. Nurs. Res. 41 (4), 242–246.

Gilbert, C., 2003. Clinical application of breathing regulation: beyond anxiety management. Behav. Modif. 27, 692–709.

Gill, J.S., 2008. Biomedical links between cognitions and behaviour. In: Donaghy, M., Nicol, M., Davidson, K. (Eds.) Cognitive Behavioural Interventions in Physiotherapy and Occupational Therapy. Butterworth-Heinemann Elsevier, Edinburgh.

Gloaguen, V., Cottraux, J., Cucherat, M., et al., 1998. A meta-analysis of the effects of cognitive therapy in depressed patients. J. Affect. Disord. 49, 59–72.

Goldberg, D., Huxley, P., 1992. Common Mental Disorders: A Biosocial Model. Routledge, London pp 83–113.

Goldfried, M.R., 1971. Systematic desensitization as training in self-control. J. Consult. Clin. Psychol. 37, 228–234.

Goleman, D., 1996. Emotional Intelligence: Why It Can Matter More Than IQ. Bloomsbury, London.

Gorman, J.M., 2003. Treating generalized anxiety disorder. J. Clin. Psychiatry 64 (Suppl. 2), 24–29.

Gray, J., 1990. Your Guide to the Alexander Technique. Gollancz, London.

Greenberger, D., Padesky, C.A., 1995. Mind Over Mood: Change How You Feel by Changing the Way you Think. Guilford, New York.

Gregerson, M., Roberts, I., Amiri, M., 1996. Absorption and imagery locate immune responses in the body. Biofeedback Self Regul. 21, 149–165.

Greist, J.H., Klein, M.H., Eischens, R.R., Faris, J.W., Gurman, A.S., Morgan, W.P., 1979. Running as a treatment for depression. Compr. Psychiatry 20, 41–54.

Grimshaw, G.M., Stanton, A., 2006. Tobacco cessation interventions for young people. Cochrane Database Syst. Rev. Issue 4. Art. No.: CD003289. DOI: 10.1002/14651858.CD003289.pub4.

Guercio, J.M., Ferguson, K.E., McMorrow, M.J., 2001. Increasing functional communication through relaxation training and neuromuscular feedback. Brain Inj. 15 (12), 1073–1082.

Gunaratana, B.H., 2002. Mindfulness in Plain English. Wisdom, Somerville, MA.

Guzman, J., Ezmail, R., Karjalainen, J., Malmivaara, A., Irvin, B., Bombadier, C., 2001. Multidisciplinary rehabilitation for chronic low back pain: systematic review. Br. Med. J. 322, 1511–1516.

Halpin, L.S., Speir, A.M., Capobianco, P., Barnett, S.D., 2002. Guided imagery in cardiac surgery. Outcomes Manag. Nurs. Pract. 6 (3), 132–137.

Hambrick, J.P., Weeks, J.W., Harb, G.C., et al., 2003. Cognitive-behavioral therapy for social anxiety disorder: supporting evidence and future directions. Cent. Nerv. Syst. Spectr. 8 (5), 373–381.

Han, J.N., Stegen, E., de Valck, C., Clement, J., van de Woestijne, K.P., 1996. The influence of breathing therapy on anxiety and breathing patterns in patients with hyperventilation syndrome and anxiety disorders. J. Psychosom. Res. 41 (5), 481–493.

Hanh, T.N., 1991. The Miracle of Mindfulness. Rider, London.

Harris, A., Cronkite, R., Moos, R., 2006. Physical activity, exercise, coping and depression in a 10-year cohort study of depressed patients. J. Affect. Disord. 93, 79–85.

Hartland, J., 1971. Medical and Dental Hypnosis and its Clinical Applications, second ed. Baillière Tindall, London.

Hay, P.J., Bacaltchuk, J., Stefano, S., 2004. Psychotherapy for bulimia nervosa and binging. Cochrane Database Syst. Rev. Issue 3. Art. No.: CD000562. DOI: 10.1002/14651858.CD000562.pub2.

Health Education Authority, 1995. Health Update 5: Physical Activity. Health Education Authority, London.

Heimberg, R.G., 2002. Cognitive-behavioural therapy for social anxiety disorder: current status and future directions. Biol. Psychiatry 51, 101–108.

Hendler, C.S., Redd, W.H., 1986. Fear of hypnosis: the role of labelling in patients' acceptance of behavioural interventions. Behav. Ther. 17, 2–13.

Henry, M., de Rivera, J.L.G., Gonzales-Martin, I.J., Abreu, J., 1993. Improvement of respiratory function in chronic asthmatic patients with autogenic therapy. J. Psychosom. Res. 37, 265–270.

Heptinstall, S.T., 1995. Relaxation training. In: Everett, T., Dennis, M., Ricketts, E. (Eds.) Physiotherapy in Mental Health. Butterworth-Heinemann, Oxford, pp. 188–208.

Herbert, R.D., de Noronha, M., 2007. Stretching to prevent or reduce muscle soreness after exercise. Cochrane Database Syst. Rev. Issue 4. Art. No.: CD004577. DOI: 10.1002/14651858.CD004577.pub2.

Herbert, R.D., Gabriel, M., 2002. Effects of stretching before and after exercising on muscle soreness and risk of injury: systematic review. Br. Med. J. 325, 468–470.

Heron, J., 1977. Catharsis in Human Development Human Potential Research Project. University of Surrey, Guildford.

Higgins, J.E., Endler, N., 1995. Coping, life stress and psychological and somatic distress. Eur. J. Pers. 9, 253–270.

Hillenberg, J.B., Collins, F.L., 1982. A procedural analysis and review of relaxation training research. Behav. Res. Ther. 20, 251–260.

Hollon, S.D., de Rubeis, R.J., Shelton, R.C., et al., 2005. Prevention of relapse following cognitive therapy vs medications in moderate to severe depression. Arch. Gen. Psychiatry 62, 417–422.

Holloway, E.A., Ram, F.S.F., 2004. Breathing exercises for asthma. Cochrane Database Syst. Rev. Issue 1. John Wiley, Chichester.

Holloway, E.A., West, R.J., 2007. Integrated breathing and relaxation training (the Papworth method) for adults with asthma in primary care: a randomized controlled trial. Thorax 62, 1039–1042.

Holmes, M.D., Chen, W.Y., Feskanich, D., Kroenke, C.H., Colditz, G.A., 2005. Physical activity and survival after breast cancer diagnosis. J. Am. Med. Assoc. 293, 2479–2486.

Holmes, T.H., Rahe, R.H., 1967. The social readjustment rating scale. J. Psychosom. Res. 11, 213–218.

Homme, L.E., 1965. Perspectives in psychology: XX1V control of coverants; the operants of the mind. Psychol. Rec. 15, 501–511.

Hoppes, K., 2006. The application of mindfulness-based cognitive interventions in the treatment of co-occuring addictive and mood disorders. Cent. Nerv. Syst. Spectr. 11 (11), 829–851.

Hough, A., 2001. Physiotherapy in Respiratory Care: An Evidence-Based Approach to Respiratory and Cardiac Management, third ed. Nelson Thornes, Cheltenham.

Hui, P.N., Wan, M., Chan, W.K., et al., 2006. An evaluation of two behavioral rehabilitation programs, qigong versus progressive relaxation, in improving the quality of life in cardiac patients. J. Altern. Complement. Med. 12 (4), 373–378.

Hunot, V., Churchill, R., Teixeira, Silva da Lima, M., 2007. Psychological therapies for generalized anxiety disorder. Cochrane Database Syst. Rev. Issue 1. Art no. CD00 1848 DO1 10.1002/14651858 CD00 1848 pub4.

Huntley, A., White, A.R., Ernst, E., 2002. Relaxation therapies for asthma: a systematic review. Thorax 57 (2), 127–131.

Innocenti, D.M., 1983. Chronic hyperventilation syndrome. In: Downie, P.A. (Ed.), Cash's Textbook of Chest, Heart and Vascular Disorders for Physiotherapists, third ed. Faber and Faber, London.

Innocenti, D.M., Troup, F., 2008. Dysfunctional breathing. In: Pryor, J., Prasad, A. (Eds.) Physiotherapy for Respiratory and Cardiac Problems, fourth ed. Churchill Livingstone, Edinburgh, pp. 529–549.

Irwin, M.R., Cole, J.C., Nicassio, P.M., 2006. Comparative meta-analysis of behavioral interventions for insomnia and their efficacy in middle-aged adults and in older adults 55+ years of age. Health Psychol. 25 (1), 3–14.

Jackson, T., 1991. An evaluation of the Mitchell method of simple physiological relaxation for women with rheumatoid arthritis. Br. J. Occup. Ther. 54, 105–107.

Jacobson, E., 1934. Electrical measurements concerning muscular contraction (tonus) and the cultivation of relaxation in man: relaxation times of individuals. Am. J. Physiol. 108, 573–580.

Jacobson, E., 1938. Progressive Relaxation, second ed. University of Chicago Press, Chicago.

Jacobson, E., 1964. Anxiety and Tension Control. J B Lippincott, Philadelphia.

Jacobson, E., 1970. Modern Treatment of Tense Patients Including the Neurotic and Depressed, with Case Illustrations, Follow-Ups and Emg Measurements. Charles C Thomas, Springfield, IL.

Jacobson, E., 1976. You Must Relax. Souvenir Press, London.

James, A., Soler, A., Weatherall, R., 2005. Cognitive behavioural therapy for anxiety disorders in children and adolescents. Cochrane Database Syst. Rev. Issue 4. Art. No.: CD004690. DOI: 10.1002/14651858.CD004690.pub2.

Jefferies, W.M., 1991. Cortisol and immunity. Med. Hypotheses 34, 198–208.

Johnson, U., 2000. Short-term psychological intervention: a study of long-term injured competitive athletes. J. Sport Rehabil. 9 (3), 207–218.

Johnson, U., Ekengren, J., Andersen, M.B., 2005. Injury prevention in Sweden: helping soccer players at risk. J. Sport Exerc. Psychol. 1, 32–38.

Johnstone, M., Wright, S., Weinman, J., 1995. Stress, emotion and life events. In: Measures in Health Psychology: A User's Portfolio. NFER-Nelson, Windsor.

Johnstone, R., Donaghy, M., Martin, D., 2002. A pilot study of a cognitive-behavioural therapy approach to physiotherapy for acute low back pain patients who show signs of developing chronic pain. Adv. Physiother. 4 (4), 182–188.

Jones, C., Cormac, I., Silveiro da Mota Neto, J.I., et al., 2004. Cognitive behaviour therapy for schizophrenia. Cochrane Database Syst. Rev.

Jorm, A.F., Christensen, H., Griffiths, K.M., et al., 2004. Effectiveness of complementary and self-help treatments for anxiety disorders. Med. J. Aust. 181 (Suppl. 7), S29–S46.

Jorm, A.F., Morgan, A.J., Hetrick, S.E., 2008. Relaxation for depression. Cochrane Database Syst. Rev. Issue 4. Art. no:CD007142.D01:10.1002/14651858.CD007142.pub2.

Jung, C.G., 1963. Memories, Dreams, Reflections. Vintage Books, New York.

Kaapa, E.H., Frantsi, K., Sarna, S., et al., 2006. Multidisciplinary group rehabilitation versus individual physiotherapy for chronic non-specific low back pain: a randomized trial. Spine 31 (4), 371–376.

Kabat-Zinn, J., 2003. Mindfulness-based interventions in context: past, present and future. Clin. Psychol. Sci. Pract. 10, 144–156.

Kabat-Zinn, J., Wheeler, E., Light, T., et al., 1998. The influence of a mindfulness intervention on rates of skin clearing in patients with moderate to severe psoriasis undergoing phototherapy and photochemotherapy. Psychosom. Med. 60 (5), 625–632.

Kanji, N., White, A.R., Ernst, E., 1999. Antihypertensive effects of autogenic training: a systematic review. Perfusion 12, 279–282.

Kanji, N., Ernst, E., 2000. Autogenic training for stress and anxiety: a systematic review. Complement. Ther. Med. 8, 106–110.

Kanji, N., White, A.R., Ernst, E., 2004. Autogenic training reduces anxiety after coronary angioplasty: a randomized clinical trial. Am. Heart J. 147 (3), E10.

Kanji, N., White, A.R., Ernst, E., 2006. Autogenic training for tension-type headaches: a systematic review of controlled trials. Complement. Ther. Med. 14 (2), 144–150.

Kanner, A.D., Coyne, J.C., Schaefer, C., Lazarus, R.S., 1981. Comparison of two modes of stress management: daily hassles and uplifts versus major life events. J. Behav. Med. 4, 1–3.

Kaptchuk, T.J., Kelley, J.M., Conboy, L.A., et al., 2008. Components of the placebo effect: a randomized controlled trial in patients with irritable bowel syndrome. Br. Med. J. 336, 999–1003.

Karjalainen, K., Malmivaara, A., van Tulder, M., 2007. Biopsychosocial rehabilitation for upper limb repetitive strain injuries in working age adults. CochraneDatabase Syst. Rev. Issue 3.

Kaushik, R., Kaushik, R.M., Mahajan, S.K., et al., 2005. Biofeedback-assisted diaphragmatic breathing and systematic relaxation versus propanolol in long-term prophylaxis of migraine. Complement. Ther. Med. 13 (3), 165–174.

Kazarian, L., 1975. Creep characteristics of the human spinal column. Orthop. Clin. North Am. 6 (1), 3–15.

Keable, D., 1997. The Management of Anxiety: A Manual for Therapists, second ed. Churchill Livingstone, Edinburgh.

Keefe, F.J., Rumble, M.E., Scipio, C.D., Giordano, L.A., Perri, L.C.M., 2004. Psychological aspects of persistent pain: current state of the science. J. Pain 5, 195–211.

Kellett, C., Mullan, J., 2002. Breathing control techniques in the management of asthma. Physiotherapy 88 (12), 751–758.

Kermani, K.S., 1990. Autogenic Training. Souvenir Press, London.

Kerr, K.M., 2000. Relaxation techniques: a critical review. Crit. Rev. Phys. Rehabil. Med. 12, 51–89.

Kessler, R.C., Sonnega, A., Bromet, E., et al., 1995. Posttraumatic stress disorder in the national co-morbidity. Surv. Arch. Gen. Psychiatry 52, 1048–1060.

Kessler, R.S., Patterson, D.R., Dane, J., 2003. Hypnosis and relaxation with pain patients: evidence for effectiveness. Semin. Pain Med. 1 (2), 67–78.

King, M.S., Carr, T., D'Cruz, C., 2002. Transcendental meditation, hypertension and heart disease: a review. Aust. Fam. Physician 31 (2), 164–168.

Kirk, A., Barnett, J., Mutrie, N., 2007. Physical activity consultation for people with type 2 diabetes: evidence and guidelines. Diabet. Med. 24 (8), 809–816.

Klein, M.J., Griest, J.H., Gurman, A.S., et al., 1985. A comparative outcome study of group psychotherapy vs. exercise treatments for depression. Int. J. Ment. Health 13, 148–177.

Knols, R., Aaronson, N.K., Uebelhart, D., et al., 2005. Physical exercise in cancer patients during and after medical treatment: a systematic review of randomized and controlled clinical trials. J. Clin. Oncol. 23 (16), 3830–3842.

Kobasa, S.C., 1982. The hardy personality. In: Sanders, G., Suls, J. (Eds.) The Social Psychology of Health and Illness. Lawrence Erlbaum, New Jersey.

Kokoszka, A., 1992. Relaxation as an altered state of consciousness: a rationale for a general theory of relaxation. Int. J. Psychosom. 39, 4–9.

Kosslyn, S.M., 1983. Ghosts in the Mind's Machine. WW Norton, New York.

Koszicki, D., Benger, M., Schlik, J., et al., 2007. Randomized trial of a mindfulness-based stress reduction programme and cognitive behaviour therapy in generalized social anxiety disorder. Behav. Res. Ther. 45 (10), 2518–2526.

Kovacs, M., 2007. Stress and coping in the workplace. The Psychol. 20 (9), 548–550.

Krisanaprakornkit, T., Krisanaprakornkit, W., Piyavhatkul, N., et al., 2006. Meditation therapy for anxiety disorders. Cochrane Database Syst. Rev. Issue 1. CD 004 998.

Kwekkeboom, K.L., Gretarsdottir, E., 2006. Systematic review of relaxation interventions for pain. J. Nurs. Sch. 38 (3), 269–277.

La Forge, R., 1995. Exercise-associated mood alteration: a review of interactive neurobiological mechanisms. Med. Exerc. Nutr. Health 4, 17–32.

Lamarche, L.J., de Koninck, J., 2007. Sleep disturbance in adults with post-traumatic stress disorder: a review. J. Clin. Psychiatry 68 (8), 1257–1270.

Lampinen, P., Hiekkinin, R.L., Kauppinen, M., Hiekkinin, E., 2006. Activity as a predictor of mental well-being among older adults. Ageing Ment. Health 10, 454–466.

Langer, E.J., 1989. Mindfulness. Da Capo, Cambridge.

Larkin, D.M., 1988. Therapeutic suggestion. In: Zahourek, R.P. (Ed.), Relaxation and Imagery: Tools for Therapeutic Communication and Intervention. WB Saunders, Philadelphia.

Larsson, B., Carlsson, J., Fichtel, A., et al., 2005. Relaxation treatment of adolescent headache sufferers: results from a school-based replication series. Headache 45 (6), 692–704.

Larun, L., Nordheim, L.V., Ekeland, E., Hagen, K.B., Heian, F., 2006. Exercise in prevention and treatment of anxiety and depression among children and young people. Cochrane Database Syst. Rev. Issue 3. Art. No.: CD004691. DOI: 10.1002/14651858.CD004691.pub2.

Lau, M.A., Shelley, F., McMain, S.F., 2005. Integrating mindfulness meditation with cognitive and behavioural therapies: the challenge of combining acceptance- and change-based strategies. Can. J. Psychiatry 50 (13), 863–869.

Laurion, S., Fetzer, S.J., 2003. The effect of two nursing interventions on the postoperative outcomes of gynecologic laparoscopic patients. J. Peri-Anesth. Nurs. 18 (4), 254–261.

Lazarus, R.S., 1991. Cognition and motivation in emotion. Am. Psychol. 46, 352–367.

Lazarus, R.S., Folkman, S., 1984. Stress, Appraisal and Coping. Springer, New York.

Lazarus, R.S., Cohen, J.B., Folkman, S., Kanner, A., Schaefer, C., 1980. Psychological stress and adaptation: some unresolved issues. In: Selye, H. (Ed.), Selye's Guide to Stress Research, vol. 1. Van Nostrand Reinhold, New York, pp. 90–117.

Lee, C., Russell, A., 2003. Effects of physical activity on emotional well-being among older Australian women: cross-sectional and logitudinal analyses. J. Psychosom. Res. 54 (2), 155–160.

Lehrer, P.M., 1982. How to relax and how not to relax: a re-evaluation of the work of Edmund Jacobson. Behav. Res. Ther. 20, 417–428.

Lehrer, P.M., 1996. Varieties of relaxation methods and their unique effects. Int. J. Stress Manag. 3, 1–15.

Lehrer, P.M., Batey, D.M., Woolfolk, R.L., Remde, A., Garlick, T., 1988. The effect of repeated tense-release sequences on EMG and self-report of muscle tension: an evaluation of Jacobsonian and post-Jacobsonian assumptions about progressive relaxation. Psychophysiology 25, 562–567.

Leibowitz, J., Connington, B., 1990. The Alexander Technique. Souvenir Press, London.

Levy, R.L., Langer, S.L., Whitehead, W.E., 2007. Social learning contributions to the etiology and treatment of functional abdominal pain and inflammatory bowel disease. World J. Gastroenterol. 13 (17), 2397–2403.

Ley, R., 1988. Panic attacks during relaxation and relaxation-induced anxiety: a hyperventilation interpretation. J. Behav. Ther. Expe. Psychiatry 19, 253–259.

Lichstein, K.L., 1988. Clinical Relaxation Strategies. John Wiley, New York.

Lichstein, K.L., Sallis, J.F., Hill, D., Young, M.C., 1981. Psycho-physiological adaptation: an investigation of multiple parameters. J. Behav. Assess. 3, 111–121.

Lindsay, W.R., Hood, E.H., 1982. A Cognitive Anxiety Questionnaire. Unpublished, University of Sheffield.

Lindsay, W.R., Morrison, F.M., 1996. The effects of behavioral relaxation on cognitive performance in adults with severe intellectual disabilities. J. Intellect. Disabil. Res. 40 (4), 285–290.

Lindsay, W.R., Pitcaithly, D., Geelen, N., Buntin, L., Broxholme, S., Ashby, M., 1997. A comparison of the effects of four therapy procedures on concentration and responsiveness in people with profound learning disabilities. J. Intellect. Disabil. Res. 41 (3), 201–207.

Little, P., Lewith, G., Webley, F., et al., 2008. Randomized controlled trial of Alexander Technique lessons, exercise and massage for chronic and recurrent back pain. Br. Med. J. 337, 438.

Loder, E., Rizzoli, P., 2008. Tension-type Headache. Br. Med. J. 336, 88–92.

Logsdon-Conradsen, S., 2002. Using mindfulness meditation to promote holistic health in individuals with HIV/AIDS. Cogn. Behav. Pract. 9 (1), 67–71.

Long, A.F., Dixon, P., Hall, R., Carr-Hill, R.A., Seldon, T.A., 1993. The outcomes agenda: contribution of the UK clearing house on health outcomes. Qual. Health Care 2, 49–52.

Longabaugh, R., Donovan, D.M., Karno, M.P., et al., 2005. Active ingredients: how and why evidence-based alcohol behavioural treatment interventions work. Alcohol. Clin. Exp. Res. 29 (2), 235–247.

Looker, T., Gregson, O., 1989. Stresswise: A Practical Guide for Dealing With Stress. Hodder and Stoughton, London.

Lucic, K.S., Steffen, J.J., Harrigan, J.A., Stuebing, R.C., 1991. Progressive relaxation training: muscle contractions before relaxation? Behav. Ther. 22, 249–256.

Lum, L.C., 1981. Hyperventilation and anxiety state. J. R. Soc. Med. 74, 1–4.

Luskin, F.M., Newell, K.A., Griffith, M., et al., 2000. A review of mind–body therapies in the treatment of musculoskeletal disorders with implications for the elderly. Altern. Ther. 6 (2), 46–56.

Luthe, W. (Ed.), 1965. Autogenic Training: Psychosomatic Correlations. Grune and Stratton, New York.

Luthe, W., 1970. Research and theory. In: Luthe, W. (Ed.), Autogenic Therapy, fourth ed. Grune and Stratton, New York.

Lyman, B., Bernadin, S., Thomas, S., 1980. Frequency of imagery in emotional experience. Percept. Mot. Skills 50, 1159–1162.

Lynn, S.J., Rhue, J.W., 1977. Hypnosis, imagination and fantasy. J. Ment. Imagery 11, 101–113.

Ma, S.H., Teasdale, J.D., 2003. Mindfulness-based cognitive therapy for depression: replication and exploration of differential relapse-prevention effects. J. Consult. Clin. Psychol. 72, 31–40.

Madders, J., 1981. Stress and Relaxation: Self-Help Ways to Cope With Stress and Relieve Nervous Tension, Ulcers, Insomnia, Migraine and High Blood Pressure, third ed. Martin Dunitz, London.

Maddison, R., Prapavessis, H., 2005. A psychological approach to the prediction and prevention of athletic injury. J. Sport Exerc. Psychol. 27, 289–310.

Maisel, E., 1969. The Alexander Technique. Thames and Hudson, London.

Mantle, J., Haslam, J., Polden, M., 2004. Physiotherapy in Obstetrics and Gynaecology, second ed. Butterworth-Heinemann, Oxford.

Manzoni, G.M., Pagnini, F., Castelnuovo, G., Molinari, E., 2008. Relaxation training for anxiety: a ten years' systematic review with meta-analysis. Bio.-Med. Cent. Psychiatry 8, 41.

Margolin, A., Schuman-Oliver, Z., Beitel, M., et al., 2007. A preliminary study of spiritual self-schema (3-S+) therapy for reducing impulsivity in HIV positive drug users. J. Clin. Psychol. 63 (10), 979–999.

Marine, A., Ruotsalainen, J.H., Serra, C., Verbeek, J.H., 2006. Preventing occupational stress in healthcare workers. Cochrane Database Syst. Rev. Issue 4. Art. No.: CD002892. DOI: 10.1002/14651858.CD002892.pub2

Marsden, E., Kirk, A., 2005. Becoming and staying physically active. In: Nagi, D. (Ed.), Exercise and Sport in Diabetes. Wiley, London, pp. 181–192.

Marshall, S., Turnbull, J., 1996. Cognitive-Behaviour Therapy: An Introduction to Theory and Practice. Baillière Tindall, London.

Martin, D., McLeod, L., 2008. Chronic pain. In: Donaghy, M., Nicol, M., Davidson, K. (Eds.) Cognitive-Behavioural Interventions in Physiotherapy and Occupational Therapy. Butterworth-Heinemann Elsevier, Edinburgh, pp. 121–134.

Martinez-Devesa, P., Waddell, A., Perera, R., Theodoulou, M., 2007. Cognitive behavioural therapy for tinnitus. Cochrane Database Syst. Rev. Issue 1. Art. No.: CD005233. DOI: 10.1002/14651858.CD005233.pub2.

Martinsen, E.W., 1990. Physical fitness, anxiety and depression. Br. J. Hosp. Med. 43, 194–199.

Matchim, Y., Armer, J.M., 2007. Measuring the psychological impact of mindfulness meditation on health among patients with cancer: a literature review. Oncol. Nurs. Forum 34 (5), 1059–1066.

Matsumoto, M., Smith, J.C., 2001. Progressive muscle relaxation, breathing exercises and ABC relaxation theory. J. Clin. Psychol. 57 (12), 1551–1557.

Matthews, G., Deary, I.J., Whiteman, M.C., 2003. Personality Traits, second ed. Cambridge University Press, Cambridge.

McCance, K., Heuther, S., 1998. Patho-Physiology: The Biologic Basis for Disease in Adults and Children, third ed. Mosby, St Louis.

McGuigan, F.J., 1971. Covert linguistic behaviour in deaf subjects during thinking. J. Comp. Physiol. Psychol. 75, 417–420.

McGuigan, F.J., 1981. Calm Down: a Guide for Stress and Tension Control. Prentice-Hall, Englewood Cliffs, NJ.

McGuigan, F.J., 1984. Progressive relaxation: origins, principles and clinical applications. In: Woolfolk, R. L., Lehrer, P.M. (Eds.) Principles and Practice of Stress Management. Guilford Press, New York.

McKee, J., Warber, S.L., 2005. Integrative therapies for menopause. South. Med. J. 98 (3), 319–326.

Mead, G.H., 1934. Mind, Self and Society. Chicago University Press, Chicago.

McPherson, K., 2009. Do patients' preferences matter? Editorial. Br. Med. J. 338, 59–60.

Mead, G.E., Morley, W., Campbell, P., Greig, C.A., McMurdo, M., Lawlor, D.A., 2008 Exercise for depression. Cochrane Database Syst. Rev. Issue 4. Art. No.: CD004366. DOI: 10.1002/14651858.CD004366. pub3.

Mead, G.H., 1934. Mind, Self and Society. Chicago University Press, Chicago.

Melzack, R., Wall, P.D., 1965. Pain Mechanisms: A New Theory. Science 150, 971–979.

Melzack, R., Wall, P.D., 1983. The Challenge of Pain. Penguin, London.

Mendelson, W.B., 2007. Combining pharmacologic and nonpharmacologic therapies for insomnia. J. Clin. Psychiatry 68 (Suppl. 5), 19–23.

Mental Health Foundation, 2005. Up and running: exercise therapy and the treatment of mild or moderate depression in primary care. www.mentalhealth.org. uk/campaigns/mhaw/exercise-and-depression/

Meuret, A.E., Wilhelm, F.H., Ritz, T., et al., 2003. Breathing retraining for treating panic disorder: useful intervention or impediment? Behav. Modif. 27 (5), 731–754.

Meuret, A.E., Ritz, T., Wilhelm, F.H., et al., 2005. Voluntary hyperventilation in the treatment of panic disorder: functions of hyperventilation, their implications for breathing training and recommendations for standardization. Clin. Psychol. Rev. 25 (3), 285–306.

Miller, K.M., Perry, P.A., 1990. Relaxation techniques and postoperative pain in patients undergoing cardiac surgery. Heart Lung 19 (2), 136–145.

Miller, M.A., Rahe, R.H., 1997. Life changes scaling for the 1990s. J. Psychosom. Res. 43 (3), 279–292.

Miller, W.R., Hester, R.K., 1995. Treatment for alcohol problems: towards an informed eclecticism. In: Hester, R.K., Miller, W.R. (Eds.) Handbook of Alcoholism Treatment Approaches: Effective Alternatives, second ed. Allyn & Bacon, Needham Heights, MA, pp. 1–11.

MIND Survey, 2002. http://news.bbc. co.uk/2/hi/health/1338145stm

Mitchell, L., 1987. Simple Relaxation: The Mitchell Method for Easing Tension, second ed. John Murray, London.

Mobily, K.E., Rubenstein, L.M., Lemke, J.H., O'Hara, M. W., Wallace, R.B., 1996. Walking and depression in a cohort of older adults: the Iowa 65+ Rural Health Study. J. Aging Phys. Act. 4, 119–135.

Montgomery, P., Dennis, J.A., 2003. Cognitive behavioural interventions for sleep problems in adults aged 60+. Cochrane Database Syst. Rev. Issue 1. Art. No.: CD003161. DOI: 10.1002/14651858.CD003161.

Morgan, W.P., 1981. Psychophysiology of self-awareness during vigorous physical activity. Res. Q. Exerc. Sports 52, 385–427.

Morgenthaler, T., Kramer, M., Alessi, C., et al., 2006. Practice parameters for the psychological and behavioral treatment of insomnia: an update. An American Academy of Sleep report. Sleep 29 (11), 1415–1419.

Morley, S., 2004. Process and change in cognitive behaviour therapy for chronic pain. Pain 109, 205–206.

Morley, S., Eccleston, C., Williams, A., 1999. Systematic review and meta-analysis of randomized controlled trials of cognitive behaviour therapy and behaviour therapy for chronic pain in adults, excluding headache. Pain 80, 1–13.

Motl, R.W., Birnbaum, A.S., Kubik, M.Y., Dishman, R.K., 2004. Naturally occurring changes in physical activity are inversely related to depressive symptoms during early adolescence. Psychol. Med. 66, 336–342.

Motl, R.W., Konopack, J.F., McAuley, E., Elavsky, S., Jerome, G.J., Marquez, D.X., 2005. Depressive symptoms among older adults: long term reduction after a physical activity intervention. J. Behav. Med. 28, 385–394.

Mutrie, N., Faulkner, G., 2003. Physical activity and mental health. In: Everett, T., Donaghy, M., Feaver, S. (Eds.) Interventions for Mental Health. Butterworth-Heinemann, Oxford, pp. 82–98.

Mutrie, N., Campbell, A.M., Whyte, F., et al., 2007. Benefits of supervised group exercise for women being treated for early stage breast cancer: a pragmatic randomized controlled trial. Br. Med. J. 334 (7592), 517–520B.

National Institute for Clinical Excellence, 2003. Depression: NICE Guideline 2nd consultation. National Institute for Clinical Excellence, London.

Neimeyer, R.A., 1985. Personal constructs in clinical practice. In: Kendall, P.C. (Ed.), Advances in Cognitive-Behavioural Research and Therapy. Academic Press, Orlando, FL.

Newman, M.G., Borkovec, T.D., 2002. Cognitive behaviour therapy for worry and generalized anxiety disorder. In: Simos, G. (Ed.), Cognitive Behaviour Therapy: A Guide for the Practising Clinician. Brunner-Routledge, East Sussex, pp. 150–172.

Norton, M., Holm, J.E., McSherry, W.C., 1997. Behavioral assessment of relaxation: the validity of a behavioral rating scale. J. Behav. Ther. Exp. Psychiatry 28 (2), 129–137.

O'Kearney, R.T., Anstey, K.J., von Sanden, C., 2006 Behavioural and cognitive behavioural therapy for irritable bowel syndrome in children and adolescents. Cochrane Database Syst. Rev. Issue 4, Art. CD004 856 D01.

Olton, D.S., Noonberg, A.R., 1980. Biofeedback: Clinical Applications in Behavioural Medicine. Prentice-Hall, Englewood Cliffs, NJ.

Oman, D., Hedberg, J., Thoresen, C.E., 2006. Passage meditation reduces perceived stress in health professionals: a randomized controlled trial. J. Consult. Clin. Psychol. 74 (4), 714–719.

Öst, L.-G., 1987. Applied relaxation: description of a coping technique and review of controlled studies. Behav. Res. Ther. 25, 397–407.

Öst, L.-G., 1988. Applied relaxation versus progressive relaxation in the treatment of panic disorder. Behav. Res. Ther. 26, 13–22.

Öst, L.-G., Breitholtz, E., 2000. Applied relaxation versus cognitive therapy in the treatment of generalized anxiety disorder. Behav. Res. Ther. 38 (8), 777–790.

Ostelo, R.W.J.G., van Tulder, M.W., Vlaeyen, J.W.S., Linton, S.J., Morley, S., Assendelft, W.J.J., 2005. Behavioural treatment for chronic low-back pain. Cochrane Database Syst. Rev. Issue 1. Art. No.: CD002014. DOI: 10.1002/14651858.CD002014.pub2.

Ott, M.J., Norris, R.L., Bauer Wu, S.M., 2006. Mindfulness meditation for oncology patients: a discussion and critical review. Integr. Cancer Ther. 5 (2), 98–108.

Oyle, I., 1976. Magic, Mysticism and Modern Medicine. Celestial Arts, Millbrae, CA.

Paffenbarger, R.S., Lee, I.M., Leung, R., 1994. Physical activity and personal characteristics associated wih depression and suicide in American college men. Acta Psychiatr. Scand. 89 (S377), 16–22.

Paivio, A., 1985. Cognitive and motivational functions of imagery in human performance. Can. J. Appl. Sport Sci. 10, 22S–28S.

Paul, G.L., 1969. Physiological effects of relaxation training and hypnotic suggestion. J. Abnorm. Psychol. 74, 425–437.

Paykel, E.S., 1997. The Interview for Recent Life Events. Psychol. Med. 27 (2), 301–310.

Payne, R.A., 1989. Glad to be yourself: a course of practical relaxation and health education talks. Physiotherapy 75, 8–9.

Payne, R.A., 2004. Relaxation techniques. In: Kolt, G.S., Andersen, M.B. (Eds.) Psychology in the Physical and Manual Therapies. Churchill Livingstone, Edinburgh, p. 112.

Payne, R.A., Rowland Payne, C.M.E., Marks, R., 1985. Stress does not worsen psoriasis. A controlled study of 32 patients. Clin. Exp. Dermatol. 10, 239–245.

Pennebaker, J.W., 1990. Opening Up: The Healing Power of Confiding in Others. William Morrow, New York.

Peveler, R., Carson, A., Rodin, G., 2002. Depression in medical patients. Br. Med. J. 325, 149–152.

Picardi, A., Mazzotti, E., Gaetano, P., et al., 2005. Stress, social support, emotional regulation and exacerbation of diffuse plaque psoriasis. Psychosomatics 46, 556–564.

Pinney, S., Freeman, L.J., Nixon, P.G.F., 1987. Role of the nurse counsellor in managing patients with the hyperventilation syndrome. J. R. Soc. Med. 80, 216–218.

Polden, M., Mantle, J., 1990. Physiotherapy in Obstetrics and Gynaecology. Butterworth-Heinemann, Oxford.

Pomeroy, V.M., 2007. Facilitating independence, motivation and motor learning. Editor. Physiother. 93 (2), 87.

Poppen, R., 1998. Behavioural Relaxation Training and Assessment, second ed. Sage, Thousand Oaks, CA.

Poppen, R., Maurer, J., 1982. Electromyographic analysis of relaxed postures. Biofeedback Self Regul. 7, 491–498.

Pothongsunun, P., 2006. Wellness programmes in the community. Editor. Physiother. 92 (3), 133–134.

Potter, M., Grove, J.R., 1999. Mental skills training during rehabilitation: case studies of injured athletes. N. Z. J. Physiother. 27 (2), 24–31.

Powell, T.J., Enright, S.J., 1990. Anxiety and Stress Management. Routledge, Taylor and Francis, London.

Price, J.R., Couper, J., 1999. Cognitive-Behaviour Therapy for Chronic Fatigue Syndrome in Adults. The Cochrane Library, Issue 2, John Wiley, Chichester.

Price, J.R., Couper, J., 2003. Cognitive-Behaviour Therapy for Chronic Fatigue Syndrome in Adults (Cochrane Review). The Cochrane Library, Issue 4, John Wiley, Chichester.

Priest, J., Schott, J., 1991. Leading Antenatal Classes: A Practical Guide. Butterworth-Heinemann, Oxford.

Prigatano, G.P., 2005. Impaired self-awareness after moderately severe to severe traumatic brain injury. Acta Neurochir. 93 (Suppl.), 39–42.

Proctor, M.L., Murphy, P.A., Pattison, H.M., et al., 2007. Behavioural interventions for primary and secondary dysmenorrhoea. Cochrane Database Syst. Rev. Issue 3. CD002248.

Project MATCH. Matching alcohol treatments to client heterogeneity: Project MATCH 3-year drinking outcomes 1998. Alcohol. Clin. Exp. Res. 22 (6), 300–311.

Puskarich, C.A., Whitman, S., Dell, J., Hughes, J.R., Rosen, A.J., Hermann, B.P., 1992. Controlled examination of effects of progressive relaxation training on seizure reduction. Epilepsia 33 (4), 675–680.

Quick, J.C., Quick, J.D., 1984. Organizational Stress and Preventative Management. McGraw Hill, New York.

Rachman, J., 2003. Eysenck and the development of cognitive-behavioural therapy. The Psychol. 16 (11), 588–591.

Rahe, R.H., 1975. Epidemiological studies of life change and illness. Int. J. Psychiatr. Med. 6, 133–146.

Rains, J.C., Penzien, D.B., McCrory, D.C., et al., 2005. Behavioural headache treatment: history, review of the empirical literature and methodological critique. Headache 45 (Suppl. 2), S92–S109.

Ralston, G.E., 2008. Cognitive behavioural therapy for anxiety. In: Donaghy, M., Nicol, M., Davidson, K. (Eds.) Cognitive Behavioural Interventions in Physiotherapy and Occupational Therapy. Butterworth-Heinemann Elsevier, Edinburgh, pp. 75–90.

Rankin, J., 2002. Effects of antenatal exercise on psychological well-being in pregnancy and birth outcomes. Whurr, London.

Rasid, Z.M., Parish, T.S., 1998. The effects of two types of relaxation training on students' levels of anxiety. Adolescence 33 (129), 99–101.

Reich, J., Noyes, R., Troughton, E., 1987. Dependent personality disorder associated with phobic avoudance in patients with panic disorder. Am. J. Psychiatry 144, 332–336.

Remocker, A.J., Storch, E.T., 1992. Action Speaks Louder: A Handbook of Structured Group Techniques, fifth ed. Churchill Livingstone, Edinburgh.

Richardson, A., 1969. Mental Imagery. Springer, New York.

Rief, W., Weise, C., Kley, N., et al., 2005. Psychophysiologic treatment of chronic tinnitus: a randomized clinical trial. Psychosom. Med. 67 (5), 833–838.

Ritz, T., 2001. Relaxation therapy in adult asthma: is there new evidence for its effectiveness? Behav. Modif. 25 (4), 640–666.

Rodebaugh, T.L., Holaway, R.M., Heimberg, R.G., 2004. The treatment of social anxiety disorder. Clin. Psychol. Rev. 24 (7), 883–908.

Roffe, L., Schmidt, K., Ernst, E., 2005. A systematic review of guided imagery as an adjuvant cancer therapy. Psycho-Oncol. 14 (8), 607–617.

Rosa, K.R., 1976. Autogenic Training. Victor Gollancz, London.

Roth, A., Fonagy, P., 1996. What Works for Whom? A critical Review of Psychotherapy Research. Guilford Press, New York.

Rotter, J.B., 1966. Generalized expectancies for internal versus external control of reinforcement. Psychol. Monogr. 80, 609.

Rowbottom, I., 1992. The physiotherapy management of chronic hyperventilation. J. Assoc. Chart. Physiothera. Respir. Cond. 21, 9–12.

Roykulcharoen, V., Good, M., 2004. Systematic relaxation to relieve post-operative pain. J. Adv. Nurs. 48 (2), 140–148.

Ryman, L., 1994. Relaxation and visualization. In: Wells, R.J., Tschudin, V. (Eds.) Wells' Supportive Therapies in Health Care. Baillière Tindall, London.

Ryman, L., 1995. Relaxation and visualization. In: Rankin-Box, D. (Ed.), The Nurses' Handbook of Complementary Therapies. Churchill Livingstone, Edinburgh.

Safran, M.R., Seaber, A.V., Garrett, W.E., 1989. Warm-up and muscular prevention. Sports Med. 8, 239–249.

Salkovskis, P.M., 2002. Empirically grounded clinical interventions: cognitive-behavioural therapy progresses through a multi-dimensional approach to clinical science. Behav. Cogn. Psychother. 30, 3–9.

Salt, V.L., Kerr, K.M., 1997. Mitchell's simple physiological relaxation and Jacobson's progressive relaxation techniques: a comparison. Physiotherapy 83 (4), 200–207.

Samuels, M., Samuels, N., 1975. Seeing with the Mind's Eye: The History, Technique and Uses of Visualization. Random House, Toronto.

Schaffer, S.D., Yucha, C.B., 2004. Relaxation and pain management: the relaxation response can play a role in managing chronic and acute pain. Am. J. Nurs. 104 (8), 75–76, 78–79, 81–82.

Schilling, D.J., Poppen, R., 1983. Behavioural relaxation training and assessment. J. Behav. Ther. Exp. Psychiatry 14, 99–107.

Schneider, R.H., Alexander, C.N., Staggers, F., et al., 2005. Long-term effects of stress reduction on mortality in persons > or = 55 years of age with systematic hypertension. Am. J. Cardiol. 95 (9), 1060–1064.

Scholz, J., Campbell, S., 1980. Muscle spindles and the regulation of movement. Phys. Ther. 60, 1416.

Schott, J., Priest, J., 2002. Leading antenatal classes: a practical guide, second ed. Books for Midwives, Oxford.

Schultz, J.H., Luthe, W., 1969. Autogenic Methods. Grune and Stratton, New York.

Schwartzer, R., 1992. Self-efficacy in the adoption and maintenance of health behaviours: theoretical approaches and a new model. In: Schwartzer, R. (Ed.), Self-Efficacy: Thought Control of Action. Hemisphere, Washington, DC, pp. 217–243.

Scottish Intercollegiate Guidelines Network, 2009. Non-pharmacological Management of Mild to Moderate Depression. Scottish Intercollegiate Guidelines Network, Edinburgh.

Scully, D., Kremer, J., Meade, M.M., Graham, R., Dudgeon, K., 1998. Physical exercise and psychological well-being: a critical review. Br. J. Sports Med. 32, 111–120.

Sealey, C., 1999. Two common pitfalls in clinical audit: failing to complete the audit cycle and confusing audit with research. Br. J. Occup. Ther. 62 (6), 238–243.

Segal, Z.V., Teasdale, J.D., Williams, M.G., 2004. Mindfulness-based cognitive therapy: theoretical rationale and empirical status. In: Hayes, S.C., Follette, V.M., Linehan, M.M. (Eds.) Mindfulness and Acceptance: Expanding the Cognitive Behavioral Tradition. Guilford Press, New York.

Seligman, M.E.P., 1975. Helplessness. Freeman, San Francisco.

Seligman, M.E.P., Csikszentmihalyi, M., 2002. Positive psychology: an introduction. Am. Psychol. 55 (1), 5–14.

Selye, H., 1956. The Stress of Life. McGraw-Hill, New York.

Shaw, K., O'Rourke, P., Del Mar, C., et al., 2005. Psychological interventions for overweight or obesity. Cochrane Database Syst. Rev. Issue 2. CD003818.

Shone, R., 1982. Autohypnosis: a Step by Step Guide to Self-Hypnosis. Thorsons, Wellingborough.

Shone, R., 1984. Creative Visualization. Thorsons, Wellingborough.

Sibbald, B., Addington-Hall, J., Brenneman, D., Freeling, P., 1993. Counsellors in English and Welsh general practices: their nature and distribution. Br. Med. J. 306, 29–33.

Siev, J., Chambless, D.L., 2007. Specificity of treatment effects: cognitive therapy and relaxation for generalized anxiety and panic disorders. J. Consult. Clin. Psychol. 75 (4), 513–522.

Sim, J., 1999 March. Randomized controlled trials. In: Frontline. Clinical Effectiveness Supplement. Chartered Society of Physiotherapy, London, pp. 12–13.

Sim, J., Adams, N., 2002. Systematic review of randomized controlled trials of non-pharmacological interventions for fibromyalgia. Clin. J. Pain 18, 324–336.

Simkin, P., Bolding, A., 2004. Update on non-pharmacologic approaches to relieve labor pain and prevent suffering. J. Midwifery Women's Health 49 (6), 489–504.

Simonton, O.C., Matthews-Simonton, S., Creighton, J.L., 1986. Getting Well Again. Bantam, London.

Skelly, M., 2003. Stress and mental health. In: Everett, T., Donaghy, M., Feaver, S. (Eds.) Interventions for Mental Health. Butterworth-Heinemann, Oxford.

Skelly, M., 2008. Fibromyalgia management using cognitive-behaviour principles: a practical approach for therapists. In: Donaghy, M., Nicol, M., Davidson, K. (Eds.) Cognitive-Behavioural Interventions in Physiotherapy and Occupational Therapy. Butterworth-Heinemann, Edinburgh.

Skinner, B.F., 1938. The Behavior of Organisms. Appleton-Century Crofts, New York.

Sloman, R., 2002. Relaxation and guided imagery for anxiety and depression control in community patients with advanced cancer. Cancer Nurs. 25 (6), 432–435.

Slonim, N.B., Hamilton, L.H., 1976. Respiratory Physiology, third ed. Mosby, St Louis, MO.

Smeaton, J., 1995. Exercise and mental health. In: Everett, T., Dennis, M., Ricketts, E. (Eds.) Physiotherapy in Mental Health. Butterworth-Heinemann, Oxford.

Smith, E., Wilks, N., 1988. Meditation. Optima, London.

Smith, J.E., Richardson, J., Hoffman, C., et al., 2005. Mindfulness-based stress reduction as supportive therapy in cancer care: a systematic review. J. Adv. Nurs. 52 (3), 315–327.

Smith, J.F., 2006. Is Exercise Beneficial in the Rehabilitation of Drug Users? MPhil dissertation, University of Strathclyde, Glasgow.

Snyder, M., 1985. Independent Nursing Interventions. John Wiley, New York.

Sordoni, C., Hall, C., Forwell, L., 2002. The use of imagery in athletic injury rehabilitation and its relationship to self-efficacy. Physiother. Can. 54 (3), 177–185.

Speca, M., Carlson, L., Goodey, E., et al., 2000. A randomized wait-list controlled trial: the effects of a mindfulness-based stress reduction programme on mood and symptoms of stress in cancer outpatients. Psychosom. Med. 62, 613–622.

Spence, S.H., Sharpe, L., Newton-John, T., Champion, D., 1995. Effect of electromyographic biofeedback compared to applied relaxation training with chronic, upper extremity cumulative trauma disorders. Pain 63 (2), 199–206.

Spielberger, C.D., 1980. Manual for the State–Trait Anxiety Inventory. Consulting Psychologists Press, Palo Alto, CA.

Stallibrass, C., Sissons, P., Chalmers, C., 2002. Randomized controlled trial of the Alexander technique for idiopathic Parkinson's disease. Clin. Rehabil. 16, 705–718.

Stefano, G.B., Esch, T., 2005. Integrative medical therapy: examination of meditation's therapeutic and global medicinal outcomes via nitric oxide. Int. J. Mol. Med. 16 (4), 621–630.

Stenstrom, C.H., Arge, B., Sundbom, A., 1996. Dynamic training versus relaxation training as home exercise for paients with inflammatory rheumatic diseases: a randomized controlled study. Scand. J. Rheumatol. 25, 28–33.

Stetter, F., Kupper, S., 2002. Autogenic training: a meta-analysis of clinical outcome studies. Appl. Psychophysiol. Biofeedback 27 (1), 45–98.

Stevens, A., Price, J., 1996. Evolutionary Psychiatry: A New Beginning. Routledge, London.

Stevens, J.O., 1971. Awareness: Exploring, Experimenting, Experiencing. Real People Press, Moab, UT.

Strawbridge, W.J., Deleger, S., Roberts, R.E., Kaplan, G.A., 2002. Physical activity reduces the risk of subsequent depression for older adults. Am. J. Epidemiol. 156, 328–334.

Stricker, C., Drake, D., Hoyer, K., Mock, V., 2004. Evidence-based practice for fatigue management in adults with cancer: exercise as an intervention. Oncol. Nurse Forum 31 (5), 963–976.

Stulemeijer, M., de Jong, L.W.A.M., Fiselier, T.J.W., Hoogveld, S.W.B., Bleijenberg, G., 2005. Cognitive behaviour therapy for adolescents with chronic fatigue syndrome: randomized controlled trial. Br. Med. J. 330, 14–17.

Sudsuang, R., Chentanez, V., Veluvan, K., 1991. Effect of Buddhist meditation on serum cortisol and total protein levels, blood pressure, pulse rate, lung volume and reaction time. Physiol. Behav. 50, 543–548.

Tacon, A.M., 2003. Meditation as a complementary therapy in cancer. Fam. Community Health 26 (1), 64–73.

Takaishi, N., 2000. A comparative study of autogenic training and progressive relaxation as methods for teaching clients to relax. Sleep Hypn. 2 (3), 132–137.

Tatrow, K., Montgomery, G.H., 2006. Cognitive behavioural therapy techniques for distress and pain in breast cancer patients: a meta-analysis. J. Behav. Med. 29 (1), 17–27.

Teasdale, J.D., Segal, Z.V., Williams, J.M.G., et al., 2000. Prevention of relapse recurrence in major depression by mindfulness-based cognitive therapy. J. Consult. Clin. Psychol. 68, 615–623.

Thomas, P.W., Thomas, S., Hillier, C., et al., 2006 Psychological interventions for multiple sclerosis. Cochrane Database Syst. Rev. Issue 1. CD004431.

Thomas, S., 2004. Buteyko: a useful tool in the management of asthma? Int. J. Ther. Rehabil. 11 (10), 476–480.

Tindle, H.A., Barbeau, E.M., Davis, R.B., 2006. Guided imagery for smoking cessation in adults: a randomized pilot trial. Complement. Health Pract. Rev. 11 (3), 166–175.

Titlebaum, H., 1988. Relaxation. In: Zahourek, R.P. (Ed.), Relaxation and Imagery: Tools for Therapeutic Communication and Intervention. WB Saunders, Philadelphia.

Toneatto, T., Nguyen, L., 2007. Does mindfulness meditation improve anxiety and mood symptoms? A review of the controlled research. Can. J. Psychiatry 52 (4), 260–266.

Tsatsoulis, A., Fountoulakis, S., 2006. The protective role of exercise on stress system dysregulation and comorbidities. Ann. N. Y. Acad. Sci. 1083, 196–213.

Tschudin, V., 1991. Beginning with Awareness: a Learner's Handbook. Churchill Livingstone, Edinburgh.

Tusek, D.L., Cwynar, R.E., 2000. Strategies for implementing a guided imagery programme to enhance patient experience. Adv. Pract. Acute Crit. Care 11 (1), 68–76.

Twomey, L.T., 1993. Lumbar biomechanics and physical therapy. J. Organ. Chart. Physiother. Priv. Pract. 70, 14–19.

Twomey, L.T., Taylor, J.R., 1987. Physical Therapy of the Low Back. Churchill Livingstone, New York.

United States Department of Health and Human Service, 1999. Mental Health: A Report from the Surgeon General, US Department of Health and Human Services, Substance Abuse and Mental Health Services Administration, Centre for Mental Health Services, National Institutes of Health, National Institute of Mental Health, Rockville, MD.

US Preventive Services Task Force, 1989. Exercise counselling. In: Guide to Clinical Preventive Services. Williams and Wilkins, Baltimore, MD. US Preventive Services Task Force.

van Dixhoorn, J., Duivenvoorden, J.A., 1989. Breathing awareness as a relaxation method in cardiac rehabilitation. In: Stress and Tension Control 3. Plenum, New York, pp. 19–36.

van Dixhoorn, J., White, A., 2005. Relaxation therapy for rehabilitation and prevention in ischaemic heart disease: a systematic review and meta-analysis. Eur. J. Cardiovasc. Prev. Rehabil. 12 (3), 193–202.

van Doorn, P., Colla, P., Folgering, H., 1982. Control of end-tidal PCO_2 in the hyperventilation syndrome: effects of biofeedback and breathing instructions compared. Bull. Eur. Physiopathol. Respir. 18, 829–836.

van Gool, C.H., Kempen, G.I., Penninx, B.W., Deeg, D.J., Beekman, A.T., van Eijk, J.T., 2003. Relationship between changes in depressive symptoms and unhealthy lifestyles in late middle aged and older persons: results from the Longitudinal Ageing Study, Amsterdam. Age Ageing 32, 81–87.

van Rooijen, A.J., Rheeder, P., Eales, C.J., et al., 2004. Effect of exercise versus relaxation on haemoglobin A1C in black females with type 2 diabetes mellitus. Qld J. Med. 97 (6), 343–351.

van Tulder, M.W., Ostelo, R.W.J.G., Vlaeyen, J.W.S., Linton, S.J., Morley, S.J., Assendelft, W.J.J., 2000. Behavioural treatment for chronic low back pain (Cochrane Review). Cochrane Libr. Issue 2. Update Software, Oxford.

Vazquez, M.I., Buceta, J.M., 1993. Effectiveness of self-management programmes and relaxation training in the treatment of bronchial asthma: relationships with trait anxiety and emotional attack triggers. J. Psychosom. Res. 37 (1), 71–81.

Verhagen, A.P., Damen, L., Berger, M.Y., et al., 2005. Conservative treatments of children with episodic tension-type headache. A systematic review. J. Neurol. 252 (10), 1147–1154.

Vissing, Y., Burke, M., 1984. Visualization techniques for health care workers. J. Psychosoc. Nurs. Ment. Health Serv. 22, 29–32.

Vlaeyen, J.W.S., Morley, S., 2005. Cognitive-behavioural treatments for chronic pain: what works for whom? Clin. J. Pain 21, 1–8 Special Topic Series: Cognitive-behavioural Treatment for Chronic Pain.

Wade, J.E., Kosinski, M., Dewey, J.E., 2000. How to Score Version 2 of the SF 36 Health Survey. Quality Metric Incorporated, Lincoln, RI.

Wallace, J.M., 1980. Muscular relaxation. In: Look After Yourself. Health Education Authority, London.

Walton, K.G., Schneider, R.H., Nidich, S., et al., 2002. Psychosocial stress and cardiovascular disease, part 2: effectiveness of the transcendental meditation programme in treatment and prevention. Behav. Med. 28 (3), 106–123.

Walton, K.G., Schneider, R.H., Nidich, S., 2004. Review of controlled research on the transcendental meditation program and cardiovascular disease. Risk factors, morbidity and mortality. Cardiol. Rev. 12 (5), 262–266.

Warburton, D.E.R., Nicol, C.W., Bredin, S.S.D., 2006. Health benefits of physical activity: the evidence. Can. Med. Assoc. J. 174 (6), 801–809.

Ware, J.E., Sherbourne, C.D., 1992. The MOS 36–item short form health survey (SF–36) 1. Conceptual framework and item selection. Med. Care 30, 473–483.

Waugh, A., Grant, A., 2006. Ross & Wilson Anatomy and Physiology in Health and Illness, tenth ed. Churchill Livingstone Elsevier, Edinburgh.

Welz, K.H., 1991/2000. Autogenic Training: A Practical Guide in Six Easy Lessons. c/o HSCTI, PO Box 1298, Woodstock, GA 30188.

West, M.A. (Ed.), 1987. The Psychology of Meditation. Oxford Science Publications, Oxford.

Wetherell, J.L., Sorrell, J.T., Thorp, S.R., et al., 2005. Psychological interventions for late-life anxiety: a review and early lessons from the CALM study. J. Geriatr. Psychiatry Neurol. 18 (2), 72–82.

Weydert, J.A., 2006. Evaluation of guided imagery as treatment for recurrent abdominal pain in children: a randomized controlled trial. BMC Pediatr. 6, 29.

Weyerer, S., 1992. Physical inactivity and depression in the community: evidence from the Upper Bavarian Field Study. J. Sports Med. 13, 492–496.

White, P., Naish, V., 2001. Graded exercise therapy for chronic fatigue syndrome: an audit. Physiotherapy 87 (6), 285–288.

Whitfield, H.J., 2006. Towards case-specific applications of mindfulness-based cognitive behavioural therapies: a mindfulness-based rational emotive behaviour therapy. Couns. Psychol. Q. 19 (2), 205.

Williams, D.A., 2003. Psychological and behavioural therapies in fibromyalgia and related syndromes. Best Pract. Res. Clin. Rheumatol. 17 (4), 649–665.

Wilson, K.J.W., 1990. Ross and Wilson Anatomy and Physiology in Health and Illness, seventh ed. Churchill Livingstone, Edinburgh.

Wolpe, J., 1958. Psychotherapy by Reciprocal Inhibition. Stanford University Press, Stanford, CA.

Wolpe, J., Lazarus, A.A., 1966. Behaviour Therapy Techniques. Pergamon Press, New York.

Woolfolk, R.L., Lehrer, P.M. (Eds.), 1984. Principles and Practice of Stress Management. Guilford Press, New York.

World Health Organization, 2001. ICF checklist: version 2: a clinician's form for international classification of functioning in disability and health. www.who.int/classification/icf/checklist/icf–chechlist.pdf.

World Health Organization, 2004. Global strategy on diet, physical activity and health. www.who.int/dietphysicalactivity/strategy/eb11344/strategy–english–web.pdf.

Wright, L.D., 2006. Meditation: a new role for an old friend. Am. J. Hosp. Palliat. Care 23 (4), 323–327.

Wulf, G., 2007. Self-controlled practice enhances motor learning: implications for physiotherapy. Physiotherapy 93 (2), 96–101.

Yorke, J., Fleming, S., Shuldam, C., 2005. Psychological Interventions for Children With Asthma. Cochrane Database Syst. Rev. Issue 4. CD003272.

Young, A., Dinan, S., 2005. Activity in later life. Br. Med. J. 330, 189–191.

Yung, P., French, P., Leung, B., 2001. Relaxation training as complementary therapy for mild hypertension control and the implications of evidence-based medicine. Complement. Med. Nurs. Midwifery 1 (2), 59–65.

Yung, P., Fung, M.Y., Chan, T.M.F., et al., 2004. Relaxation training methods for nurse managers in Hong Kong: a controlled study. Int.J. Ment. Health Nurs. 13 (4), 255–261.

Zahourek, R.P. (Ed.), 1985. Clinical Hypnosis and Therapeutic Suggestion in Nursing. Grune and Stratton, Orlando, FL.

Zahourek, R.P. (Ed.), 1988. Relaxation and Imagery: Tools for Therapeutic Communication and Intervention. WB Saunders, Philadelphia.

Zigmond, A.S., Snaith, R.P., 1983. The Hospital Anxiety and Depression Scale. Acta Psychiatr. Scand. 67, 361–370.

Index